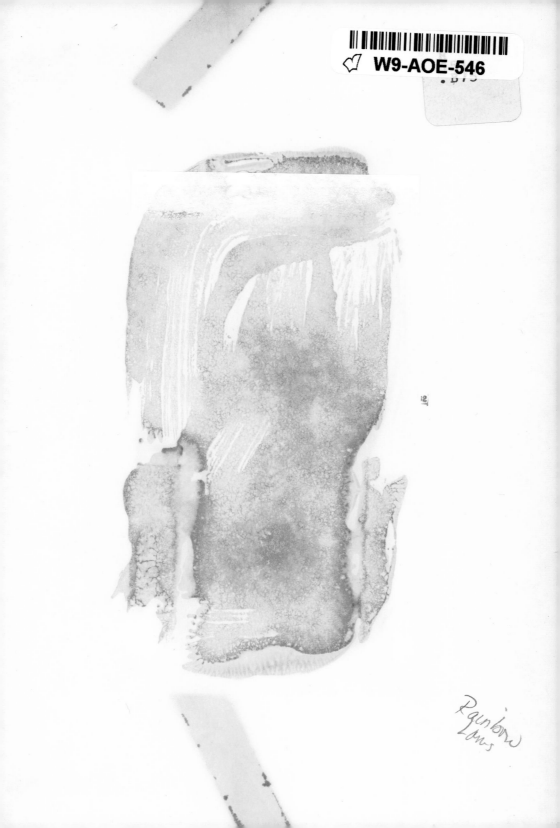

Rainbow
Lows

Medical America in the Nineteenth Century

Medical America in the Nineteenth Century

Readings from the Literature

edited by
Gert H. Brieger

The Johns Hopkins Press
Baltimore and London

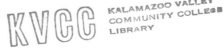

The Johns Hopkins Press, Baltimore, Maryland 21218
The Johns Hopkins Press Ltd., London

Library of Congress Catalog Card Number 76-165053
International Standard Book Number 0-8018-1237-2

CONTENTS

Preface ix

I **Medical Education**

Introduction 3
Daniel Drake: Practical Essays on Medical Education and the
    Medical Profession in the United States 8
Andrew Boardman: An Essay on the Means of Improving
    Medical Education and Elevating Medical Character 24
Annual Catalogue of the College of Physicians and Surgeons,
    in the City of New York, 1849–50 37

II **Medical Literature**

Oliver Wendell Holmes: Report of the Committee on Medical
    Literature 45

III **The Medical Profession**

Introduction 57
F. Campbell Stewart: The Actual Condition of the Medical
    Profession in This Country; with a Brief Account of Some
    of the Causes Which Tend to Impede Its Progress, and
    Interfere with Its Honors and Interests 62
Edwin L. Godkin: Orthopathy and Heteropathy 75

IV **Medical Practice**

Introduction 87
Benjamin Rush: On the Causes of Death in Diseases That
    Are Not Incurable 90
Jacob Bigelow: On Self-limited Diseases 98
Nathaniel Chapman: Remarks on the Chronic Fluxes of
    the Bowels 107

Elisha Bartlett: An Inquiry into the Degree of Certainty in
    Medicine; and into the Nature and Extent of Its Power
    over Disease 115
Nathan S. Davis: Nature and Art. Their Relative Influence
    in the Management of Diseases. Are They Antagonistic or
    Co-operative? 127
Austin Flint: Conservative Medicine 134
Edouard Seguin: Clinical Thermometry 143
Francis Delafield: Some Forms of Dyspepsia. 152

V Surgery

Introduction 163
Ephraim McDowell: Three Cases of Extirpation of Diseased
    Ovaria 166
Henry J. Bigelow: Insensibility during Surgical Operations
    Produced by Inhalation. 169
Edmund Andrews: The Surgeon 176
John Eric Erichsen: Impressions of American Surgery 182
Samuel D. Gross: The Factors of Disease and Death after
    Injuries, Parturition, and Surgical Operations 190
Robert F. Weir: On the Antiseptic Treatment of Wounds,
    and Its Results 198
Stephen Smith: The Comparative Results of Operations in
    Bellevue Hospital 201

VI Psychiatry

Introduction 213
Pliny Earle: A Glance at Insanity, and the Management of the
    Insane in the American States 215
S. Weir Mitchell: Address before the Fiftieth Annual Meeting
    of the American Medico-Psychological Association 222

VII Hospitals

Introduction 233
John Jones: Appendix to *Plain Concise Practical Remarks on
    the Treatment of Wounds and Fractures*, "Camp and
    Military Hospitals" 237
W. H. Rideing: Hospital Life in New York 242

VIII Hygiene

Introduction 253
Robert Tomes: Why We Get Sick 256
Stephen Smith: New York the Unclean. 263
Frederick A. P. Barnard: The Germ Theory of Disease and Its
  Relations to Hygiene 278
Dorman B. Eaton: The Essential Conditions of Good Sanitary
  Administration 293
John Shaw Billings: The Registration of Vital Statistics 301

IX Announcement of The Johns Hopkins Medical School 313

Index 331

PREFACE

An increasing interest in the development of medicine in America makes the need for a source-book apparent. I have, therefore, collected a series of papers to illuminate various aspects of the historical development of the medical profession and the commitment to public health in nineteenth-century America.

The book is not intended to be a traditional collection of classical papers, although some are indeed classics, frequently cited but little read. Many well-known papers, such as J. Marion Sims's description of vesico-vaginal fistula repair, have recently been reprinted and are already available. Instead, I have included selections that highlight problems and attitudes encountered in their time, to give the reader a better appreciation of what our forebears said and thought.

This volume, then, is intended for all who wish to read, in their original form, the works of some of the important authors of the nineteenth century. It will become apparent that many problems faced by students, practitioners, and patients of that day are still being discussed. The introductions and references for each section are meant to give the entire volume some continuity, but more important, to help students find their way into a particular subject.

The great scientific advances, beginning with the germ theory and the rise of the science of bacteriology in the last two decades of the 1800's, are touched upon, but only in so far as their surgical and hygienic applications are concerned. Papers by Walter Reed, Theobald Smith, George Sternberg, and many other medical scientists will be included in another volume dealing with the rise of scientific medicine in America between *ca.* 1880 and World War II, a period when the United States began to assume a preeminent position in world medicine.

The final selection stands as a landmark of the beginning of a new era. It is also a fitting end for this volume.

I have incurred several debts in the preparation of this book. Above all, I would like to express my appreciation to Professor Richard H. Shryock for his kindness and his encouragement, as well as for his many scholarly contributions in the history of medicine. All too often, when those of us who follow him think we have a good idea, it will be found to have been clearly stated already in one of his books or papers. Saul Benison, whose friendship and help have been invaluable, has been an encouraging and kindly critic who has saved me from a number of pitfalls. I also want to thank Professors Owsei Temkin, Lloyd G. Stevenson, and Charles E. Rosenberg for their suggestions and criticisms. I have not always heeded their advice, hence imperfections and omissions are chargeable to me.

In most instances it has been necessary for me to shorten an article, and I hope my pruning will have been subtle enough so as not to be obvious. The spelling and punctuation of the essays have been modernized for easier reading. For typing and general assistance I owe thanks to Mrs. Mary Moore of the Institute of the History of Medicine, The Johns Hopkins University.

GERT H. BRIEGER

PART I

MEDICAL EDUCATION

INTRODUCTION

A glance at the section devoted to medical education in Professor Genevieve Miller's *Bibliography* reveals the extent of the interest in this aspect of the history of medicine.[1] Coupled with the truly staggering numbers of inaugural discourses and graduation orations available in the medical journals and the bound pamphlet files of many libraries, there is material for many volumes. Much of what has been written, it is true, is of local character, but certainly the history of medical education is not one of the neglected fields.

It is well known, for instance, that apprenticeship was the primary method of medical education for nearly 200 years in the American colonies. This was an efficient method for practical training and moulding the medical character, as George Corner has said, but it failed to provide systematic instruction in the principles of medicine.[2]

In the middle and latter nineteenth century an increasing number of medical schools were founded. These were sometimes an integral part of an already established college. Occasionally, groups of practitioners formed a school and then sought a college affiliation. A few medical societies sponsored schools, but, unfortunately, the largest number were proprietary in nature. In these schools the professors collected the fees and so were not eager to carefully screen students or to fail them once they began to study medicine.[3]

Until the last quarter of the nineteenth century the average student spent three or four years as an apprentice to a practicing physician. During this time the student usually attended two terms of lectures at a medical college, each lasting three to four months. The second "year" of medical school was often a repeat of the first. In addition to the prescribed apprenticeship and medical

---

[1] *Bibliography of the History of Medicine in the United States and Canada, 1939–1960* (Baltimore: The Johns Hopkins Press, 1964).

[2] George W. Corner, "Apprentice to Aesculapius," *Proc. Am. Phil. Soc.* 109 (1965): 249–58.

[3] William F. Norwood, *Medical Education in the United States before the Civil War* (Philadelphia: University of Pennsylvania Press, 1944), pp. 380–86. Norwood's is the most comprehensive secondary source available.

school matriculation, the requirements for a degree were that the candidate be
of good moral character and that he be twenty-one years of age. Some Americans completed their medical education abroad, where they walked the wards of
Europe's famous hospitals.[4]

One of the first orders of business for the newly formed American Medical
Association in 1847 was to assess the state of medical education in the country.
With this in view, a committee was appointed and given the following charge:

> ... 1st, prepare an annual report on the general condition of medical
> education in the United States, in comparison with the state of medical
> education in other enlightened nations; noticing as occasion may call for,
> 2d, the course of instruction, the practical requirements for graduation,
> the modes of examination for conferring degrees, and 3d, the reputed
> number of pupils and graduates at the several medical institutions in the
> United States during the year. Noticing 4th, the requirements of the
> United States Army and Navy Boards of Medical Examiners; 5th, the legal
> requirements exacted of medical practitioners in our several states, and
> 6th, all such measures, prospective or established, in reference to medical
> education and the reputable standing of the profession, as may be deemed
> worthy of special consideration.[5]

This broad charge summarized the existing problems. The succeeding volumes of
the *Transactions* supplied some of the answers to the questions. One point the
committee made in this first report was that our system, in general, was defective and lagged behind the great European centers. "In the United States alone,"
the committee warned, "is continued an obsolete system of teaching demonstrative science by description, of teaching the manipulations of surgery, and the art
of recognizing and healing diseases without exhibiting the practice of either, and
of explaining the movements and changes of living bodies to those who are
ignorant of the laws which govern inert matter."[6]

In the session of 1846–47, the committee found 4,192 students in 25 schools
of medicine. One must remember, though, that those were so-called "regular"
schools only. By 1849, in another survey, 39 schools appeared on the list, but a
few of these were reorganizing or had just closed. As Abraham Flexner has
shown, the greatest spurt in the number of new schools came in the final decades
of the nineteenth century. At the time of his report, in 1910, 155 schools
survived, of more than 450 that had at one time or another existed.[7]

The great issues in medical education, from John Morgan to Abraham
Flexner, are illustrated by the concerns of the A.M.A. in the nineteenth century.
The number of graduates, their qualification and regulation, and the methods

[4] See Robert P. Hudson's "Patterns of Medical Education in Nineteenth Century
America," master's essay, The Johns Hopkins University, 1966.
[5] "Report of the Committee on Education," *Trans. A.M.A.* 1 (1848): 235–47; 235–36.
[6] Ibid., p. 236.
[7] See especially the historical introduction to Abraham Flexner, *Medical Education in
the United States and Canada*, Bulletin #4, Carnegie Foundation, New York, 1910, pp.
3–19.

and levels of their training were constantly discussed and criticized. Not only was the profession examining itself by European standards but also when measured against other forms of education in this country, the physicians often expressed feelings of inferiority. Worthington Hooker, in the Report of the Committee on Medical Education of the A.M.A. in 1851 stated bluntly that, "It is a fact so papable that few are disposed to question it, that the general standard of education and attainment is much lower in the medical than it is in the other professions."[8]

One of the reasons why medical education was of uneven quality, often inferior to other forms of education, was the lack of rigid criteria for preparation of students for admission to medical schools and for planning the curricula of these schools. There was keen interest in medical education in mid-century, however, to the point that there was even a "mania for college making," according to Nathan Smith Davis. Davis, one of the moving spirits behind the A.M.A., rued the fact that so many professional men were ambitious for distinction as teachers, and so many sought professorships in medical colleges, that there was need for creation of new schools.[9]

Thirty years later Davis was no longer so concerned with the medical schools as he was with the institution of apprenticeship. The requirement that a medical graduate be twenty-one years of age, of good moral character, a graduate of an approved school, and that he spend some time with a preceptor, was standard throughout the United States. By 1876, Davis lamented, in nine cases out of ten, the apprenticeship consisted of "little more than the registry of the student's name in the doctor's office."[10]

While apprenticeship was a source of much discussion in the nineteenth century, it was an effective means of transmitting practical knowledge in the days before hospitals were widely used for teaching and when medicine was less theoretical and scientific than it is today. The preceptor, usually a physician practicing in the neighborhood, was not only a teacher but he also had the responsibility for seeing that his students were properly qualified to go on to medical school or to receive their degrees or licenses.

As one up-state New York preceptor put it: "Upon private practitioners, therefore, mainly rests the responsibility of introducing to the profession persons incapable of meeting its exigencies. We, *we* are the janitors at the temple gates of our Profession, and upon our vigilance and discrimination depend the character and usefulness of those who enter its honored portals."[11]

---

[8] *Trans. A.M.A.* 4 (1851): 409–41; 409.

[9] Nathan S. Davis, *History of Medical Education and Institutions in the United States, from the First Settlement of the British Colonies to the Year 1850* (Chicago: Griggs, 1851), p. 117.

[10] N. S. Davis, *Contributions to the History of Medical Education and Medical Institutions in the United States of America, 1776–1876* (Washington: Government Printing Office, 1877), p. 43.

[11] Caleb Green, "Qualifications for the study of medicine," *Trans. Med. Assoc. Southern Central New York* (1849): 22–35; 35.

In most schools standards of admission were very low. Charles W. Eliot remarked that when he became president of Harvard in 1869 anyone who chose could come off the street and enter the Harvard School of Medicine. Eliot proposed a number of reforms, among them lengthening the school year from four to nine months and that each candidate pass a written examination for the degree. The dean of the medical school thought these "improvements" would destroy the school. "I had to tell him," the dean is reputed to have said, "that he knew nothing about the quality of Harvard medical students. More than half of them can barely write."[12]

Despite the discouraging situation still existing around 1870, some improvements were made and many of the schools instituted laboratory studies, lengthened their terms, and imposed some standards. While the model was Europe, William Welch was optimistic when he spoke at Yale in 1888 on "Some of the Advantages of the Union of Medical School and University." On opening his address he said: "It is a hopeful and gratifying circumstance that within the last few years universities in this country and in England have shown an awakened and enlightened interest in the advancement of medical science and the promotion of higher medical education."[13]

While the Johns Hopkins University perhaps went farthest in its requirements in 1893, schools in New York, Philadelphia, Boston, Chicago, and Michigan had also been improving. It would be misleading, I think, to leave the impression that between 1850 and 1893 nothing changed until suddenly there dawned in Baltimore the new light of the future.

Bibliographical Note

John Morgan, *A Discourse Upon the Institution of Medical Schools In America*, 1765; reprinted with an introduction by Abraham Flexner, Baltimore: The Johns Hopkins Press, 1937.

Samuel Bard, *Two Discourses Dealing with Medical Education in Early New York*, New York: Columbia University Press, 1921; the discourses date from 1769 and 1819.

For conditions as they existed in the 1870's see particularly the reprint of lectures delivered by John Shaw Billings at the Johns Hopkins University shortly after its opening. The lectures were originally published in 1878, but may be conveniently found as "Two papers by John Shaw Billings on medical education," *Bull. Hist. Med.* 6 (1938): 285–359.

The most extensive secondary work is William F. Norwood, *Medical Education in the United States Before the Civil War*, Philadelphia: University of Pennsylvania Press, 1944. See also Henry B. Shafer, *The American Medical Profession, 1783 to 1850*, New York: Columbia University Press, 1936.

---

[12] Quoted by Esther Lucille Brown, *Physicians and Medical Care* (New York: Russell Sage Foundation, 1937), pp. 16–17.

[13] In William H. Welch, *Papers and Addresses*, 3 vols. (Baltimore: The Johns Hopkins Press, 1920) 3: 26–40.

A general work on the history of medical education is Theodor Puschmann, *A History of Medical Education from the Most Remote to the Most Recent Times*, E. H. Hare, trans., London: Lewis, 1891. For the British story see Charles Newman, *The Evolution of Medical Education in the Nineteenth Century*, London: Oxford University Press, 1957; and F. N. L. Poynter, ed., *The Evolution of Medical Education in Britain*, Baltimore: Williams and Wilkins, 1966.

DANIEL DRAKE

PRACTICAL ESSAYS ON MEDICAL EDUCATION AND THE MEDICAL PROFESSION IN THE UNITED STATES

Editor's Note

Daniel Drake (1785–1852) has long been a heroic figure in American medicine. His fame rests on his writings, which were voluminous and of very high quality, and on his efforts to bring good medical education to the western states. The fact that he represented the ideal frontier physician undoubtedly also enhanced his reputation. His fellow medical teacher Samuel D. Gross called him a great lecturer. "He had natural talent and genius of a high order, and would have become eminent in whatever pursuit he might have engaged."[1]

Drake has been remembered especially for his monumental *Systematic Treatise, Historical, Etiological, and Practical, on the Principal Diseases of the Interior Valley of North America*, published in two volumes in 1850 and 1854, with a total of 1,863 pages.[2] His essays on medical education are of equal interest and have become classics in their own right. They are informative because they describe so many of the conditions then existing, as well as the problems to be solved. The essays first appeared in Drake's own *Western Journal of Medical and Physical Sciences*, before he collected them into a book in 1832. One hundred and twenty years later they were reprinted as volume 5 of the *Bibliotheca Medica Americana* Series of the Institute of the History of Medicine, The Johns Hopkins University. Unfortunately, they quickly went out of print again.

Bibliographical Note

The secondary sources on Daniel Drake are extensive. He himself also wrote more on medical education. See especially his *Strictures on Some of the Defects and Infirmities of the Intellectual and Moral Character in Students of Medicine*, Louisville: Prentice & Weisinger, 1847.

For recent descriptions and evaluations of Drake and his work see particularly:

James Thomas Flexner, *Doctors on Horseback*, New York: Viking, 1937, reprinted by Dover, 1969.

Emmet F. Horine, *Daniel Drake, 1785–1852; Pioneer Physician of the Midwest*, Philadelphia: University of Pennsylvania Press, 1961.

Cincinnati: Roff & Young, 1832; reprinted by The Johns Hopkins Press, 1952.

[1] S. D. Gross, *Autobiography*, 2 vols. (Philadelphia: Barrie, 1887) 2: 261–74.

[2] Selections from this have recently been reprinted by the University of Illinois Press, Norman D. Levine, ed., 1964.

D. A. Tucker, Jr., "Daniel Drake and the origin of medicine in the Ohio Valley," *Ohio Archives of History* 44 (1935): 451–68.

See also the introduction by Norman D. Levine, in the reprint cited above, and Henry D. Shapiro and Zane L. Miller, eds., *Physician to the West, Selected Writings of Daniel Drake on Science and Society*, Lexington: University of Kentucky Press, 1970.

ESSAY I

SELECTION AND PREPARATORY EDUCATION OF PUPILS

Of the various occupations in society, scarcely one requires greater talent and knowledge than the medical profession. This is especially true in the United States, where almost every practitioner must be, at the same time, physician, surgeon, and apothecary. Obvious as this proposition is to many, its truth, unfortunately, is not generally perceived by those who are about to dedicate their sons to the profession—in other words, by the persons who above all others should feel and acknowledge its reality. Hence, it results that the ranks of the profession are in a great degree filled up with recruits, deficient either in abilities or acquirements—too often indeed in both—who thus doom it to a mediocrity, incompatible with both its nature and objects. Other causes contribute to its degradation, but this I am persuaded is one of the most frequent and most difficult to obviate. Still, much might be done if those who have the power would open their eyes to the evil and exert their influence in its suppression.

Few of those who are put to the study of medicine can be aware of the magnitude of the undertaking or of the insufficiency of their capacity and preparation; for the obvious reason that they are, in general, young and inexperienced. There are, however, two classes of persons who might be expected to judge more correctly and have much in their power. These are parents and physicians, both of whom, rather than our sons, should feel responsible to society on this subject; and to them I beg leave respectfully to address myself.

In the selection of boys for the study of medicine, many circumstances, entirely disconnected with their fitness, too often exert a dominant influence; when their sway should be kept subordinate or even regarded as entirely inadmissible. A neighboring physician wants a student to reside in his office; or one son of the family is thought too weakly to labor on the farm or in the workshop; he is indolent and averse to bodily exertion; or addicted to study, but too stupid for the Bar or too immoral for the Pulpit; the parents wish to have one gentleman in the family, and a *doctor* is a *gentleman*:—these and many other extraneous considerations not unfrequently decide the choice and swell the numbers while they impair the character of the profession.

Both parents and physicians should know that boys of feeble frame and unsound constitution cannot endure close study and are best strengthened by hard labor; they should not, indeed, even be put to the learned professions, unless they chance to possess extraordinary genius. Every physician must have seen many who dragged out the whole period of their brief and reluctant pupilage with dyspepsia, a pain in the breast, or hypochondraism; conditions which either preclude all intense and successful application or render it the cause of some other distressing malady which terminates in premature death.

But it is not sufficient that boys selected for the study of medicine should have good constitutions, they ought, equally, to be endowed with vigorous and inquiring minds. Without these, whatever may be the appearances of success, they must at last make incompetent physicians. It is especially and indispensably necessary that they possess, in a high degree, the faculties of observation and judgment, without which they can neither comprehend the principles of the science nor apply them correctly in the treatment of diseases. Notwithstanding this obvious fact, hundreds are put to the study of medicine whose utmost grasp of intellect never encompasses the rudiments of the profession. As a matter of course they slur over every difficult proposition, and afterwards grope their way for forty years, unconsciously committing "sins of omission or commission," thoughout the whole of that long period. It is in vain to rely on society to correct this great evil by discriminating among the candidates for their confidence; for the knowledge necessary to a correct selection does not exist among them. In the other learned professions this species of empyricism cannot produce the same mischief. The incompetent Divine at most but occupies the place of an abler teacher, and the superficial Lawyer is either driven from the Bar by the exposure of his errors or they are rendered harmless by the skill of competent associates. But the physician who has passed through the usual forms of a professional education, without the capacity to improve by his opportunities, is presumed by the people to be qualified for every emergency and sometimes even preferred to the ablest practitioners.

The student of medicine should not only be of sound understanding but imbued with ambition. A mere love of knowledge is not to be relied upon, for the greatest lovers of knowledge are not unfrequently deficient in executive talents and go on acquiring without learning how to appropriate. Let parents, therefore, not be misled by the signs which indicate a fondness for study, unless the desire involves a feeling of emulation. A thirst for fame is indeed a safer guarantee than a taste for learning, as it generates those executive efforts which are indispensable to the successful practice of the profession.

Further, the temperament of the youth should be that of industry and perseverance, without which he will balk at every difficulty and require to be goaded on through all stages of his pupilage. An indolent or irresolute student, whatever may be his genius, can never figure as a physician and should, without delay, be apprenticed to some vocation in which the destruction of limbs and life will not be the inevitable consequence of idleness and discouragement.

Finally, parents who are too poor to afford their sons the necessary opportunities should not aim at making them physicians. If we now and then see one whose talents, ambition, and enterprise, have enabled him to acquire distinction, despite every obstacle, we meet with many more who all their lives remain unfinished and imperfect from want of adequate time and opportunities while engaged in their professional studies. I am the most disposed to insist on these truths because so many fathers are ignorant of what is really necessary to make their sons good physicians and place them to the study of physic before they have accurately counted the cost. Of all the causes which impede the progress of medicine in the United States, not one is more operative than this. The amiable vanity in which it originates can scarcely be condemned, but parents should be admonished to look at the *consequences* of such an indulgence of feeling. Under the most limited opportunities, a son can make acquirements that may satisfy a fond father who knows but little of the extent and complexity of the medical sciences; to be prepared, however, for the various exigencies of the profession is a much more difficult affair. Paternal affection may blind us to the errors of our sons but cannot obviate their prejudicial influence on society.

Having briefly considered the moral and physical qualities which fit young men for the study of medicine, I come now to say that a majority of those who are selected for that purpose are deficient in one or both classes of requisites. Let us enquire into the principal causes of this state of things—so unfavorable to the dignity of the profession and prejudicial to the interests of humanity.

The current opinion that men of slender abilities are competent to the practice of physic is, obviously, a great cause why so many feeble-minded boys are dedicated to its study. There never existed a time when this opinion was well founded. In past ages, when medicine could not claim a place in the ranks of philosophy, it was still a science of observation and called for an acute and discriminating mind. Though it could not rise above the grade of an experimental art, it never sank to a trade, the results of which were purely accidental, except when it fell into the hands of the imbecile or the unprincipled. At the present time, when the intricacies of the human structure have been unravelled and many of its functions are understood; when the accumulated experience of centuries has developed numerous general truths, and the spirit of inductive philosophy has arranged them into a science—imperfect it is true, but still a science—when chemistry, natural philosophy, botany and natural history have become essential preliminary branches, nothing can be more adventurous than to engage in the study of the profession without a logical and comprehensive mind.

Another cause of the evil which we deprecate is the liberal proportion of inferior men who unfortunately belong to the profession and so often succeed in acquiring business and popularity. An observation of this fact, not a little mortifying to the more talented members of the profession, encourages parents to set apart for the study of medicine those sons who are least remarkable for strength of mind; reserving the better class for pursuits which in their opinion require more vigor of intellect or promise greater distinction. Thus a degraded state of the profession is made to perpetuate itself by influencing not only the ignorant but the well informed; for when a father who has a just estimate of the strong talents necessary to the study and practice of physic apprehends that a son, of whose genius he is proud, may, on entering the arena, meet with many whose emulation is vitiated with envy, who labor to please rather than preserve their patients, or whose skill consists more in the arts of imposture than of cure, it is not unnatural for him to shrink from the anticipation of the rude struggle.

The root of this great evil is planted in society itself. Some persons are too dull to discriminate among the members of the profession, others allow themselves to be captivated by pleasant manners, and not a few call for *cheap doctoring*, all of which tend directly to elevate false pretension and depress real merit.

But there are causes which attract as well as repel young men of genius from the profession.

It will not be denied that no passion is more intense and universal than the love of gain. If not the first to be developed it is the last to be extinguished; and, taken in the aggregate, perhaps no other exercises so much sway over the course and conduct of man. But in most parts of the United States the practice of medicine offers little to gratify this desire, in comparison with commercial pursuits, and hence we find that *they* exert an influence which draws into the vortex of trade no inconsiderable part of the talents and enterprise of the nation.

Strong, however, as the attractions of commerce unquestionably are, their influence is trifling compared with those of law and politics. In no other country is the union of those two sciences so intimate as in the United States. The regular course of promotion is from the county court house to the capital of the state, thence to the halls of congress, and, finally, to the presidential palace, whose lofty entablatures, by a kind of looming, are seen with magical effect from every part of the union.

It is marvelous to see with what luster the "seals of office glitter in the eyes" of the good people of these United States. The whole world furnishes no parallel case. The number of state and federal offices is so great as to awaken political aspirations on our entire male population, and some of them are invested with sufficient emolument, power, and patronage to excite the most intense emulation—I ought rather to say the angriest rivalry. Thus are the genius and ambition of the nation drawn into the race for political glory. But for this, the law would scarcely exert stronger attractions upon the talent of the country than medicine; for its own intrinsic rewards are not of a higher order, as the problems which it offers do not require for their solution a greater amount of intellect than the practice of medicine. How long this will continue to be the case it is difficult to foresee; but as our population is progressive, while the number of political offices is nearly stationary, we may hope that the time is not distant when the proportion of talented youth who are dedicated to the study of physic will be much greater than at present.

The consequences of this deficiency of talent in the profession are of serious import to the science and to the people at large. It is unquestionably one of the causes which retard the progress of discovery and improvement. Of the thousands who annually go forth with diplomas or licenses, or without either, to engage in the practical duties of the profession, very few ever contribute a single new fact to its archives or communicate an impulse to the minutest wheel in its complicated machinery. Acting on the precepts of others, they may, it is true, do some good, but they also do much harm; while to the great work of revising and correcting the principles of the science, they are of course utterly incompetent.

But this incompetency is not the effect of inferior *talents* only, it results, perhaps, in an equal degree from want of education and mental discipline, on the extent and causes of which I shall now proceed to speak.

Although medicine is ranked with the *learned* professions, not a few of its professors are signally deficient in learning.* This is the case not only in the western states, where for obvious reasons it might be expected, but in almost every part of the union, with the exception of some of our large cities. Writing as I do for practical effect and to promote *reform*, I am constrained to say that even at this late period the profession abounds in students and practitioners who are radically defective in spelling, grammar, etymology, descriptive geography, arithmetic, and, I might add book-keeping, but that they generally apply themselves to the study of that important branch with a diligence which supplies the want of early opportunities. Grammar and spelling especially (to use the language in which I once heard a physician speak of the circulation of the blood) appear to be among the "*secret arcanums of nature which Dr. Hamilton said never would be found out.*" Nothing is more common than to commit gross violations of both, in the directions which we write for our patients; and, what is still more humbling to the pride of the profession, not a few of us never learn to spell the names, either of the medicines which we administer or the diseases which we cure. Were this confined to unauthorized members of the profession it would be an affair of little magnitude, but extending to many of the graduates of *all* our Universities it calls for unreserved exposure and unqualified reprehension. Before the Revolution, the schools of the Colonies were generally bad, and till lately those of the West were not fitted to impart a good elementary education; but at present they are so improved as to leave no excuse for the literary ignorance which disgraces the profession. The taint, however, is hereditary and may yet run through several generations, unless the authoritative members of the faculty can be moved to unite their prescriptions upon it. It would certainly not

---

*Of course, on this occasion I expect the reader to understand the word *professor* as synonymous with *practitioner* and not as referring to public teachers, whose commissions must be regarded as evidence of learning, should other proofs *happen* now and then to be wanting.

be unreasonable to require that every youth who aspires to connect himself with a liberal pursuit should first learn to spell and write his mother tongue with as much accuracy as a country schoolmaster; if either his genius or misfortunes preclude such acquirements, he had better take to some calling which does not demand them.

On reading the foregoing sentences to a friend, I found him sceptical as to their accuracy; which leads me to declare that *I* am entirely convinced of it. Nothing could be further from my heart than a desire to disparage the character of a profession to which, "man and boy," I have been attached for nearly thirty years, and to the advancement of which my humble exertions have been devoted for most of that period. During this time, I have become acquainted with the literary and professional ignorance of so many students and physicians in and of various parts of the Union that I cannot be mistaken in asserting that the majority of the profession in America are deficient in common school learning. If such be the fact, it should not be considered libelous to publish it, especially when done by one who claims no exemption from the imperfections which he deplores. So long as we "measure ourselves by ourselves and compare ourselves among ourselves" we are not likely either to perceive or supply our defects. There can be no true reformation without a consciousness of its necessity; and if these remarks should contribute, but in the slightest degree, to excite it I shall submit cheerfully to the odium which they may bring upon me from those who find recrimination more convenient than improvement.

But is the education which our common schools confer a sufficient preparation for the study of medicine? It certainly is not. To a familiar acquaintance with the branches which have been enumerated, the intended student of medicine should add a competent knowledge of the elements of physical geography, general history, the art of composition, algebra, geometry, and mechanics. If these acquirements are not made before he enters on his professional studies, he will most probably remain without them through his whole life; the effects of which will be sufficiently obvious to others, if not felt by himself. After what has been said concerning our deficiencies in the rudiments of learning, it will scarcely be supposed that our acquaintance with the sciences of this second group is such as to constitute a suitable introduction to medical studies. In truth, most of use live and die in utter ignorance of them. There *was* a time when this ignorance, particularly of mechanical philosophy, would have been thought fatal to the success of a student of medicine. Our science was then held to be a branch of general physics, and the laws of the living system a mere modification of those which govern the operations of dead matter. I would be among the last to desire the revival of these exploded errors, but that we have passed from one extreme to another, seems to me an unquestionable fact. We cannot explain the phenomena of living bodies *by* the principles of natural philosophy, but at the same time are unable to comprehend them without the aid of those principles.

The functions of seeing, hearing, locomotion, respiration, and the circulation of the blood can no more be understood without an acquaintance with the laws of natural philosophy than the movements of the atmosphere or the heavenly bodies; but their agency in the two cases is widely different. In the movements of the universe we behold *only* the influence of these principles, but in the functions of organized beings they are subordinate to a vital power, the laws of which constitute the science of life, or physiology. Thus, organized bodies present us with a case in which the general laws of matter are not repealed but subjected to modification. Among all the works of God, we meet with no others which present such a great assemblage of agencies;—so diversified, yet co-operative—so admirably balanced—so harmonious, though complex and apparently involved—so productive of striking and beautiful forms! The human system is, indeed, the great mystery of creation, offering problems of matchless intricacy and shrouded from human observation by a veil which none should attempt to draw aside without deep and varied preparation.

Suppose, what is not the fact, that to common-school attainments our students added the first principles of mathematics and the other sciences constituting an academical course, would they *then* be properly qualified? I again answer they would not; and this brings us to the consideration of the learned languages as an introduction to professional studies. I shall not attempt to travel over the whole ground.

The United States are, perhaps, the only civilized country in modern times where it has been seriously doubted whether the languages and literature of the ancients should make a part of the studies of professional men. Of the various causes which have combined to suggest this question, one of the most operative is the spirit of liberal inquiry, which originated and is cherished by our free institutions. No people are so unshackled by prejudices and precedents, none so excursive, none so experimental as the American. If they do not "try all things, and hold fast to that which is good," they try many and are strongly disposed to fix upon something new.

Another cause contributing to excite the same doubt, is the successful acquisition of business by physicians who lived and died in ignorance of Greek and Latin. With such examples before us, it was natural to ask whether the study of the dead languages should be regarded as indispensable, or even beneficial, to the candidate for the honors of the profession; and not a few have, at all times, been ready to answer in the negative. In this inquiry there has been much to lead us astray.

Our forefathers (most of whom were illiterate) emigrated to a forest which it has been the occupation of their sons to subdue. In the prosecution of this Herculean task, and the subsequent establishment of institutions—political, social, and literary—they frequently experienced a want of appropriate means and were compelled by the exigencies of their novel and trying situation to think

and act with originality. Hence arose a feeling of self-reliance, a spirit of independence, a disregard of ancient customs to which we may in a great degree ascribe
that indifference to the languages and learning of antiquity which characterizes
the majority of our citizens.

Thus physical circumstances have, indirectly, exercised a mastery over moral
causes and given a deflection to our European character which promises to
become permanent. Moral causes, however, have contributed to the same effect.
In migrating from the old world, our ancestors took leave of the institutions
devoted to classical instruction; and hence a generation, of necessity, grew up in
comparative ignorance. It would be in vain to hope that a due respect for the
learned languages, or even a conviction of their utility, could survive such a
transition; and hence we find that in the United States a want of acquaintance
with them has been no serious obstacle to the attainment of high *relative* distinction in any of the pursuits of society. How long this will be the case it is not easy
to foresee. A perception of their value appears to be returning, but I cannot
suppose that they will ever attain to the rank which they hold in the estimation
of our elder brethren of Europe.

Meanwhile, it is the duty of those who can exercise any control over public
sentiment in this respect to exert themselves; and if all who are interested in the
dignity of the medical profession could be brought to unite their efforts in favor
of a more classical preparation of young men designed for the study, it cannot
be doubted that much might be accomplished, even in a single generation.

A physician who is ignorant of the Latin and Greek languages, whatever may
be his genius and professional skill, must, to the eye of sound scholarship, appear
defective and uncultivated. For more than two thousand years these languages,
especially the former, were the vehicles of all medical knowledge, except the
little contributed by the Arabians; and till within a century our professional
ancestors wrote and prescribed and thought and lectured in Latin. It was,
indeed, to the profession a universal language; affording the means of an easy
and accurate correspondence among all the schools and physicians of Europe.
Even down to the present time, the lectures in most of the Italian and German
universities are delivered in Latin; while the examination of candidates, in many
others, is conducted in the same language. Thus it has had a most protracted and
intimate companionship with medicine; to the nomenclature of which it has
freely lent its opulent vocabulary. Many of its words no doubt, as well as those
drawn from the dialects of Greece, are intended to convey in their new situation
ideas materially different from their vernacular import; but in attempting to
understand even these, the student is greatly assisted by an acquaintance with
their primitive significations. With this knowledge of our dependence on the
languages and literature of the ancients, to deny that the study of them must be
beneficial is scarcely less absurd than to affirm, on the other hand, that every
classical scholar is of necessity a physician. . . .

ESSAY II

PRIVATE PUPILAGE

It is impossible to approach this subject without emotion. I know of no other, the free discussion of which would be so likely to agitate the profession in America. That I shall treat it without prepossession, prejudice, or passion is not probable; nor is it certain that I shall say all which should be said; but intending to write with courage and candour, I may hope to awaken, if not to guide, the spirit of reform.

To come at once to a full understanding with the reader, I shall assume the general proposition that *our system of private tuition is essentially bad*. But, in truth, we have *no system*; and it would be more correct to say that in the United States *a good system of private pupilage is imperiously required*.

In the preceding essay, on the preparatory education of students, I have endeavored to show that its errors and imperfections are permanently stamped on our *literary* character. If this be the fact, we can scarcely doubt that a defective elementary education, in medicine, must greatly retard our advancement to *professional* excellence; and whatever does this, demands the gravest attention.

The ordinary time of private instruction is so short as to require that it should be well employed. If the rudiments of the profession are not *then* acquired, they are seldom properly understood. It is not easy, afterwards, to supply the omissions or correct the errors of that period. I have never known it done. Every stage of life has its peculiar tastes and appropriate studies. In youth we acquire elementary truths; in manhood arrange them into general principles; in the meridian of life apply them to the production of practical results. Such is the law of nature; and was it inscribed on the doors of every medical library they would not so often be opened to no beneficial effect.

Having spoken at large of the selection of pupils, I come now to the choice of preceptors. This is a point of more importance than most parents suppose. Many of them, indeed, seem to act on this important subject with but little discrimination. The circumspection with which they select masters, when about to apprentice their sons to mechanical occupations, is seldom manifested when a medical education is the object. They appear indeed to feel themselves incompetent to judge in the latter case and, generally, consult economy or convenience; although in so doing they not unfrequently determine for their sons a far more imperfect and limited destiny than they intend.

1. It is not *necessary* that the preceptor should be a man of genius, but it is indispensable that he should possess a sound and discriminating judgment, otherwise he will be a blind guide. Of his qualifications in this respect, every parent with opportunities of personal intercourse may form a correct opinion. It is not requisite that he himself should be acquainted with the principles of the profes-

sion to judge of the talents and common sense of its practitioners: the most unlearned can distinguish between a clouded and an unclouded intellect.

2. A preceptor should be learned, at least in his profession. If a father wishes to make his son a skilful mechanic, he places him with a good workman—not a botch. How can a man direct the studies of a youth through the elements of several different sciences, if his own acquaintance with them is imperfect and confused? As well might architecture be taught by one who ignorantly combined in the same column the parts and proportions which belong to all the different orders. To judge of the *attainments* of professional men is a more difficult task than to estimate their *abilities*; but although a father may not be able to do this by direct inquiries, he still has much in his power in this respect. The previous opportunities of the individual whom he scrutinizes, taken in connection with his existing habits, will generally enable him to come to a correct conclusion. If the former have been limited and the latter are idle, he may safely conclude that the requisite attainments are wanting and look elsewhere for the aid which is indispensable to a rapid and logical prosecution of studies.

3. It is not sufficient that a private preceptor has talents and learning. He must be devoted to his profession, jealous of its character, and ambitious of its honors. With such feelings, he will awaken high aspirations in the bosom of the youth whose destiny is committed to his keeping, enamour him with the sciences whose rudiments he is to acquire, and animate him in the toil which their difficulties impose.

4. The preceptor should be conscientious in the performance of his duties; that is, he should feel the responsibilities of his office and studiously endeavor to discharge them. It is easy to deceive a father in regard to the progress of a son, in the study of a profession with which the former is unacquainted, for all his partialities coincide with the flattering reports of the master and cause them to be received with credulity. In this way many a tutor has repressed paternal anxiety and screened from paternal vigilance his inattention and neglect; inspiring high hopes at the very moment when his own criminal derelictions of duty were sowing the seeds of their future destruction.

5. The private preceptor should, if possible, be a man of business:—punctual to his pecuniary engagements, accurate in his accounts, and systematic in all his affairs. He will thus be an example for the imitation of his pupils on points in which too many students of medicine grow up with deplorable and enduring imperfections.

6. Finally, sound morals and chastened habits are not among the least of those qualifications which an anxious father would require in the man whose deportment and precepts are to exert so great an influence on the character of his son. It would be superfluous to enumerate all the vices which ought to disqualify a physician for the private tuition of boys and young men; but there are a few which from their frequency and effect deserve on every suitable occasion to be held up to the scorn of society. A want of attention to profes-

sional promises, with a consequent fabrication of excuses and apologies, is a
failure which no preceptor can habitually display with impunity to the morals of
his pupil and ought to be regarded as a disqualification, with whatever genius
and learning it might happen to be associated. Gambling is another vice, the
morbid influence of which on the plastic and imitative pupil should be still more
seriously deprecated, since, in addition to the corruption which it carries into
the youthful heart, it diverts from study, generates neglect of business, and leads
to the loss of character and fortune. Lastly, intemperance, not less than gaming,
should displace a physician from the ranks of those whom we entrust with the
tuition of young men. Intemperance, in the United States at least, has been
regarded as a prevailing vice of the profession, and it has too often happened
that boys, almost from necessity, have been apprenticed to drunken doctors. I
am proud to say that this necessity is rapidly diminishing. Nevertheless, the
number of intemperate physicians is still so great that parents should proceed
with care and caution in the choice of preceptors. One of the greatest calamities
they could inflict on a son would be to place him under the guardianship of a
drunkard: if unsusceptible of being corrupted by example, he would suffer
numerous embarrassments and mortifications—if susceptible, he must be ruined.
   It would not be easy to estimate the injury which has resulted to individuals,
to the profession, and to society at large from a want of discrimination in
parents, when about to place their sons to the study of medicine. Many a youth
has, in this manner, been sacrificed by an ignorant or thoughtless father. Irreso-
lution has sunk into moral cowardice, dullness declined into stupidity, and
genius substituted its flights and phantasies for patient analysis; ambition has
found its goal in the acquisition of premature and badly earned certificates and
diplomas; idleness relieved itself by ceaseless changes from frivolity to frivolity;
and the love of pleasure been left to luxuriate into licentiousness and vice. It is
playing at cross purposes for a father to dispense with the services of his son and
incur the expense of his professional education and, at the same time, to place
him under an unqualified or unprincipled master. It is due to themselves and
their children that parents should consider this subject seriously. It is, also, due
to the profession and the community that they discriminate on this point. When
they confide their sons to the ignorant, the indolent, or the vicious they encourage that which every member of the commonwealth is bound to discountenance,
and withhold from the learned and meritorious members of the profession one
of the legitimate rewards of their industry, zeal, and perseverance. Could no
physician hope to attain the distinction of being a preceptor without first establishing a character for sound science and good morals, not a few who are now
reckless of both would be held firmly to their acquisition.
   Another mistake which requires correction relates to the time of life when
medical studies are commenced. Essentially latitudinarian, the American people
allow themselves in this respect, as in most others, a singular degree of liberty.
Many boys are put to the study of physic at fifteen, while men of twenty five or

upwards, who have been too indolent or too unskillful to succeed in their first pursuits, are every day seen to betake themselves to this most difficult and elevated vocation without a single misgiving. Examples of success might be cited in support of both periods, but still they are extremes. When a boy begins the study at fifteen or sixteen, he generally sets up for himself at nineteen or twenty, a time of life when he lacks *judgment*, whatever may be his acuteness of parts or the extent of his information. On the other hand, he who takes his first lessons after his mind has attained maturity will seldom move with ease in the practical duties of the profession, even if his life has been spent in studies up to that period; and, if this should not have been the case, which in America is the general fact, the chances are altogether against his ever becoming useful or acquiring public confidence. Seventeen or eighteen seems to me the most proper age to commence the study. By that time, a due preparatory education may be acquired, the mind and *hands* are still so plastic as to be directed in their operations, the reasoning faculties are sufficiently developed to investigate the principles of the profession, and the period between that and twenty-one or twenty-two is about long enough to admit of the necessary acquisitions.

The youth of the United States are not only put to the study of medicine at improper ages but the period of their studies is too short. Nothing is more common than for them to enter on the practice at the end of two years or even eighteen months, and three years are thought to be a protracted and tiresome pupilage. But I do not hesitate to assert that even that term is too short and that four years should be considered as indispensable. Of the various causes which have retarded the advancement of the profession in this country and inflicted upon it such multitudes of medical practitioners who leave behind them no single monument of skill or science this is one of the most operative and universal. The blame rests, in part, on our *national* impatience to engage in practical exertions, but still more on the custom which prevails among fathers who are indigent, or but little above that condition, of assigning their sons to the profession. The term of their pupilage is thus determined not by the sciences which they ought to study but their means of support.

The situation and circumstances in which a pupil should prosecute his studies deserve to be considered. In the country and all the smaller towns of the United States, the fashion is for the student to reside and study in the *shop* or office of his preceptor, and often to become a member of his family. The latter has its advantages, as contributing to preserve him from dissipation; but his time is too often wasted in labors foreign to his studies, and he is apt to be introduced more frequently into company than is compatible with his interests as a student. Of the *office* as a place for study, "much might be said on both sides." It is the resort of many persons besides those who call for medical assistance, and the student is subjected to perpetual, if not protracted, interruptions. In this way he loses many precious hours which can never be reclaimed. At first, the effect of

these interruptions is so distracting as materially to impede his progress; but
their influence diminishes with the repetition, until at last he comes to form
habits that are not without their value in after life. . . .

The student who intends to limit himself to the practice of physic must
recollect that even in countries where the line of separation is drawn with an
absurd and unnatural precision, the physician is compelled to prescribe for a
great number and variety of cases which belong equally to the province of the
surgeon. If this be the case in Europe, it must be much more so in the United
States, where out of the large cities there are no professed surgeons. In fact, all
our physicians are surgeons likewise, and differ from the practitioners so called,
only in declining the performance of a few of the greater operations—such as
those for hernia, lithotomy, aneurysm, deep-seated tumors, cataract, and a few
others. In the reduction of dislocation and fractures, the management of ulcers,
trephining, amputating, dressing wounds, and other duties of a similar kind,
which, from their frequency, make up the mass of surgical business, every physician is presumed to be competent. The pupil then, even when engaged in his
practical studies, is by no means to limit himself to that which is technically
called physic, but, extending his inquiries to surgery, stops short of nothing but
its higher operations.

Every part of a course of medical studies abounds in difficulties and calls for
intense and sustained application; but no stage is so trying to the powers of the
student as that which may be called the *therapeutick*. Hitherto he has occupied
himself, successively, upon distinct sciences which he perceived to abound in
connections favorable to their union into a system of professional knowledge;
and that union, in reference to his own mind, he is now to effect. He is faithfully
represented by the commander, who having embodied and equipped a great
variety of separate military *corps*, has at length to consolidate them into an army
and direct its active operations.

It is difficult to furnish a student with rules for the organization of his various
attainments into a practical system, and much must necessarily be left to his
own genius and judgment. A few hints, however, may not be without their
utility.

1. If he now finds deficiencies in any of his preliminary acquirements, he
should supply them, without delay, by a recurrence to the branches in which
they are discovered to exist.

2. In ascertaining general principles, he should carefully note those which are
of a doubtful character and rest upon them as few rules of practice as possible.

3. His practical maxims, in all cases, should be logical deductions from his
principles.

4. If they do not conform to those of the great and original writers of the
profession, he should *doubt* their correctness and act upon them cautiously, but
not reject them without a trial.

5. He should recollect that the same diseases, in different countries, frequently require variations in their treatment and that he must not implicitly adopt the rules of practice that have been found successful elsewhere.

6. When he meets, in practical works, with different modes of treatment for the same disease, he should not suppose that one only can be correct and the others necessarily erroneous, for diseases may be cured by various methods. In becoming an eclectic, in these cases he must carefully examine the whole and test their merits by the great principles of pathology and therapeutics which compose his own system. When he attempts to select from among them, he should avoid uniting rules or recipes that are incompatible and would therefore countervail or neutralize each other.

7. In his practical readings, he should always prefer original works to compilations and monographs to systems.

8. He must be on his guard against the delusion of a fancied simplicity in the system which he constructs. Every complex machine is liable to a variety of irregular movements which can only be reduced to order by a corresponding diversity of means. But of all machines the human body is the most complicated, exhibits the greatest number of disordered actions, all differing from each other, and requires the greatest variety of remedial applications.

9. When arrived at this stage of his studies, he should no longer stand aloof from the practical duties of the profession, but avail himself of frequent opportunities to make an application of his knowledge. This is the end for which he has studied, and his final success will be proportionate to the facility and effect with which he can make such application. Skill in practice does not arise, however, from the number of cases he may see or treat, so much as the manner in which he contemplates them. Each one should be a study, and all things relating to it should be connected with the principles that guide him and which, in turn, they may serve to illustrate or overthrow.

Should the student intend to make Operative Surgery, his principal object, he may observe most of the foregoing suggestions, while he bestows especial attention on the following subjects:

1. The anatomy of the parts which are the seats of the greater operations of the art. With these parts, particularly such of them as cannot be cut into without danger, he should be perfectly familiar:—not merely able to enumerate the muscles, and fasciae, and nerves, and blood vessels of which they are composed, but to conceive accurately of the relative situation of those anatomical elements. He should, moreover, learn to know each part, not only by the eye but by the finger; as it will frequently happen, in deep and bloody operations, that the sense of touch is the only one he can employ.

2. He should practice the various operations on the dead subject; for by practice only, can he become adroit or acquire that confidence which gives self-possession in moments of difficulty and doubt. In this stage of his *practical* studies, he will often find it advantageous to supply this deficiency of human

subjects by a resort to dead animals; in the selection of which he will be materially aided by some acquaintance with zoology.

3. He should practise on the living or the dead subject the application of the various kinds of bandages and apparatus of surgery. For the neat and efficient discharge of this duty more experience is necessary than many persons suppose, until they come to the trial in cases of real injury when it is too late to prepare themselves.

I shall conclude this branch of the subject with a reference to obstetrics. This department of the profession is emphatically a compound of physic and surgery and, on this account not less than many others, it should be the last which a pupil studies. The healthy functions of the uterine system, however, will have been learned by him, as a portion of physiology. As to obstetrical studies, the most important observation I can make is that the young physician will be called upon to act with less of *practical* information than in any other branch of the profession, for in no stage of his pupilage can he have many opportunities of acquiring that kind of knowledge. Hence he should study the subject in books and by means of plates and models with extraordinary care and diligence. Without doing this he may be thrown into situations of responsibility most harrowing to his feelings, if not fatal to his patient.

With these intimations I shall close what it seems necessary to say concerning the method on which a course of professional studies should be conducted. . . .

ANDREW BOARDMAN

AN ESSAY ON THE MEANS OF IMPROVING MEDICAL EDUCATION AND ELEVATING MEDICAL CHARACTER

Editor's Note

Very little biographical data seem to be available on Andrew Boardman. He published a book in 1847 entitled *A Defence of Phrenology* (New York: Kearny), which would explain his remark on the first page of his essay where chemistry is compared to alchemy, astronomy to astrology, and phrenology to palmistry.[1]

Boardman's essay on medical education is of interest because it represents a frank appraisal of the way things really were. One lesson to be drawn from him is that not all that was listed in the medical school catalogs came to pass. In his case very little did, if we can believe his criticisms.

Boardman dealt with the popular problem of his day, the uncertainty in medicine (see Sections III and IV). He also dealt with one of the minor conflicts in medical education at the time—the necessity of training in the classical languages. Boardman strongly decried this remnant from a time past. Some contemporaries agreed with him, many, such as Daniel Drake, did not. The usual argument in favor of studying Latin and Greek was similar to that noted by Boardman and voiced by Dr. John Ware of Boston in 1843:

> there is a kind of improvement of the mind from liberal studies,—I refer more particularly to the study of classics . . . . I know it is fashionable, especially in our utilitarian communities, to decry these studies are useless, and account the time spent upon them as wasted. I cannot agree to this opinion. I believe the study of language to be the most fitting occupation of a certain period of life, and indeed, we may say, a necessary, or at least a very important process in the cultivation of the mind.[2]

On the problem of medical examinations and certification of physicians Boardman made some sensible suggestions, albeit against the ideals of states' rights.[3]

---

[1] The Library of Congress card for this book does not list his dates either. John D. Davies in his, *Phrenology, Fad and Science: A 19th-Century American Crusade* (New Haven: Yale University Press, 1955), mentions Boardman in connection with the *Defence*, but identifies him only as the secretary of the New York Phrenological Society.

[2] John Ware, "Medical Education in 1843," in *Discourses on Medical Education and the Medical Profession* (Boston: Munroe, 1847), pp. 51–80; 58. Ware admitted that the knowledge of Greek and Latin may be of very little use, but not so the study. He was not prepared to admit that the study of French and German would have the same effect in mental discipline (pp. 59–60).

[3] See Richard H. Shryock's *Medical Licensing in America, 1650–1965* (Baltimore: The Johns Hopkins Press, 1967).

INTRODUCTION*

The views maintained in the following thesis were formed from observation and reflection suggested by the difficulties which I had to encounter in attempting to become fitted for the practice of medicine. The inferences which I have drawn from the facts stated, and the propositions which I make may be or may not be sound; but as the facts themselves are undeniable, the necessity for reform cannot be questioned, and if the following essay has no other effect than that of increasing the interest of the profession in the momentous cause of medical reform, of directing to the subject minds better fitted for the investigation, and of eliciting views more in accordance with sound principles, I shall deem myself repaid a hundredfold.

I have stated that my own experience prompted the investigation of which the following essay is the result; and as facts accurately stated are to the philosophic mind of the utmost value and importance, I respectfully invite attention to a few of the items of that experience.

On formally commencing my medical studies, I attended a private course of anatomical lectures delivered by a gentleman of fine talents and of great professional zeal. With this course I was much pleased and benefited. Everything was described and demonstrated most clearly and satisfactorily; and the descriptions and demonstrations were repeated by the students, subject to the correction of the instructor. In this class were a number who, as I learned from themselves, paid for the college ticket that they *might graduate*, but seldom attended the college lectures; and they paid for and attended the private course, that they *might learn anatomy*. I was at once struck with the injustice of making them pay for lectures which they did not attend and of counting valueless those lectures, dissections, and demonstrations which were so admirably fitted to give a thorough knowledge of the human structure. On attending college lectures myself, I was more deeply convinced of this injustice on finding, by comparison, that *caeteris paribus*, private lectures were superior to public ones as means of acquiring anatomical knowledge. In the private class everything may be seen clearly by every student. In the anatomical theater, on the contrary, the nearest students cannot see distinctly the parts alluded to, and those at a distance can hardly see them at all. I think I observed distinctly another important fact, namely, that those who depended for support on the voluntary attendance of pupils were more zealous and industrious than those who were favored and protected by a chartered monopoly. Indeed, I have paid for lectures at public institutions which would not have been tolerated from private lecturers. I paid for one course on physiology which embodied the science not as it now exists but as it existed a long time ago; and for another course which was not delivered

*It will be seen by the reader, at once, that this Introduction was written subsequently to the Dissertation which follows, and which is now published in the form in which it was presented to the Faculty of Geneva College.

I paid for one course on the theory and practice which consisted, to a great extent, of historical accounts and labored refutations of all the defunct and entombed medical absurdities of which the annals of our art speak; and for another course which consisted chiefly of verbatim extracts from Eberle's and from Mackintosh's theory and practice. I paid for a course on therapeutics in which I could accompany the professor in Eberle and Dunglison, word for word through entire lectures, the plagiarism extending to Dunglison's numerous poetical quotations. I do not wish to convey the idea that the lectures at chartered institutions are generally unworthy of patronage. I have attended lectures at such institutions which have been most able and beneficial and which have afforded almost unmixed and unanimous satisfaction. I deem much in the present system of medical education to be unsound, but it may, by talented and zealous men, be rendered productive of gratifying results. That it is liable to great and manifold abuses, however, is undeniable, and to illustrate this still further I state the following facts, without note or comment.

I attended the lectures of Geneva College during the session of 1839–40, and graduated at the end of the term. I here introduce a comparison between the promises held out in the college circular as inducements to medical students and the mode in which those promises were fulfilled.

Promise of the Circular. That the course on chemistry should be delivered by a doctor of medicine.

Fulfilment. The chemical course was delivered by a doctor of divinity who acknowledged, in my hearing, that he had often to lecture from notes which he had not looked at for five or six years before bringing them into the lecture-room.

Promise of the Circular. That a course of lectures on medical jurisprudence should be delivered.

Fulfilment. We were not favored with a single lecture on the subject.

Promise of the Circular. That there should be a course of lectures on physiology.

Fulfilment. No such course was delivered.

Promise of the Circular. That the anatomical class should have a full supply of subjects for dissection.

Fulfilment. Not *a single subject* was provided for dissection during the *whole session*, though students deposited money for them at the rate of $40 a subject at the commencement of the term. Nor was there more than a single subject, and that a very poor one, used for demonstration during the entire anatomical course.

Promise of the Circular. That the students attending Geneva College should have the great advantage of clinical instruction at The Western Hospital, an institution connected with the medical school.

Fulfilment. The Western Hospital consisted of the second floor of an old building labeled in large letters, "Geneva Shoe Store," and during the whole session it contained *not one* medical patient and *only one* surgical patient. I was house surgeon and performed my daily rounds for a considerable time by going from one side of the bed of a quiet old negress to the other. Attracted by the reputation of the surgical professor, however, many patients came in from the surrounding country, on whom operations were performed before the class.

Promise of the Anatomical Professor. That a special diploma should be presented to the best practical anatomist of the graduating class.

Fulfilment. Such diploma with the heading "*palmam qui meruit ferat*," was made out in my favor; but no means of acquiring practical skill having been afforded and no tests of practical skill having been applied, I declined the proffered honor.

Promise of the Circular. That a gold medal should be presented to the author of the *best thesis* on any medical subject.

Fulfilment. On this subject I am not a competent witness and, therefore, take the liberty of introducing the following copy of a letter addressed by Professor Rogers to a few of his friends:

> Geneva, 20*th January*, 1840
>
> *Dear Sir,*—I sit down this evening to state briefly the cause of my resigning the chair of surgery in the Geneva Medical College, that you may be enabled to give an authentic explanation to any of my friends who may inquire concerning it.
>
> After accepting the professorship of surgery, I engaged to place annually at the disposal of the faculty a gold medal for presentation to that graduate who should produce the *best thesis* on some medical subject. During last summer I received a letter from a former student of mine (Mr. Boardman), announcing his intention of graduating at Geneva and inquiring whether the thesis would be judged of by the accordance of their views with those of the professors or by the comparative ability with which the writers maintained their opinions, and by the comparative clearness, force, and correctness of style; intimating, at the same time, that if the latter were the case, he should advocate some views adverse to the present system of medical education.
>
> With the sanction of the only collaborator then in Geneva, I replied, that we were not so illiberal as to expect that gentlemen should conform their opinions to ours and that in awarding the medal we decided exclusively on the comparative merits of the theses as literary productions.
>
> I shall not trouble you with a detailed account of intermediate proceedings, but briefly state that Mr. Boardman came to Geneva and in due time presented his thesis, that one professor immediately stated had great merit, but that a thesis maintaining such views would not be permitted to take the medal, whatever might be its intrinsic merits. The others spoke more liberally, but decided on the same grounds; thus, in fact, putting his thesis out of the pale of competition and, accordingly, notwithstanding our printed assurance, notwithstanding the personal assurance given by myself and another professor, that merit in composition and ability in writing would form the exclusive grounds of decision, the medal was awarded to a production which no member of the faculty will hazard his

MEDICAL EDUCATION

reputation by placing on an equal footing with Mr. Boardman's in these respects. The preferred thesis has merit, but there is in it nothing original, no striking views or sustained argumentation: the style is verbose, unequal, and sophomoric, full of scraps of Latin and allusions to the heathen mythology. The rejected thesis is grave, thoughtful, and argumentative, indicative of an observant and sagacious mind: the style is clear, forcible, and mature, and though the positions are bold, they are maintained with courtesy.

Under the circumstances no course was left me to pursue but that of withdrawing my name from a transaction in which there appeared to me a violation of honor and justice and an attempt to crush instead of encourage an inquiring and independent spirit.

Yours very sincerely,
D. L. ROGERS

I shall merely add to the above letter an extract from one which I addressed to another professor on the occasion of his making to me a proposition in the name of the faculty: "Immediately after presenting my thesis, I was informed by one professor that the subject would inevitably damn it without the slightest reference to its merits, and you yourself acknowledge that you took into consideration in your decision the circumstances which, I had been assured, would be left out of view. I mention these facts to show, sir, that I object not to your judgment but to your rule of judging—that I feel wronged, not because another has been preferred but because I have been put out of the pale of competition."

A medal is of small value, but justice and freedom of opinion are of paramount importance.

INAUGURAL DISSERTATION

The healing art is doubtless coëval with the breach of those laws on the observance of which immunity from disease depends, and we need no fable from the heathen mythology to account for its origin. Whoever first attempted to relieve the physical sufferings of a fellow being was the father of physic. Ignorant of internal organization and function, and to a great extent of external agents and influences, remedial efforts would at first be confined to the soothing attentions of a sympathizing spirit, a remedy which may yet be classed as not only the most agreeable but as one of the most efficient of therapeutic agents. The necessity of the healing art sprang then from the misfortunes, the ignorance, and the wickedness of man, and the art itself from what may well be called the divinity of human nature—intellect prompted to exertion by benevolence and affection.

Medical men and their profession have often been the butt of the humorist's gibes and the satirist's sarcasms, and not undeservedly in all cases. But a change has come over the profession: the days of bag-wigs, powdered heads, lengthened solemnity of visage, and inveterate technicality of phrase, are gone, we hope, forever. The time, too, has passed away, when oil from kittens boiled alive was considered an admirable application to wounds; when toads roasted alive were administered for asthma, and the hairs of mad dogs for hydrophobia; when the powdered thigh-bone of an executed felon was considered a specific in dysentery, and ointment was applied to the inflicting weapon in order to cure the wound; when physicians placed confidence in phylacteries and watched with intense anxiety the influence of black and white days and the aspects of the stars; and when they hurried their unfortunate patients to an untimely grave in attempting to quench the fires of fever and inflammation by diligently feeding the consuming flame. To confound medicine as now with medicine as then taught, would be as illiberal and unjust as to confound chemistry with alchemy, astronomy with astrology, or, I must add, phrenology with palmistry.

But though we cannot agree with the writer who defines physic to be the art of amusing the patient while nature cures the disease; nor with him who asserts that almost the only resource of medicine is the art of conjecturing, it cannot be denied that much uncertainty does in reality exist. The talented editor of the *Medico-Chirurgical Review* recently asserted (April, 1839) that "one-half of our practice is guess work"; and if he meant his remark to apply not to the art itself but to the art as practiced, many, doubtless, will subscribe to its truth.

Much, however, that has been *popularly* said of the uncertainty of medicine, has arisen from misconceiving its true objects. When a beloved parent or child is lying on the bed of sickness, or a friend who has gilded the pathway of life with the blessed light of affection is on the brink of the grave, grief, in its unreasoning paroxysms, asks why our art is not omnipotent; forgetting that it is not for man to set aside the laws of nature, rejuvenate the old, and restore the broken constitution to healthy vigor. Physic possesses not, nor does it look for, an elixir of immortality: it merely claims to be the application of such means as accumulated experience, cautious observation, and sound judgment have proved efficacious in ameliorating or curing disease; and its perfection would consist in a knowledge of the most certain, ready, and least painful mode of restoring health when restoration is possible, and of the means of soothing pain and prolonging life to the utmost when restoration is impossible. In view of this definition, it is not too much to say that our art may yet approximate closely to perfection; and even now it may be questioned whether uncertainty is not much more in physicians than in physic.

This word uncertainty is often employed as though it were relative not to man's ignorance but to nature's operations. In these, however, whether on the most minute or expanded scale, there is no uncertainty, indefiniteness, or chance-play. Whenever, therefore, it is said that, on any point, uncertainty exists, it merely shows that on that point our knowledge of nature is incomplete. There was a time when the motions of the comets were considered irregular and lawless as those of the winds are now commonly considered, but our knowledge has been enlarged, and we can calculate their revolutions with perfect precision; and the time may come, it seems, indeed, near at hand, when it shall be demonstrated that every movement of the air, whether in the form of a zephyr, a gale, or a tornado, depends for its course, intensity, and duration on laws as invariable as those which buoy the sun upon nothing and give speed and invariableness to the wingless and compassless comets. In medicine, the physician's assertion that anything is uncertain is, in truth, an acknowledgment that on that point his knowledge is only partial. No disease occurs which has not a certain adequate cause, though of that cause we may be ignorant, which has not its chief seat in some definite part of the system, though of that seat we may be unable to satisfy ourselves, which has not produced at any given time a precise amount of functional derangement or organic change, though our idea of that amount may be most erroneous; and for which there exists not, in the nature of things, a remedial course, the most appropriate that can be pursued, though we, in our ignorance, may honestly pursue a course much less efficacious, or which shall even aggravate instead of ameliorating or curing.

If then there is no uncertainty in nature, we must seek for its sources in man alone, and these may be reduced to three.

1. *The imperfection of existing knowledge.*—The present resources of our art are immense. How quickly and surely do diseases quit or relax their grasp when encountered by learning, experience, and judgment. Then is it demonstrated beyond controversy how much the healing art can achieve. Still it must be owned that if the present collective knowledge of the profession were centered in one man of the greatest experience and soundest judgment, he would sometimes be in unpleasant dilemmas from lack of more knowledge. For this we have no remedy but that of winning further discoveries from nature by careful observation and rigid induction.

2. *Our constitutional incapacities*—There are great constitutional differences in the mental fitness of men for the practice of medicine. It needs in the intellect a combination of the observing and reflecting faculties, and in the moral nature a union of caution, courage, and sympathy which is not common. Against mental incapacity the profession might, in some degree, protect itself by rendering the conditions of admission into its ranks such as would exclude those who possess not a fair share of the requisite intellectual qualities.

3. *Our lack of such knowledge as exists, and our inability to reduce to practice such knowledge as we possess.*—Over the first source of uncertainty we have no present control; our control over the second is limited; over this, however, it is great, and as the subject of medical education occupies at present the attention of practitioners throughout the union, as everywhere such education is acknowledged to be imperfect and propositions of reform are made, I shall dwell chiefly in the present essay on the deficiency, inappropriateness, and reformation of medical education.

I am aware that what I am about to advance may, at first, appear ultra and visionary, but being profoundly convinced of the truth and importance of my views, I pray that they may not be disregarded, because of the humble source whence they emanate. I adduce facts and invite scrutiny, arguments, and beg for calm and serious consideration. I am merely an inquirer, desirous of taking my stand on the broad foundations of human and external nature and of asking the opinions and practices which I consider the *why* of their existence.

The two most prominent propositions which have been made for the purpose of elevating medical character, and improving medical education, are:

1. The requirement of a knowledge of Greek and Latin, as a prerequisite to a medical degree.

2. One year's extension of the prerequisite period of study. . . .

It is true that there is a technical language employed by medical men derived principally from the dead tongues. But that is learned at the time a knowledge of the things signified is learned, and neither Hellenist nor Latinist can learn it in any other way; and though the classical scholar would often be aided in the recollection of terms by his previous education, yet it is undeniable that the derivation of our technical words often affords no clue whatever to their meaning. What aid does the student derive from knowing that sacrum is derived from *sacer*, sacred; fibula from *figo*, to fasten; clavicle from *clavis*, a key; tartar from *tartaros*, infernal; ranula and ranunculus from *rana*, a frog; scrofula from *scrofa*, a swine; artery from *aer*, air, and *tereo*, to keep. Nay, there are many diseases so named that he who understands the derivation of the words used in naming them, is more likely to misconceive their true nature than he who merely knows their names as the exponents of certain pathological conditions. For instance the words typhus and gonorrhea; also cholera, as applied to the late epidemic; nyctalopia and hemeralopia, as commonly employed. But then the elegance, the euphony of these languages! Let these qualities be admitted to their fullest extent—what then? I answer that they will be most necessary to the physician when he has to talk in Greek or Latin periods, or to write his prescriptions in hexameters, but that that time has not yet arrived.

But, say the advocates of this proposition, the study of these languages is useful in training the mind. I do not deny this, but maintain, that as a preparation for the practice of medicine, the mind might be much better and more usefully trained by a thorough study of our native tongue; by the study of mental and moral philosophy, political economy, the general principles of law, and various branches of natural history. But even admitting that the study of languages should be insisted upon as a prerequisite of practice, the question—what languages? would necessarily be suggested; and the preference could not be given on any grounds of utility, to the Greek and Latin over the French and German. In the two latter, new works of great value are continually appearing; whereas, in the two former, hardly any new work, either literary or scientific, is now published. . . .

From these considerations I conclude, that whatever may be the desirableness of a knowledge of the dead languages, as a prerequisite to other pursuits, to insist on such knowledge as a prerequisite to the practice of medicine would be unjust and irrational.

Let us now examine the second proposition; namely, an extension of the time of study from three to four years. This might be efficacious, could its adoption secure a greater amount of study and observation; but in this it would most probably fail. It is true, indeed, that a man can obtain more knowledge and practical skill in four years than in three; but it is also true that he may merely proceed with his studies more lazily and leisurely and thus impair the power of concentrated attention. We want some better test of a man's fitness for a medical degree than that he has had his name on a physician's book, three, four, or any other number of years. Indeed, this proposition is founded on the erroneous notion that man's acquirements are in the direct ratio of the time they may be studying or pretend to be studying; but it is matter of common observation that of two who are equally assiduous, one can acquire knowledge and skill much more rapidly than the other, and that of two who have equal capacity and equal facility of acquirement, the one may be much more assiduous than the other. To subject all capacities and all degrees of assiduity to the same unbending rule of time is, I think, unjust; it breaks down all the natural distinctions between lassitude and energy, indolence and industry, talent and imbecility.

Having given my reasons for believing the proposed changes to be inadequate and inappropriate, I proceed to survey the present mode and extent of medical education and prerequisite qualifications of a graduate, and to explain my views of what medical education should be and what prerequisites should constitute the *sine qua non* of graduation.

By collating the circulars of the various medical schools throughout the United States, it will be found that each has professorships separate or conjoint for the teaching of—1. Anatomy. 2. Physiology. 3. Theory and Practice. 4. Materia Medica. 5. Surgery. 6. Obstetrics. 7. Chemistry. 8. Medical Jurisprudence. And that in each the prerequisites of a diploma are: 1. Three years study with a regular practitioner. 2. Attendance on the lectures of some chartered school during two sessions. 3. The presentation of a thesis on some medical subject. 4. The approval, after examination, of the medical professors whose lectures the candidate has attended.

To the physician, as such, man is the center of the universe. He should study the human frame in health and disease and then study all things which relate to or have an influence upon it. He should be so acquainted with the human body as to see with conception's eye all its various parts in their true relative position. This constitutes anatomical knowledge. He should be acquainted with the operations of these various parts, their modes and purposes of action; this constitutes physiological knowledge. He should be acquainted with the influence of all physical and moral agents on healthy man; with the properties of the *materia alimentaria*, of air, temperature, occupation; with the influence of location, seasons and emanations; that he may know how to keep the whole organization in a state of health; this constitutes hygienic knowledge. Anatomy, physiology, and hygiene form the group of studies which have for their object a knowledge of what man is, and of what he should be, and of the mode of keeping his organs in healthy and harmonious play. They are the foundation of all correct knowledge and practice, making known as they do those standards in human and external nature, to remedy or obviate departures from which is the peculiar object of our art. The physician should earnestly direct attention to derangements of function, alterations of structure, the aberrations from hygienic laws on which such derangements and alterations depend, and to the remedial means required to restore the body to physical soundness. All knowledge relating directly to these things is comprised under the terms pathology and therapeutics. He should be acquainted with the properties, relations, and mode of preparing remedial agents. Materia medica, pharmacy and, to a certain extent, the collateral sciences are, therefore, important branches of study. He should be acquainted, too, with whatever relates to operative surgery, obstetrics, and medical jurisprudence.

By comparing the subjects taught at our medical schools with the above exposition of the attainments necessary to constitute an accomplished practitioner, it will be seen that the objects sought to be attained are almost sufficiently comprehensive. There is, indeed, one important omission, that is, of Hygiene, which comprises knowledge of the utmost importance to the practitioner and ought, therefore, to form an essential branch of medical education. If, then, the objects sought to be attained are almost sufficiently comprehensive, the inefficiency of medical education must be looked for in the mode in which it is conducted. To this point, then, let us now turn our attention.

The examination which a candidate has to undergo previous to receiving the highest medical honor, and being pronounced most learned and most worthy, is simply of the following nature. During the college terms the professors say certain things, and at the examination they ask certain questions, in order to ascertain whether what they have said be recollected by the candidates, and he who can say back the sayings of the professors with the most accuracy and readiness passes with the greatest applause, notwithstanding that this is a feat performable by men who are unfit both by mental constitution and education to undertake the treatment of disease. It is not necessary that it should appear in proof that the candidate is an accurate observer and sound reasoner; that he can dissect, can discriminate disease in the sick room, or that he can even apply pressure to an artery, or a bandage to a limb. All that is required is that he should be a good echo. It is true that the candidate has to show certificates of having had his name on a physician's book during three years, but there is no test applied to ascertain whether the time has been profitably spent. It is true, also, that practical observation is recommended, but so long as opportunities for such observation are not afforded, so long as the education is not practical and the examinations are not practical, such recommendation can have but small weight or value. There are many medical schools to which no clinical chairs are attached, and in those to which they are attached they are considered as merely collateral and subordinate. Even dissection itself is practically treated with neglect, so much so, indeed, that three medical schools, at least, as if expressly to warn students from the dissecting room, state in their circulars that it is optional whether the pupil dissect or not; thus, that of one medical school for 1838, says, "The dissecting ticket may be taken or omitted at the option of the student, as it is not required to constitute a full course." It is not absolutely required, I believe, in *any* of the medical schools; but expressly to mention the fact as an inducement to students, shows a reprehensible disregard of true educational principles. . . .

There are two great but opposite evils prevalent in society. The mechanic learns the practical part of his calling without learning the scientific principles on which his practice is founded. The physician learns the science without learning the practice of his art. The one can make a piece of mechanism without being able to explain the theory of its construction. The other can explain principles and theories, but cannot reduce them to operation. The education of the one is useful, of the other learned; in both it is defective, but especially in the latter. The artisan may be said to have the fruit without the flower; the young physician to have the flower without the fruit: the former, indeed, are the most beautiful, but the latter the most substantial. It is by the union of theory and practice alone, that man becomes both able and accomplished; and for lack of this union the practitioner often finds himself in such a dilemma as the artisan would experience who, after hearing lectures on cabinet-making, should receive a certificate of his learning and ability and be set to construct sofas before having handled a tool.

The present neglect of whatever is practical in education may be well illustrated by reference to the plan of a medical college not long since issued by the University of the city of New York. This was adopted after long deliberation and consultation, by letters, with the most eminent practitioners throughout the union; it was intended to surpass that of every other school in the United States; therefore, if we have a right to look for perfection in anything it is surely in this plan. But what do we find? That the professorships are divided into a graduate group, consisting of one for anatomy, one for physiology, one for theory and practice, one for surgery, one for obstetrics, one for chemistry, and for materia medica; and an extra-graduate group comprising a professorship for *clinical* medicine, one for *clinical* surgery, one for clinical midwifery, one for pathological anatomy, and one for operative surgery and surgical anatomy. On the graduate group of professors the student *must* attend; on the extra-graduate professors he *might* attend if he chose, or let it alone if he chose. That is, this plan provided that the student, before obtaining a diploma, *must* attend such professors as merely *describe* diseases and operations: he may absent himself from those who would take him to the operating table and show him how to operate; to the subject, and let him operate for himself; to *post mortem* examinations, and let him see the pathological conditions attendant on various diseases; to the bedside, and let him observe from day to day the indications and treatment of disease. Is this the way to make able practitioners?

Having shown the defective nature of medical education, it will not be difficult to point out, in a general way, the means of reformation. Physicians must be more attentive to their students; lecturers more laborious and practical. The dissecting room must be turned into a classroom; and, instead of receiving an occasional visit from the professor, it must be the chief arena of his labors. Every subject should, in the first place, be used by the student for the performance of such operations as would not mar it for dissection, and this under the eye of the surgical professor. Hospitals should be turned into and connected with medical schools; and besides having daily clinical instruction from able and experienced men, each student should be allowed to visit for himself, once a day at least, a certain number of cases, the history of which he should be required to write down in a notebook, which should be daily examined and commented on by the clinical professor. . . .

The plan, then, which I recommend for the reformation of medical education, and the elevation of medical character, may be comprised in a few propositions.

1. Insist on no qualification, as a pre-requisite to a medical diploma, which is not necessary to the practitioner of medicine, and insist on every qualification which is necessary.

2. Regulate the whole course of medical education in accordance with what should be its objects, namely, to so instruct and train a set of men as to impart to them practical skill to fulfil the duties of physicians and surgeons.

3. To secure such qualification, confer the diploma on no man who does not show, on a rigid examination, that he possesses the necessary ability as well as the necessary learning.

4. To secure zealous and masterly training, take from medical colleges the exclusive right of medical instruction, and subject them to the rivalry of individual talent and enterprise.

5. To secure the door of the profession from being opened by kindness, favoritism, or interest, take from the medical teachers the power of conferring diplomas and vest it in a board of examiners appointed for that purpose.

6. To secure examiners of the first ability, let them be appointed by the profession at large, through their representatives, at the state medical societies, and let their office be considered as the most honorable in the profession. To secure disinterestedness in the examiners, allow them to have no connection with the business of education during their term of office, and let no part of their remuneration depend on the number of candidates which they may pass.

7. To secure union among medical men and uniformity in medical examinations, let the members of the profession throughout the country unite in one

body, to be called the Medical University or College of the United States, by sending delegates from each state to a yearly medical congress, the members of which shall first regulate everything relating to the general welfare of the profession, and then form themselves into boards of examination and proceed to all the states of the Union for the purpose of examining candidates, and conferring diplomas.

Such is the outline of a plan which would, I humbly believe, be found not only perfectly practicable but perfectly just and in the highest degree efficacious for the attainment of the desired ends.

ANNUAL CATALOGUE OF THE COLLEGE OF PHYSICIANS AND SURGEONS, IN THE CITY OF NEW YORK, 1849–50

Editor's Note

The College of Physicians and Surgeons, one of two regular medical schools in New York in 1850, was a descendant of King's College, the site of the second medical school founded in the American colonies. Its successor is the medical school of Columbia University, which celebrated its 200th anniversary in 1967.

In 1850 the school occupied a three-story brick building. Despite rather good facilities, one medical editor wondered how the college maintained a respectable existence: "It is no small thing to pack from two to four hundred persons six hours a day, for four or five months in these places, neither well heated nor ventilated; and the pale face and haggard countenance of many a student that goes out from them in the spring, is to be attributed to such causes rather than hard study."[1]

The members of the faculty in 1850 were leading practitioners and medical authors. They were also innovative in their teaching as witnessed by the introduction of clinical instruction directly into the medical college curriculum and the use of the microscope in physiology.[2]

Thomas Bond gave clinical lectures in Philadelphia a century before, but most schools still used a purely didactic form of teaching. When James P. White introduced medical students into the delivery room in Buffalo in 1850, the resulting medical and public outcry was not stilled for some time.[3]

Around 1841, Willard Parker introduced the clinic at Physicians and Surgeons. Private pupils had been going to hospitals and dispensaries where they could observe their teachers treating patients. Parker thought it would be useful to bring the patients to the students, so he arranged to examine selected cases in the amphitheater before the entire class. Soon the system was used in obstetrics and medicine as well. Paradoxically, the clinical teaching in the medical school itself seemed to reduce the total clinical instruction the students received, for they now no longer crowded the hospital wards as they had before 1841. One

---

[1] Editorial, "Medical Colleges,—our ideas of what they should be," *New York Register of Med. and Pharm.* 2 (1851): 8–10; 9.

[2] Unlike Andrew Boardman's case, the catalog promises seem to have been fulfilled at Physicians and Surgeons. One of the members of the class of 1850 later recalled, "the most novel and interesting feature of the course of lectures was the exhibition by Professor Alonzo Clark of the circulation of the blood in the frog's foot, with a single small microscope." Stephen Smith, "Random recollections of a long medical life," *Med. Record* 79 (1911): 891–97; 892.

[3] See Carl T. Javert, "James Platt White, a pioneer in American obstetrics and gynecology," *J. Hist. Med.* 3 (1948): 489–506.

solution was the establishment of hospital medical schools as used in Europe. The medical schools at Long Island Hospital and Bellevue Hospital were thus begun in 1860 and 1861.[4]

Bibliographical Note

For additional information about the faculty members see any of the standard biographical dictionaries and particularly:

John C. Dalton, *History of the College of Physicians and Surgeons*, New York: Columbia College, 1888;

Edward Delafield, "Sketch of the history of the College of Physicians and Surgeons of the University of the State of New York," *New York J. Med.* 2 (1857): 163–82.

Thomas M. Gallagher, *The Doctors' Story*, New York: Harcourt, Brace, World, 1967.

John Shrady, ed., *The College of Physicians and Surgeons, New York, and its Founders, Officers, Instructors, Benefactors, and Alumni*, 2 vols., New York: Lewis, 1902.

James J. Walsh, *History of Medicine in New York*, 5 vols., New York: National Americana Society, 1919, vol. 2, pp. 413–51.

The matriculated class for the present session is one of the largest that has ever been in the college, and the faculty cannot but congratulate themselves and the profession upon this tangible evidence that they are sustained in having been among the first to respond to the wishes of the profession, as expressed by the American Medical Association, for a prolonged course, increased facilities in teaching, a larger number of teachers, and a higher standard of qualification for graduation.

The faculty of the college in issuing their Annual Catalogue, take pleasure in informing their numerous friends and graduates of the continued prosperity of the institution. In addition to the matriculated class, a large number of gentlemen have been in attendance upon one or more of the courses, who being graduates of the college, or from other causes, are not required to matriculate, and whose names, therefore, do not appear on the album or the catalogue. The best return that the faculty can make to those gentlemen, both at home and abroad, who have shown their approval of the character and present course of the college by sending to it those in whose professional education they are

---

[4]Several pages from the original catalog containing names of the Board of Regents, the faculty, and the currently enrolled class of 208 students have not been reprinted. The list of graduates does appear, primarily to show the thesis topics chosen by the students. Since the graduates are included in the original, the catalog must have been printed late in the academic year. An alternative explanation would be that these pages were later bound with this catalog, but originally appeared in the catalog of the following year.

interested, is by an earnest perseverance in increasing the material and facilities for a thorough and sound acquisition not only of theoretical but also of practical knowledge of a most responsible and honorable profession. The great object of the faculty is to make the several courses of instruction as demonstrative and practical as possible, and in this object they are warmly sustained by the trustees of the college; hence the means of illustration have been increased—the facilities for a rigid knowledge of practical anatomy are great; and through the kind co-operation of medical friends, the college clinique has assumed a degree of importance that could hardly have been anticipated at its origin.

The faculty respectfully solicit from the graduates and other friends of the college, donations of anatomical, pathological, and natural history specimens, etc. It is well known that every practitioner meets with specimens of great value in the museum of a medical college, which are comparatively useless when isolated. The trustees have appointed Dr. Isaacs "curator of the college museum," and all donations sent to him will be properly put up and placed in the museum, with the name of the donor.

The course on physiology and pathology has been a very important addition to the regular course of instruction and is the only course of the kind given in this country. The lectures on physiology embrace the minute anatomy of the tissues and are amply illustrated by magnified drawings, and by frequent demonstrations under the microscope. The course on pathology is equally full and is constantly enriched by the exhibition and demonstration of recent specimens illustrating the various changes produced in tissues and organs by disease.

It is now beyond controversy, that New York is without a rival in the abundance of means for practical and clinical instruction, and that those means are being rapidly developed. In the college clinique a great number and variety of cases are presented to the class, and frequently the students are called upon to make the diagnosis and to take charge of the patient. The obstetrical clinique gives to the advanced students the opportunity to practice in that important branch. Besides the clinical instruction given in the college, the students resort to the New York Hospital, which is open daily for that purpose, and where they see disease in its graver and more acute forms, both medical and surgical, hospital fee $8 per annum.

The New York Eye Infirmary is one of the most valuable practical schools in the country, where students may study every variety of disease to which the eye is liable, and profit by the experience of able and willing teachers. This infirmary is open three days in the week, without fee.

Since the opening of the present session, the medical board of Bellevue Hospital have made arrangements, by which that institution is accessible to students, and clinical instruction is given regularly to all who wish to attend—without fee.

New York Hospital.—*Physicians.*—Drs. Joseph M. Smith, John H. Griscom, John A. Swett, Henry D. Bulkley. *Surgeons.*—Drs. J. Kearny Rodgers, John C. Cheesman, Gurdon Buck, Jr., Richard K. Hoffman, Alfred C. Post, John Watson.

New York Eye Infirmary.—*Surgeons.*—Drs. George Wilkes, Abraham Dubois.

Bellevue Hospital.—*Physicians.*—Drs. Alonzo Clark, Thomas F. Cock, S. Conant Foster, Chandler R. Gilman, Benjamin W. Macready, John T. Metcalf. *Surgeons.*—Drs. S. Russell Childs, Isaac Greene, Willard Parker, John O. Stone, William H. Van Buren, James R. Wood.

LECTURES

The regular course of lectures for the session of 1849–50, was commenced on Monday, 15th October, 1849, and will be continued until the second Thursday in March, 1850.

In addition to the regular course, and not interfering with it, a course of lectures was commenced on Monday, 1st October, and continued until 15th October, on the following subjects:

Hygiene, by Dr. Smith

Anatomy of the Heart and Large Vessels, by Dr. Watts

Diseases of the Male Genital Apparatus, by Dr. Parker

Organic Diseases of the Uterus, by Dr. Gilman

FEES:—Matriculation fee, *$5.*

Fees for the full course of lectures by all the professors, $96; but students are not required to take out all the tickets during one session.

Graduation fee, $25.

Board, average $3 per week.

Students who have attended two full courses of lectures in this college, or one full course in some other regularly established medical school, and one full course in this college, are admitted to subsequent courses free of expense, except the matriculation fee.

Graduates of this college are admitted without fee; Graduates of other schools, who have been in practice three years, and *theological students*, are admitted on general ticket by paying the matriculation fee.

Practical Anatomy.—The trustees of the college have added another story to the rear of the college building, for the express purpose of providing a large and commodious apartment for practical anatomy. It is admirably lighted and ventilated and abundantly supplied with gas and Croton water; and it is confidently believed that it is at least equal in the convenience and comfort of its arrangements, to any dissecting room in this country. It will be opened early in October and continue open until the following April.

Material for dissection is supplied in abundance, and at a low rate, so that every student can go through with a thorough course of dissection. Demonstrator's ticket, $5, which admits the student to the dissecting room.

Graduation.—There are two periods for conferring the degrees; one, the *Annual Commencement* in March—the other at the opening of the regular course. Candidates for the degree of Doctor of Medicine must have attended two full courses of lectures, the *last* in this college; they must also have studied medicine three years, including the attendance upon lectures, under the direction of a regular physician, and have attained the age of twenty-one. Each candidate is required to write a thesis on some subject connected with the science of medicine and to deposit it with the secretary of the faculty. Full and formal certificates of time and age must be furnished.

The examination of candidates takes place semi-annually. That for graduation in the spring, early in March; and that for graduation in the fall, on the second Tuesday in September.

College of Physicians and Surgeons
67 Crosby Street, New York.

N. B.–Gentlemen wishing information about the college, lectures, etc. are requested to direct their letters to the Secretary of the Faculty, Dr. Watts, at the College, No. 67 Crosby Street.

Students are requested, on their arrival in the city, to call upon the janitor, Mr. James Knox, who resides in the college buildings, 67 Crosby Street, who will direct them to the residences of the faculty and will aid them in obtaining boarding places.

The faculty deem it highly desirable that students should arrive in the city early in October, so as to attend the preliminary course and to establish themselves for the winter, before the regular courses are commenced.

GRADUATES

of the

COLLEGE OF PHYSICIANS & SURGEONS

For the Year 1850

NAMES	RESIDENCE	INAUGURAL THESES
George Post Bissell	Connecticut	Typhus Fever
William Brodie, junr.	Monroe Co., N.Y.	Abortion
Pelatiah Brooks	Broome Co., N.Y.	History and Treatment of Croup
John Law Campbell, A.M.	New York City	Treatment of Syphilis in the Blackwell's Island Hospital
Joseph Manning Cleaveland, A.B.	New York City	Diabetes
James Harvey Crain	Ohio	Indications of Treatment in Inflammation
Joseph Creamer	Nova Scotia	Affections of the Eye-Lids
Isaac Van Deventer Culbertson	Livingston Co., N.Y.	Tubercle
Frederick Deyns	New York City	Concussion and Compression of the Brain
John Doherty	Canada West	Acute Pleuritis
Carroll Dunham, A.B.	Brooklyn	Digestion of Amylon
James Dunlap	Massachusetts	Anoemic Coma
James Woodward Elliot	New York City	The Contagion of Plague
Joseph Feeny	Richmond Co., N.Y.	Erysipelas
James Thorburn Gibbs, A.B.	New York City	The Value of Correctly Appreciating Therapeutical Indications

Gabriel Grant, A.M.	New Jersey	On Certain Reparative Processes of Nature
Desault Guernsey	New York City	Amaurosis
Levant Emery Hackley	Genesee Co., N.Y.	Peritonitis
William Smiley Halsey	Orange Co., N.Y.	Catalepsy
John Jacob Higgins, A.M.	New York City	The Lithic Acid Diathesis
Arthur Harper Jackson, A.M.	Connecticut	Morbus Coxarius
John Couse Johnson	New Jersey	Diabetes
James Galloway Junkin	Pennsylvania	Mental Excitement a Cause of Disease
Everet Hoffman Kimbark	New York City	Injuries of the Head, Including Concussion
Frederick Gebhard Leroy, A.B.	New York City	Tetanus and its Treatment by Antispasmodics and Stimulants
Oliver Sherwin Lovejoy	Massachusetts	Adhesive and Suppurative Phlebitis
Henry Martin Lyons, A.B.	Illinois	Iritis
John Jefferson Milhau	New York City	Gun-shot Wounds
Isaac Little Millspaugh	Orange Co., N.Y.	De Strictura Urethiae Virilis
George Washington Miner	New York City	Hydrocele
Joseph Augustus Monell	Orange Co., N.Y.	Dyspepsia
John Moneypenny, A.B.	New York City	
Neal Morrison	New York City	Asiatic Cholera
Edward Mulliken	Massachusetts	Scarlatina
Frederick Nash, A.M.	New York City	Hydrops
Isaac A. Nichols	New Jersey	Therapeutical Uses of Cold Water
Joseph Jerome O'Reilly	New York City	Emetics
Moses Pierson	Ulster Co., N.Y.	Diagnosis
Daniel Pratt Putnam	New Hampshire	The Use of Water as a Prophylactic and Curative Agent
Thomas Howe Rice	New York City	Hernia
James Rodgers Romeyn, A.M.	New York City	Treatment of Fractures
*Samuel Rose	Suffolk Co., N.Y.	Tetanus
Edward Rotton [?]	Williamsburgh	The Lungs, Respiration and Some of the Phenomena Connected Therewith
Isaac Jacob Senior, A.B.	Curaçoa	Water a Therapeutic Agent
Spencer Stephen Sloat	Rockland Co., N.Y.	Synovitis
Stephen Smith	Onondaga Co., N.Y.	Fractures
Richard Stebbins, A.B.	Massachusetts	Atmospheric Agency in Disease
Hiram Fairchild Stevens	Vermont	Peritonitis
Henry Morrill Stone	Vermont	Acute and Epidemic Dysentery
Richard Albert Terhune	New Jersey	Hernia
Robert Clark Thomson	New Brunswick	
Henry Topping	Orange Co., N.Y.	Dysentery
Morris Miller Townsend, A.B.	Maryland	Properties and Therapeutical Effects of Emetics
David Uhl	New York City	Dysentery
Henry Sergeant West	Broome Co., N.Y.	Acute Pericarditis
John Wellington Wilkin	New Jersey	Pleurisy

TOTAL 56

*Graduated March, 1850
Died, August, 1850.

PART II

MEDICAL LITERATURE

OLIVER WENDELL HOLMES

REPORT OF THE COMMITTEE
ON MEDICAL LITERATURE

Editor's Note

Oliver Wendell Holmes (1809–94) is probably best known as a writer and as the father of an eminent Associate Justice of the Supreme Court of the United States. For many years, however, the elder Holmes was professor of anatomy at Harvard. A thorough and popular teacher, he was one of the first Americans to stress the use of the microscope to his students. Today he is frequently cited for his 1843 essay on "The Contagiousness of Puerperal Fever." Unfortunately, this has met with much more approval from historians a century later than it did from his fellow physicians at the time it was written.

"Besides his duties to his patients, the physician is under certain obligations to contribute, by way of interest, his quota to the common stock of medical knowledge from which he has drawn so freely." With these words John Shaw Billings, one of the nineteenth century's most gifted and versatile physicians, opened his centennial report on our medical literature.[1]

Although he wrote nearly thirty years after the first A.M.A. Committee on Literature report, Billings shared many of the concerns of his earlier colleagues. In 1876 he still needed to point out that medical journalism was not yet a profession in the United States. "With one or two exceptions, our medical editors are engaged in practice and lecturing, and their labor in connection with the journals is not directly remunerative, nor is it in the main object of their thoughts."[2]

Very few American journals of the nineteenth century were able to reach a ripe age. The *Boston Medical and Surgical Journal*, founded as the *New England Journal of Medicine and Surgery and the Collateral Branches of Science*, in 1812, and the *American Journal of the Medical Sciences*, founded as the *Phila-*

Trans. A.M.A. 1 (1848): 249–88.

[1] "A century of American medicine, 1776–1876, IV. Literature and Institutions," *Am. J. Med. Sci.* 72 (1876): 439–80; 439. All four essays appeared in book form in E. H. Clarke, ed., *A Century of American Medicine, 1776–1876* (Philadelphia: Lea, 1876, recently reprinted).

[2] Ibid., p. 467. This is not to say, though, that by the last third of the century American journals had not improved considerably, both in quantity and in quality. A look at any list of medical journals, both in this country and elsewhere, immediately reveals numerous titles but short life spans. As W. R. Lefanu has pointed out, "The periodical form provides an economic answer to the demand by the growing army of scientists for prompt publication of their newest work, but the high infant mortality among journals points to the difficulties which the publisher may anticipate." "British periodicals of medicine," *Bull. Hist. Med.* 5 (1937): 735–61, 827–55; 735.

delphia Journal of the Medical and Physical Sciences by Nathaniel Chapman in 1820, are two notable exceptions. By and large, economic vicissitudes, owing in part no doubt to lack of reader interest, led to the demise of many journals. Periods of depression or unrest such as the Civil War caused particularly heavy casualties.

Apathy among medical men regarding reading of medical periodicals, and particularly their apparent unwillingness to pay for them, was bemoaned by many nineteenth-century editors. But the man who wished to keep abreast of advances had to depend upon medical journals, and this is no less true today. Besides being the medium of communication between members of the profession, journals were thought to play an important role in the advancement of medicine. They often aired questions of morality and thus helped elevate the tone of the profession. On the other hand, squabbles among opposing editors or antagonistic schools of thought were also common. Often the public pointed to these controversies when the low image of the mid-nineteenth-century physician was discussed.

For the period 1797–1878 Billings counted 250 regular medical journals, 196 of which had folded by the latter date. These figures did not include 114 homeopathic, botanic, and eclectic journals founded during the same period. Ninety-six of these were gone by 1878. As might be expected from the numbers of physicians, New York, Pennsylvania, and Ohio were the homes of most journals, but Georgia, Kentucky, Louisiana, Maryland, and Missouri had also produced a significant number.[3]

The journals provide one of the richest sources of materials for the historian of medicine in America, for they most clearly reflect the medical thought of a period. Most of the articles in the book first appeared in medical journals, and many who wrote books, or who write them today, first put forward their ideas in a journal circulated among their colleagues. It was not mere chance, then, that the American Medical Association, in its first year, appointed a committee on medical literature. A number of the subsequent annual volumes of the *Transactions* contain a report similar to the following selection.[4]

One must remember, that at mid-century the medical profession in this country was still heavily dependent on the old world for medical training, medical literature, and medical advances. The A.M.A. committee reporting in 1863 was pleased to note that the papers in American journals were becoming shorter and more practical in nature. "All this indicates improvement, and if the same progress goes on for a few years longer, we shall hope to reach the perfection of French medical journalism, where nothing but what is new is allowed to see the light."[5]

This change, noticed by Charles A. Lee in 1863, was an important one, for fifteen years earlier the committee had noted with some despair that the same articles seemed to reappear in different journals. The 1848 report charged that, "the ring of editors sit in each other's laps . . . with a wonderful saving in the article of furniture."

---

[3] See John Shaw Billings, "The Medical journals of the United States," *Boston Med. Surg. J.* 100 (1879): 1–14, recently reprinted in F. B. Rogers, comp., *Selected Papers of John Shaw Billings* (Chicago: Medical Library Association, 1965), pp. 90–114.

[4] Medical literature, however, was broadly interpreted. It included books, translations, as well as periodicals.

[5] Charles A. Lee, "Report of the Committee on Medical Literature," *Trans. A.M.A.* 14 (1864): 97–116; 99.

Most historians have agreed that Oliver Wendell Holmes, whose name appears first in the list of seven committee members, was the author of the 1848 report. There is a certain flair and flavor that Holmes, the writer, demonstrated in his many works that is also very much in evidence in this report. Witness his terse characterization of the various national medical minds: "the Frenchmen considers most in disease what there is to see about it, the German what there is to think about it, the Anglo-American what there is to do about it." Whether or not the thought was original with Holmes, the expression is typical of his piercing style.

In this report, as in many inaugural lectures, annual medical society orations, and graduation addresses of the time the concern is with the making of an independent American mind. Americans, the prevailing sentiment claimed, were perfectly capable of original work. As Holmes put it, we should stop merely setting "English portraits of disease in American frames." Notice, too, in this frequently quoted exhortation and in the lines above how closely he allied American medicine with that of Great Britain.

Bibliographical Note

The Billings pieces cited in the text above are useful. See also Myrl Ebert, "The rise and development of the American medical periodical, 1797–1850," *Bull. Medical Library Assoc.* 40 (1952): 243–76. Miss Ebert covers the history of the early journals, includes a full list of them, and gives the reader a useful bibliography of secondary sources.

Although outside the field of medical history, Frank Luther Mott's *A History of American Magazines*, 5 vols., Cambridge: Harvard University Press, 1957–68, is important because he includes medical and scientific journals.

James Eckman in his "Anglo-American hostility in American medical literature of the nineteenth century," *Bull. Hist. Med.* 9 (1941): 31–71, has discussed the problem of American medical independence. His section on the furor caused by Sydney Smith's 1820 question, "What does the world yet owe to American physicians and surgeons?", is particularly illuminating. Nathaniel Chapman went so far as to prominently display Smith's taunt on the title page of the *Philadelphia Journal*.

For the reader who is interested in heavier doses of Oliver Wendell Holmes, his collected *Medical Essays, 1842–1882*, Boston: Houghton, Mifflin, 1891, are highly recommended. For the controversy engendered by Holmes's report, see Mary Louise Marshall, "Dr. Holmes and American medical literature," *Bull. Hist. Med.* 22 (1948): 227–87. For biographical details see John T. Morse, *Life and Letters of Oliver Wendell Holmes*, 2 vols., Boston: Houghton, Mifflin, 1896; and Eleanor M. Tilton, *Amiable Autocrat: A Biography of Dr. Oliver Wendell Holmes*, New York: Schuman, 1947.

AMA Transactions
1848

The Committee on Medical Literature was appointed to prepare "an annual report on the general character of the periodical medical publications of the

United States, in reference to the more important articles therein presented to the profession, on original American medical publications, on medical compilations and compends by American writers, on American reprints of foreign medical works, and on all such measures as may be deemed advisable for encouraging and maintaining a national literature of our own."

In presenting the first report upon this subject to the association, the committee thought it desirable to take a summary retrospect of what has been done in the several branches brought under their consideration, before proceeding to examine the more recent labors in the same department. It has seemed to the committee that the duties of those who should succeed them in after years would be rendered more useful and at the same time less onerous by this general survey of the whole field which has been traversed. Much of the tediousness of the long array of names which have been unavoidably enumerated would be avoided in the future annual summaries, and many points would, doubtless, be developed which the length of this report, if no other reason, has supressed or crowded into narrow limits. It is proper to state that the materials within the reach of the committee were by no means complete, especially in what relates to periodical literature, and that with every disposition to do impartial justice they have not always had the means of obtaining complete series of journals and have sometimes been reduced to a few disconnected numbers.

PERIODICAL MEDICAL PUBLICATIONS OF THE UNITED STATES

The plan of the first medical periodical publication which appeared in this country was conceived by Dr. Elihu H. Smith of New York. He associated in his enterprise Dr. Edward Miller and Dr. Samuel L. Mitchell, and in August, 1797, the first number of the new journal appeared under the name of the *New York Medical Repository*. In the hands of different editors it continued to be published for many years, until it reached its twenty-third volume. In its pages are contained most of the writings of Dr. Miller, one of the most original thinkers and observers which this country has produced, whose eulogy has been written at length by the most renowned among the medical theorists of the present century. Here, too, are many of the productions of the originator of the enterprise, who, at the early age of twenty-seven, fell a victim of the disease he had illustrated, leaving a name which might have rewarded a long life of honorable exertion. Although a considerable portion of the *Medical Repository* is occupied by chemical disquisitions which no longer possess anything but historical value, still it will be always consulted with profit for its accounts of the diseases of this country during the period of its publication, especially of yellow fever, of spotted fever, and of typhoid pneumonia. The chemist will remember it as having been honored by many contributions from Priestley; and the obstetrician will not soon forget that a letter from Dr. Stevens, in its eleventh volume, introduced to the world the wonderful properties of ergot.

In speaking of this, the first of our medical periodicals, the expressions of Dr. Thacher may be adopted as doing justice to the pioneer journal of the western hemisphere:

> The commencement of this publication undoubtedly forms an era in the literary and medical history of our country. No work of a similar kind had ever appeared in the United States. Its influence in exciting and recording medical inquiries and in improving medical science soon became apparent. It led to the establishment of other and similar works in different parts of our own country, as well as of Europe; and may thus, with great truth, be said to have contributed more largely than any other single publication to that taste for medical investigation and improvement which has been, for a number of years, so conspicuously and rapidly advancing on this side of the Atlantic. . . .

The general plan of the original periodical publications is very similar. The first part of each number is devoted to original articles, consisting of essays, histories of epidemics and endemics, series of cases and single cases, and accounts of operations. Occasionally a more detailed and comprehensive history of some disease is introduced under the name of *monograph*, and not unfrequently extensive statistical tables are given, bearing especially upon surgical and obstetrical practice. Then follow *Reviews* or formal examinations of works recently published, usually analytical in character and having for their principal object the book rather than the general subject of which it treats. To this division succeeds a miscellaneous and heterogeneous assemblage of *bibliographical notices*; the sweepings of the critical *atelier*; the rinsings and heeltaps of the critical banquet; a necessary part of the editor's prospectus, but one which is least gratifying to minute inspection. Here the importunate friend receives his expected compliment, the dull dignitary is pacified with his scanty morsel of eulogy, the Maecenas is paid in fair words for his patronage; the book which must be noticed and has not been read, is embalmed in safe epithets and inurned in accommodating generalities. Lastly, a considerable part of the number is made up of selections, either taken promiscuously from other journals and recently published works or, in the better managed periodicals, classified so as to present a summary of the recent progress of science in its several departments.

The proportion allotted to these several divisions varies very much. Taking into consideration the usual difference of type in the original and borrowed matter and the very liberal extracts which the reviewers commonly make from the work before them it will be found that a very large part of all the journals is made up of quotations; and to a considerable extent of the same quotations, whatever may be the particular journal examined. The committee have been struck with the fact that the same articles have been presented over and over again to their notice in many different periodicals, each borrowing from its neighbors the best papers of the last preceding number, so that the perusal of many is not so much more laborious than that of a single one, as would be anticipated. The ring of editors sit in each other's laps, with perfect propriety, and great convenience it is true, but with a wonderful saving in the article of furniture.

In making these remarks, it is not intended to undervalue the great amount of intelligence and industry embodied in these periodicals, or to make any return of ingratitude to the faithful servants of science and humanity, who, in the midst of innumerable distractions and often at an absolute sacrifice of their material interests, are giving their time and health and substance to the demands of this most exacting department of mental labor. The task of filling a vessel which had no bottom, used to be thought a severe punishment enough for regions where the art of torture was a science, but to fill a quarterly or monthly or weekly receptacle with the pure distillation of two or three brains which have been tapped once, thrice, or a dozen times a quarter for an indefinite period, is more than mortal stamina can support. The natural inference is, that no journal should be established which has not a pretty wide intellectual constituency to support it, unless it wishes to live upon the common stock without contributing a fair proportion in its turn. . . .

In the course of half a century from the establishment of the first of the medical journals, their number has been gradually rising, until at the present time at least twenty are known to be in existence. Some principle in addition to the wants of the reading community must exist to account for such inordinate fecundity in this particular department. This is to be found in the homely fact that a medical journal is a convenient ally and advertising medium for public institutions and publishing establishments, and that by the *help yourself* system, so generally established, it is not necessarily much harder to edit a medical journal than to furnish the "notes and additions" to the work of a British author. Still, the general character of these journals is respectable and, of several among them, highly creditable to the state of medical science. Every year shows that exact observation is more and more valued and that a better literary standard is becoming gradually established. The committee would not discharge an important duty, if they neglected to point out what appear to them the most obvious defects noticeable in this important department. The first is a tendency to speculate and very often to dispute, about the ultimate causes of diseases, instead of thoroughly investigating their phenomena. This is a point which has been made the subject of controversy elsewhere. Whether the true version be "don't think but try" or "think, *and* try," it very certainly is *not* "think, *instead of trying*," or "instead of observing." Yet, this is the way in which an incalculable amount of time and paper has been wasted by men of ingenious minds placed in the very midst of pathological occurrences which had never been properly studied in their character of phenomena, and this it is which gives such a gaseous and unsubstantial character to many of our magazine articles, that even the greedy Abstracts and the cannibal Retrospects, pass them by as diet fit only for the chameleon! Another and sorer cause of complaint, of occasional but not frequent occurrence, is to be found in the liberties allowed to anonymous writers—not so much with regard to each other, for if "Medicus" and "Senex" were to succeed in reciprocal annihilation, the loss might not be serious—but with regard to their neighbors at large and to things in general. An editor is responsible that nothing shall be admitted into his pages, the essential character of which is hostile and inflammatory, on the same principle that he is bound to be courteous in his common intercourse. Some errors of this kind are doubtless owing to want of careful supervision on the part of the editor. That such negligence is very general there can be no dispute; there is hardly one of the journals whose fair features are not marked with the *acne* of typographical inaccuracies— and as the editors are educated men the inference is inevitable that they have not read their own pages. Some years since, a leading American journal remarked of the report of the Massachusetts Insane Hospital, "on page 79, is a very important typographical error—the word *chains* occurs twice when it should be *chairs*. No chains have ever been used in the institution." But, within a few months the same journal allowed the following words to stand upon its pages as Latin: "*mulierem uteres gerentum morta quopiam acuto corripi iefbale*"; and speaks in its January number of a disease as being "imminently curable."

The committee have no intention of furnishing a list of errata to the periodical works in question, although they have almost involuntarily accumulated the means of so doing. The most unpardonable are those which mangle and distort the names of our medical authorities—"Laennec," "Boerhaave," "Bonelli," "Shenk," and many more, have suffered this kind of mutilation or martyrdom. On the other hand, some new honors have been awarded by a similar mechanism and, what is still more remarkable, new authorities in science have been created by the same agency. "Baron Louis" received his title in Boston (Nov. 3d, 1847); "Sir John Hunter" was knighted in New York (Jan. 1848), and *Hives*, the inventor of "Hives' Syrup," was born a full-grown therapeutist at Philadelphia (April 1842).

The advertising portion of the journals seems to be considered by some editors as beyond the jurisdiction of medical ethics. It is to this opinion, or more probably to mere inadvertence, that the physician owes the privilege of reading, before he opens one of the prominent journals, the notice of one Dr. Beach's Medical Works, "for which he has received numerous gold medals from the various crowned heads of Europe, and diplomas from the most learned colleges in the Old World" (July 1847).

In connection with periodical literature, it seems proper to allude to the "Introductory Lectures," of which so large a number are delivered and printed annually. They must not be judged too harshly, for they are delivered to young men, who like high seasoning, and they naturally partake somewhat of the character of advertisements. Many of them are agreeable and appropriate performances, but others are open to severe comment. Turgid and extravagant attempts at eloquence, a fondness for effete Latin quotations, a parade of scholastic terms where simple ones only are called for, an inclination to adopt the cant phrases of political and literary writers are the common faults of these productions. The physican should remember that his style has no more occasion for pomp of oratory and glitter of epithet than his costume for the gold lace and feathers which belong to the military chieftain. Nothing is more offensive than an attempt to tell that which should be said plainly and decently in high flown language. It vitiates the taste of the student who listens to it or reads it and exposes the profession to derision from those who cannot value the important truths disguised by such ill chosen finery.

Here, too, a few words may be added on the subject of the Theses, of which many hundreds are annually presented by the candidates for graduation. It is to be feared that they would compare ill with those produced in the great European schools, very many of which have taken their place as permanent scientific documents and heralded the future celebrity of their authors. Yet a more careful attention would probably show that some theses are brought forward every year which would do credit to the institutions from which they proceed and to the country. Such a dissertation as that of Dr. Kane, on Kiesteine, or that of Dr. Porcher on the Plants and Ferns of St. John's (S.C.), forms the best possible introduction of a young man into the ranks of the profession and is an actual accession to the treasures of science. It has occurred to the committee, that some measures might be taken to elevate the character of these exercises and encourage a generous emulation throughout the country in respect to their merit.

In different parts of the country prizes have been frequently offered for the best dissertations upon certain specified subjects. Many interesting essays have been called out in this way, which would probably never have seen the light but for some such active stimulus. In some instances, a permanent fund is devoted to this object. One of the best known of these endowments is the Boylston Prize Fund, which has offered and generally awarded premiums to the amount of a hundred dollars annually for a long series of years. The Fisk Prize Fund of Rhode Island is a more recent foundation of similar character.

The original works on medical subjects produced in this country are almost all of them general treatises, intended especially for students. The national practical tendency shows itself in the best of these to good advantage. To contrast the American mind and its prototype, the English, with that of some other nations, it might be said that the Frenchman considers most in disease what there is to see about it, the German what there is to think about it, the Anglo-American what there is to do about it. The object of these works sufficiently accounts for their generally elementary character, and for the fact that few of them pretend to do more than serve a temporary purpose, and then give place to newer compilations. A few exceptions have already been referred to as of more permanent value, but it must be confessed that the part of our present medical literature most likely to reach posterity is in the form of fragmentary contributions to science rather than of any more formally and elaborately organized productions. The *Translations* made in this country are, with few exceptions, from the French and have naturalized many of the best practical authors of that country. Many of the higher class of works remain yet untouched; those of Rayer on Diseases of the Kidneys, and of Grisolle on Pneumonia, may be mentioned as examples. The three great dictionaries have proved too formidable for transfusion, and the incomparable *Compendium de Médecine*, a work which has more erudition and more actual intellectual outlay employed in its construction than would furnish forth twenty "Practices of Medicine," is absolutely ignored, as far as the committee are aware, with a single exception, by all the writers of this country.

It cannot be denied that the great *forte* of American medical scholarship has hitherto consisted in "*editing*" the works of British authors. The committee are not disposed to disguise the fact that this business has been carried on in a very cheap and labor-saving fashion. A tacit alliance between writers and publishers has infused the spirit of trade into the very heart of our native literature. The gilt letters of the book-binder play no inconsiderable part in the creation of our literary celebrities. Sometimes the additions by the "American editor" have been real and important, oftener nominal and insignificant. The following calculation of the proportion added to different recently published works, taken at random, will show the average amount of material so contributed. The editor's proportion was, in two instances, one-fourth; in two more, one-eighth; in one, one-ninth; in another, one-tenth; in others, one-fifteenth, one-seventeenth, one-nineteenth, one-twentieth, one-twenty-eighth, one-fifty-ninth, one-sixty-fifth, one-ninetieth, one hundred and seventh, and, in one instance, such a sprinkling as a single penful of ink might furnish and leave enough to spare for a flourishing autograph. The fairest fruits of British genius and research are shaken into the lap of the American student, and the great danger seems to be that in place of the genuine culture of our own fields the creative energy of the country shall manifest itself in generating a race of *curculios* to revel in voracious indolence upon the products of a foreign soil!

In viewing the great branches of anatomy, physiology, surgery, obstetrics, and practical medicine, it will be seen at once that the four first are essentially the same to the American student that they are to his European models. As might be expected in a new country, the practical branches have almost exclusively occupied the attention of the professional student. The contributions to anatomy and physiology have been few and, for the most part, insignificant compared with those which have emanated from the countries of Hunter, of Bichat, and of the Meckels. Of all the practical branches, operative surgery, a most important and attractice pursuit, but still, as its name (chirurgery) literally imports, a *handicraft*, has been the favorite, and whatever credit belongs to boldness, ingenuity, and dexterity, may be claimed, without fear of dispute, for its American practitioners.

But the higher problems of medicine have been, as yet, comparatively imperfectly investigated. Two fatal influences have acted not merely on medical science but on all natural science in this country. The first is the habit of indolence generated by the easy acquisition of a foreign literature which seems to answer every necessary purpose. The second is the habit of negligence which springs from the curious fact of a constant parallelism, which is not identity, in most natural objects and phenomena of the New World, with something of the older continent. In literature this has enfeebled the relation between words and realities; in science it has induced the same laxity and incoherence. The American constitution must be studied by itself—it differs from the European in outline, in proportions, in the obvious characters of the skin and hair—why should it not differ in the susceptibilities which, awakened, become disease? The American climate remoulds the European, and casts a new die of humanity—will it not generate causes of disease different from those of the Old World? Over this virgin soil a new Flora is weaving her long web of tapestry, flowing from the lichens of Katahdin to the myrtles of Cape Sable; is there no undiscovered healing in any of its leafy and blossoming folds? Here is the true field for the American medical intellect; not to set English portraits of disease in American frames; not to trust for immortality to a little more or less of manual adroitness or questionable hardihood; but to co-operate with that fast-gathering band of students who, in other departments of science, are studying what nature has done with her American elements, and teach us what disease is here, how it is generated, and what kindly antidotes have been sown in the same furrows with its fatal seeds.

The committee are not prepared to propose to the association any special organized mode of operation for encouraging and maintaining a national literature of our own. It is by indirect means rather than by direct contrivances that this desirable object is to be promoted; by elevating the standard of education; by the stern exclusion of unworthy articles from medical journals; by the substitution of original for parasitical authorship; and by introducing such a tone of general scholarship and scientific cultivation that the finer class of intellects may be drawn toward the ranks of the medical profession.

OLIVER WENDELL HOLMES
ENOCH HALE
G. C. SHATTUCK, JR.
D. DRAKE
JOHN BELL
AUSTIN FLINT
W. SELDEN

PART III

THE MEDICAL
PROFESSION

INTRODUCTION

The Oxford *New English Dictionary* defines profession as "The occupation which one professes to be skilled in and to follow. A vocation in which a professed knowledge of some department of learning or science is used in its application to the affairs of others or in the practice of an art founded upon it." The first listed use of the word in this sense dates from 1541 when Copland, in discussing Galen, noted "The parties of the art of Medycyne ... cannot be separated one from the other without the dammage and great detryment of all the medicynall professyon." And in these terms the problem is still being discussed more than 300 years later.

One usually assumes that the professions have been held in high esteem because their esoteric body of wisdom impressed outsiders and because their usefulness was obvious to all. Basic to professional conduct, we tend to assume independence or freedom from lay direction and the obligation to apply knowledge in a useful manner. The many thoughtful nineteenth-century physicians who wrote and editorialized about the status of their profession in American society were well aware of these presuppositions, and their problems centered around such expectations. They had repeatedly to ask themselves the basic questions: Is medicine a science? and, Is there any certainty in medicine? The questions are important, not only for the image which the profession was trying to achieve (or which it was accorded by an often skeptical public) but also because they were central to the doctor's work, especially the treatment of disease.[1]

The problem of medicine's imperfection, intimately tied to its certainty, was already a subject for discussion in the early stages of the formation of a medical profession in the United States. In 1801 Benjamin Rush, for instance, enumerated twenty-four causes which be believed "retarded the progress of our science." The reasons went from undue credulity of physicians, their unwillingness to study diseases closely and to classify them properly, to governmental

---

[1] Thus we shall encounter the subject again in Section IV in an essay by Elisha Bartlett, "An Inquiry into the Degree of Certainty in Medicine."

interference in prohibiting the use of certain remedies. "Let us strip our profession of everything that looks like mystery and imposture," Rush recommended, "and clothe medical knowledge in a dress so simple and intelligible, that it may become a part of our academical education in all our seminaries of learning."[2]

Rush also warned that the public image of the medical profession should not be viewed only from the patients' side. Most writers on the subject, from Thomas Percival on, were concerned with the duties of patients to physicians, as well as with the reverse. There were, after all, many sources of vexations which plagued the doctor. In a delightful introductory lecture to his students in 1803, Rush drew up quite a list.[3] Not only did the physician have to endure false judgments of his character, his talents, and his drugs, he also had to submit to the call of his patients no matter whether he was in bed, at the dinner table, or in company. Depending on the integrity and diligence of the physician, Rush summarized, the moral and intellectual pleasures of medicine could, however, far outweigh the pains.

The status of the physician at any given time is closely tied to internal as well as external factors. Within medicine the primary problem facing the nineteenth-century practitioner was his effectiveness, or lack of it. On the question of therapeutics hinged many a battle and most reputations. Heavy dosing with purgatives such as calomel, so commonly employed did not necessarily endear the physicians to their patients. Yet when the drug was officially removed from the army supply table in 1863, many physicians were incensed.[4] Certainly a large measure of the popularity accorded to the homeopaths was due to their renunciation of bleeding and purges.

The great want of the medical profession, the Connecticut physician Worthington Hooker wrote, was for the strict and minute observation of remedies. Physicians were too ready to adopt new remedies, he warned.[5]

Hooker also implicated the abuse of specialties when related to remedies for a prevalent disease. The physician who made a hobby of one specialty, Hooker believed, may have gained wealth and popularity, but then so did the quack for similar reasons. "As the quack gives his remedy to many more than really require it, so does the medical hobby rider apply his treatment to many to whom it is not properly applicable."[6]

---

[2] "Upon causes which have retarded the progress of medicine, and the means of promoting its certainty and greater usefulness," in *Sixteen Introductory Lectures* (Philadelphia: Bradford & Innskeep, 1811), pp. 141–65; 154.

[3] "On the pains and pleasures of a medical life," in ibid., pp. 210–31.

[4] See my "Therapeutic conflicts and the American medical profession in the 1860's," *Bull. Hist. Med.* 41 (1967): 215–22.

[5] "The present mental attitude and tendencies of the medical profession," *New Englander* 10 (1852): 548–68; 562.

[6] Ibid., p. 565.

Other writers, such as Louis Bauer (see Bibliographical Note below), disagreed with the idea that specialism was necessarily detrimental. The argument, however, was academic, because at mid-century few men actually practiced as specialists. Those who concentrated their work in surgery, happened also to be those who were most often exempt from public scorn of the profession.[7]

Suffice it to say, that in the period known to American historians as the "Jacksonian" or "Age of the Common Man," egalitarian ideals led to the unsettling of many American institutions, medicine being only one. The spirit of freedom led to rescinding of licensing laws, and every man was held to be free to practice medicine or to choose his practitioner from diverse groups. As Harvey Young has succinctly summarized it: "During the early nineteenth century, from the patient's point of view, the arduous impact of disease was aggravated by the arduous impact of therapy." And, "in the atmosphere of Jacksonian democracy . . . the common man sought common relief for his common ailments."[8]

It is readily apparent, then, that the place occupied by the medical profession throughout the nineteenth century, whether one of esteem and affection or of ridicule and scorn, was closely allied to the way medicine was practiced. Particularly important were the therapeutic measures used or available for use.

The nineteenth-century medical profession was divided in opinion on most issues, including the question of the image which it presented to the public. While most writers who examined the subject—with increasing frequency after the 1830's—bemoaned their state, some were optimistic. One of the influential men in the latter group was the New York physician John W. Francis. In an anniversary address to the New York Academy in 1847, Francis told his audience that they were living in momentous times, in an age of progress and reform. While admitting there were problems remaining to be solved, he nevertheless wished "to disprove the declaration that the profession is behind the age, reluctant of improvement, fearful of new principles, and contented with the knowledge of our forefathers."[9] Not until about forty years later, when advances in public health and surgery were becoming increasingly evident, did the public seem to agree with him.[10]

Visitors from Europe often made very harsh assessments of American achievements, including those in the field of medicine. George Combe, the Scottish lawyer and phrenologist was one such observer of the American scene. In his

---

[7]The external factors, so important in any consideration of the medical profession, have been discussed in the articles by Rosenberg and Shryock.

[8]James Harvey Young, "American medical quackery in the age of the common man," *Miss. Valley Hist. Rev.* 47 (1961): 579–93; 579.

[9]*Anniversary Discourse* (New York: Ludwig, 1847), p. 35.

[10]Professor Shryock, in his *Development of Modern Medicine* (New York: Knopf, 1947) has very aptly entitled one chapter "Public Confidence Lost," and a later one, "Public Confidence Regained."

Notes on the United States (1841) he wrote: "The profession of law and medicine in the rural districts, comprising nineteen-twentieths of the whole United States, stand in need of large accessions in knowledge to bring them to a par with the same professions in the enlightened countries of Europe."[11] Only about thirty years later the verdict was usually much more favorable, as seen by Sir John Eric Erichsen's remarks in Section V.

Bibliographical Note

In addition to the references cited above, the following will be useful. It is only a small fraction of a large body of literature available.

Louis Bauer, "On the declining relations of the medical profession to the public," *Cincinnati Med. Observer* 2 (1857): 97–106.

Thomas N. Bonner, "The social and political attitudes of mid-western physicians 1840–1940: Chicago as a case history," *J. Hist. Med.* 8 (1953): 133–64.

Daniel H. Calhoun, *Professional Lives in America: Structure and Aspiration, 1750–1850*, Cambridge: Harvard University Press, 1965.

A. M. Carr-Saunders and P. A. Wilson, *The Professions*, Oxford: Clarendon Press, 1933.

Rodney M. Coe, *Sociology of Medicine*, New York: McGraw-Hill, 1970, ch. 7, "The Professionalization of Medicine."

Nathan Smith Davis, "The mutual relations and consequent duties of the medical profession and the community," *Chicago Med. Examiner* 1 (1860): 321–33.

John Duffy, "The Changing image of the American physician," *J.A.M.A.* 200 (1967): 136–40.

Editorial, "Doctors," *Harper's Monthly* 20 (1859–60): 839–43.

Editorial, "The relations of medical men to each other, and the public," *Buffalo Med. Surg. J.* 4 (1864): 111–15.

Eliot Freidson, *Profession of Medicine, A Study of the Sociology of Applied Knowledge*, New York: Dodd, Mead, 1970.

Worthington Hooker, "On the respect due to the medical profession, and the reasons that it is not awarded by the community," *Proc. Conn. Med. Soc.* (1844): 25–48.

Joseph F. Kett, *The Formation of the American Medical Profession, The Role of Institutions, 1780–1860*, New Haven: Yale University Press, 1968.

Kenneth S. Lynn, ed., "The Professions," *Daedalus* (Fall, 1963).

David Mechanic, *Medical Sociology*, New York: The Free Press, 1968.

"Medical Etiquette," *The Nation* 3 (1866): 54–55; 94–95.

W. J. Reader, *Professional Men. The Rise of the Professional Classes in Nineteenth-Century England*, London: Weidenfeld & Nicolson, 1966.

Charles E. Rosenberg, "The American medical profession: mid-nineteenth century," *Mid-America* 44 (1962): 163–71.

_____, *The Cholera Years*, Chicago: University of Chicago Press, 1962.

Richard H. Shryock, "Public relations of the medical profession in Great Britain and the United States: 1600–1870," *Annals Med. Hist.* 2 (1930): 308–39.

---

[11] In Carl Bode, ed., *American Life in the 1840's* (New York: Anchor, 1967), pp. 294–307; 302.

_____, "The American physician in 1846 and in 1946, a study in professional contrasts," *J.A.M.A.* 134 (1947): 417–24; reprinted in *Medicine in America*, Baltimore: Johns Hopkins Press, 1966, pp. 149–76.

R. C. Word, "Obligations of the public to the medical profession," *Southern Med. Surg. J.* 1 (1866–67): 623–29.

Sanford C. Yager, "The medical profession and its standing in society," *Cincinnati Lancet and Observer* 9 (1866): 585–95.

F. CAMPBELL STEWART

THE ACTUAL CONDITION OF THE MEDICAL PROFESSION IN THIS COUNTRY; WITH A BRIEF ACCOUNT OF SOME OF THE CAUSES WHICH TEND TO IMPEDE ITS PROGRESS, AND INTERFERE WITH ITS HONORS AND INTERESTS

Editor's Note

Ferdinand Campbell Stewart (1815–99) was one of the founders of the New York Academy of Medicine, in 1847, and a well-known New York teacher and clinician when he wrote the essay that follows. After completing his medical training at the University of Pennsylvania, in 1837, he spent several more years studying abroad, mainly in Edinburgh and Paris. In 1843 Stewart, who was eminently qualified to draw comparisons between the medical professions of Europe and America, published *The Hospitals and Surgeons of Paris.*

Stewart wrote at a time when many members of the medical profession, especially in the Eastern states, were very much concerned with standards and position. As he noted in the opening paragraph of the following essay, the initial organizing meeting for what would be the American Medical Association was only a few months away. The A.M.A. took up the fight for better medical education, one of Stewart's main concerns, as a primary order of business.

The social standing of the physician Stewart proudly declared, was high—loftier, in fact, than in any other country. This elevated position was attracting perhaps too many to the ranks of medicine. But what then of the profession as a whole? Here the story was different, for, as he said, the profession was held in low esteem, often ridiculed. This was a common theme of a number of the authors already mentioned.

It is of interest that today the argument still rages. On October 16, 1966, in an article in the *New York Times Magazine* entitled "The Doctor's Image Is Sickly," Walter Goodman observed many of the same things that agitated Stewart over a century ago. In the last half decade a spate of books critical of the medical profession have appeared. The problems they describe are not all new.[1]

New York J. Med. 6 (1846): 151–71.

[1] See for instance Martin L. Gross, *The Doctors* (New York: Random House, 1966); and Roul Tunley, *The American Health Scandal* (New York: Harper & Row, 1966).

AN ANNIVERSARY ADDRESS DELIVERED
BEFORE THE NEW YORK MEDICAL AND SURGICAL SOCIETY,
ON THE 3d OF JANUARY, 1846

Gentlemen of the Medical and Surgical Society: At a period when the attention of the profession has been called to the subject by a recommendation from our State Medical Society, that a convention of representatives from all the medical corporations throughout the country should assemble in this city in the month of May, for the purpose of considering its wants and endeavoring to remedy the evils by which our profession is surrounded, I conceive that I cannot better fulfil the duty with which you have honored me than by asking your attention to this matter, and endeavoring to lay before you an exposition of what I believe to be the actual condition of the medical profession in this country, and the causes which tend to impede its progress or interfere with its honors and interests.

But before proceeding to discuss this subject, I wish distinctly to state, lest some of the remarks that I may have occasion to make may be misinterpreted, that it is not my aim nor my desire to attack individual associations. Occupying a strictly neutral position, bound by no alliance with cliques or parties, and feeling that I am influenced by none other than the purest motives, I shall, whilst disclaiming all feelings of prejudice or partiality, consider myself at liberty to discuss the question that I have raised in all its bearings—in a frank and free spirit, and without fear or hindrance.

First, then, what is the actual condition of the profession in this country and what is its relative position here as compared with that which it occupies in other countries?

In considering this subject we must draw a distinction between the social standing of the profession—the position which its members are allowed to occupy in society—and that which is accorded to it as a profession and in consideration of its claims and intrinsic merits.

In its social relations to the community, I am proud to declare that the medical profession of the United States occupies a more elevated and lofty station than that enjoyed in any other country of the world. Here, owing to the nature and tenor of our institutions, members of the learned professions occupy the first rank in general society; and in the absence of all hereditary distinctions, physicians, with lawyers, hold an enviable position and are regarded by the community in so favorable a light as to be second only in its estimation to the pious and educated divine. The road to honors and distinction in every department of the public service, and in every station in life, is open to us as well as to others; and we often see members of our profession occupying distinguished political situations of emolument and trust, from which in the older countries of Europe they are, for the most part, from the simple fact of their being medical men, almost wholly excluded.

Here, in all parts of the country, we are individually honored and esteemed; in the smaller towns and settlements, we are looked up to on important occasions for assistance and counsel, and our opinions and advice ever command the most respectful attention and consideration. Our society is everywhere courted by the intelligent and honest citizen; and we are always regarded in the light of honored family friends by those who employ us and place a degree of confidence and reliance in our honor and integrity, which, whilst most flattering and grateful, should lead us to contemplate seriously the nature and extent of the obligations which it forces us to incur and which it should be our duty and pleasure to render ourselves capable of discharging in a becoming and proper manner.

In some parts of the old world, so low is the condition of our profession in its relation to the general community that physicians are considered rather in the light of hired menials than as gentlemen and scholars, entitled by education to be regarded as on a footing of perfect equality with the most accomplished members of every civilized and refined society. Abroad, the medical man belongs to a caste which is considered comparatively low, and, although sometimes tolerated by his supposed superiors belonging to the higher circles, he is but rarely received either in England or France on a footing of acknowledged equality by the higher aristocracy, and in some parts of Italy and other portions of the Continent he occupies a position almost degrading.

Here, on the contrary, we claim and receive from the community the high consideration to which we conceive ourselves to be entitled, and which, notwithstanding occasional attempts to injure us collectively, we always find freely accorded to us in our individual capacities.

It is this flattering and honorable social position which we occupy that contributes materially to excite the ambition of many of the thousand applicants for admission to our ranks, some of whom thus see a road opened for access to a society which it might be much more difficult for them to reach by other more laborious and circuitous routes.

Such then is the relation of medical men individually to general society; but what is the relation that they bear to it collectively? How is the *profession* regarded by the public at large?

That there is a great want of respect and regard for what is called the regular profession is, I think, abundantly manifested by the unconcealed and open efforts to injure it, as evinced both by the encouragement of quackery in all its multiplied forms and varieties, and by a constant endeavor to find fault with, condemn, and ridicule the art and those who practise it.

The action of the representatives of the people in the legislatures of some of our states, proves likewise that our profession is not held in high estimation; these gentlemen seem, by their course of action, to desire to cast down and destroy every barrier of protection which had been raised by their predecessors and considered by them to be quite as essential to the welfare of the people generally as to our interests. In some instances they have succeeded in throwing the practice of medicine open, and making it free to all who choose to engage in it, without requiring from them any guarantee of their capability to treat disease, or affording to the people the slightest protection from impostors who, by arrogating the title of physician, may with impunity pursue a course of chance practice calculated to produce the most serious consequences to their health and endanger the lives of those who submit themselves to their care.

The evils resulting, not to us, but to the public, from the application of the principles of free-trade to the practice of medicine are numerous and most serious, but it is not my intention to indicate them at present, and I will only reiterate the assertion that as a *profession* we are not held in high estimation in this country. . . .

Let us now examine the question, whether we are really entitled by our intrinsic merits to the same scientific consideration as our professional brethren in other parts of the world! In a word, is our standard of learning and acquirement as high as it should be to entitle us to consider ourselves as on a footing of scientific equality with the physicians of other countries, and such as to justify us in demanding, as a matter of right, an unbounded confidence from those who employ us and place faith in our professions of capability?

This is a most delicate question and demands a careful and attentive examination. We are all, for the most part, unwilling to admit our inferiority in anything to which we have devoted a special attention and in which we desire to be considered proficients: it is only natural and to be expected, that we should hold ourselves equal to others of the same calling; and it is but very rarely that we can bring ourselves to admit, particularly in the cases of professional men, that we have superiors.

At the threshold of this investigation, I am bound to acknowledge that, in science at least, the profession in this country is far behind the medical communities of other countries, and this I think is wholly owing to the wrong and faulty system of medical education established amongst us; a system so defective as not only to have attracted the attention of foreigners, but to have led to a loud call from the disinterested and well-informed portion of our own faculty, for a thorough remodelling.

With the exception of some few attempts to support the present system, originating with parties whose position is such as to warrant the conclusion that they must be more or less influenced by personal interest in advocating it, I believe that the feeling may be considered as almost universal in favor of the adoption of a more extensive course of general and professional instruction and the establishment of a higher standard of medical acquirement.

To aid us in investigating this subject, I will present a statement of what is required by our Medical Colleges of their students, before they will allow them to apply for an examination or accord them the honors of a degree, and by comparing these with the requirements exacted by the medical boards of other countries, we shall be able to see in what the difference consists, and why it is that our physicians, at least at the period when they first become such, are not entitled to be considered on an equal scientific footing with those of other parts of the world.

At most, if not all, the chief Medical Schools of the United States it is exacted from students who apply for degrees that they shall produce evidence,

1st. Of their having studied in the office of a practitioner.

2d. Of their having attended during two courses of lectures at a medical college.

3d. That they shall have composed a thesis; and

4th. That they shall have complied with some minor general regulations.

There is no preliminary examination, and no means are resorted to for ascertaining whether a young man is capable, by previous preparation, of profiting by the lessons of his instructors, or likely to make hereafter a competent and useful physician. He may be thoroughly well grounded in the various branches of science, and his general knowledge may be most extensive; or he may be, as I have known, so ignorant and illiterate as to be unable to write his own language, or translate the Latin of the diploma which he is striving to obtain. He is not put to the proof, and no evidence is exacted of his having complied even with these few rules, other than his simple assertion, or at most the exhibition of his tickets, which is rather required as a proof of his having paid for them, than as any evidence that he has attended the lectures to which they give him admission.

Having fulfilled these obligations, he is admitted to an examination, and receives his degree, or is rejected.

The character of this examination is generally such that a student who cannot undergo it must be woefully ignorant indeed. Hence, the rejection of candidates is, with us, a matter of exceedingly rare occurrence, and almost all who have complied with the most essential requisite of paying their teachers are sure to be honored with the title to which they aspire.

At all the principal universities and colleges in Great Britain, Ireland, and on the Continent, where medicine is taught, the courses of instruction are much more complete and perfect than with us. At London, Edinburgh, Paris, Dublin, and other seats of medical schools, students are afforded many more, and much greater facilities for acquiring a thorough medical education, and the period of study is not only much longer and the subjects taught more numerous, but the preliminary and final examinations are of a character to render it certain that the candidate who obtains their diploma must be a qualified and thoroughly well-educated physician.

The courses of instruction at our colleges embrace, for the most part, six subjects, which are professed to be taught in two years, or rather in two periods of less than four months each, so that with a moderate degree of attention and a fair share of common sense, any one, may acquire the knowledge considered as necessary for a physician and obtain a license to practice, after about *eight*

months' college study! And this too under circumstances in every respect unfavorable; such as a continual and irksome attendance on lectures on different
subjects, during a great part of every day, leaving neither time for study and
preparation, nor for relaxation or dissection. More time is devoted in other
countries to the study of the fundamental science of anatomy alone, than is
allowed to our students for perfecting themselves in all the branches of a medical
education.

Whilst for the most part, then, seven or eight months' attendance at lectures
is required by the regulations of our medical colleges, in Europe four years are
considered as scarcely sufficient; and that too after a preparatory course of
study calculated to enlarge and strengthen the mind and render it fit for receiving the more difficult and important professional knowledge which is to be
subsequently imparted.

All the more important subjects, and especially practical anatomy and clinical
medicine and surgery, are there thoroughly taught. The student is not only
required to dissect, but is examined on dissection, whereas, here a very irregular
attendance on the dissecting-room, probably during a few evenings only in each
session, is all that is expected of our pupils, and indeed, in some cases, they are
notified publicly, beforehand, that though advised to do so, they will not be
required to dissect at all. Whilst it is considered of paramount importance
abroad, and is so in reality, little or no attention to hospital practice is required
from the student here. Some of our colleges exact from him that he shall
purchase a ticket of admission to a hospital when one is convenient, but there
the matter rests. And this even is not always required; and if not obligatory on
them to do so, how can it be expected that students, when they have so much
else to attend to, will go to the expense of procuring a ticket, or after getting it
will take the trouble to attend the practice of these institutions? That they do
not do so is, I think, very evident from the fact that out of upwards of six
hundred in attendance at the New York colleges during the present session, only
about one in eight have applied for the privilege of visiting our City Hospital!
And yet this is known to be the only one here to which they can obtain access.
The all important branch of clinical instruction then is not taught to students
here, at all events in a satisfactory manner; for the cliniques attached to the
schools in this city, in Philadelphia, and elsewhere, though useful, can never
present to them the advantages that they would derive from examining patients
and following their treatment in a regular and well-organized hospital and under
the direction of qualified teachers.

Botany, medical jurisprudence, practical chemistry and pharmacy, pathology,
and some other subjects considered essential to a medical education abroad are
nowhere taught properly, or as separate branches, in the medical schools of our
country, and the student's knowledge of them, if obtained at all, must be gained
by close study and application at home, after he has gotten his diploma and left
college.

It is the want of a thorough and efficient course of education here that induces so many of our young graduates to go abroad for the purpose of gaining knowledge which they ought to be able to obtain at home; and I may venture to assert, that if proper use was made of the advantages possessed by our large cities for affording medical instruction in all its departments, and if our schools would at once adopt a high standard of professional acquirement, Paris and London would soon cease to present the superior attractions which they now do, and our young men would seek at home the information which it now costs them so much trouble and expense to obtain in foreign countries.

It is most humiliating to us to know that none of our colleges are recognized by European schools as on a footing of full equality, and that alumni here are not thought entitled to be held as equals with students there. And yet such is the fact, and most keenly do some of our spirited and high-minded young men feel it to be so. I have known them ashamed to acknowledge that they were graduates, and the M.D., so coveted, and so ostentatiously displayed at home, at least whilst it is new, I have seen erased from their cards when abroad. . . .

A system then, which is so universally admitted to be defective, must stand in need of amendment, and it appears to me that a period has now arrived when a bold step may be advantageously taken in favor of reform, and the introduction of, if not a European, at least a higher standard of medical education amongst us; and the school or schools that shall adopt it, though they may for a time experience a loss in the diminished number of their pupils, will eventually, and certainly, find their reward in the increased value that will attach to their diplomas.

We can most of us recollect the time when the Edinburgh or London degree was almost necessary for the physician who expected success in his profession; it is now almost equally necessary for those who would succeed, to have enjoyed the advantages of Paris. The public, having no other sure guide, formerly esteemed a physician in proportion as the university from which he received his degree was estimated; and now that we have so many schools, and so many incompetent physicians, and are so surrounded by quacks—renegade doctors—or those who arrogate to themselves the title, people will begin to look about them again and make inquiries as to the relative standing of the various colleges, with the view of employing those physicians who shall bear the diploma of that institution which is known to give the most full and perfect course of instruction.

It would almost seem from the course pursued by them that many of our colleges are disposed to offer bounties to young men, and entice them away from honest mechanic trades to engage in the study of medicine.* So easy and

*At some of our country medical schools, students are allowed to pay their professors with due-bills, or notes, to be redeemed at some future period, when the young men shall have accumulated enough money to enable them to cancel the obligation.

cheap, do they make it appear, is the effort necessary for gaining a license that numbers are induced to study who would never for a moment think of doing so if moderate restrictions were imposed, and they were required to devote a reasonable proportion of time to attendance on lectures.

The result of this is that hundreds gain entrance to the profession who are wholly unfitted for fulfilling the high duties devolving upon practitioners; and this evil must continue so long as the efforts of our medical schools are directed to the end of obtaining the largest classes, and sending forth the greatest number of graduates. So long as they trust for reputation on the number rather than the character of their alumni, our country will be annually flooded with imperfectly and half-educated physicians, many of whom must, from absolute necessity, be forced to resort to means for gaining a livelihood calculated to degrade them in their own and in the public estimation and to produce a ruinous influence on the profession.

I regret that time does not permit me to enter more fully into the examination of this important subject, which is worthy of the closest consideration and demands the earnest attention of medical men. I have said as much, however, as the occasion warrants, and I will now proceed to indicate some of the causes which, in my opinion, tend to interfere materially with the honor and interests of our profession.

These are of two kinds: such as are produced by the acts of the profession itself and such as are caused by the acts of the community generally, or those not belonging to our society. Of these, the first, it appears to me, are by far the most important, and productive of incalculable injury; and I think that we might find, if we examined carefully, that many of the evils of which we have cause to complain are the direct consequence of the suicidal course pursued by the profession itself; and that in fact most of the difficulties by which we are surrounded are occasioned by ourselves.

Can all members of our faculty conscientiously assert that they have ever acted with the view, and in a manner to promote the interests of the profession to which they belong? And are all guiltless of having at times pursued indirectly, if not directly, a course calculated both to impair the credit of the general body and lessen the estimation in which it should be held by the public at large? It cannot be expected of anyone that he should admit the charge openly, and yet we all know that there are numbers who feel, and who are obligated to admit to themselves, that they have too often pursued a course in furtherance of their own individual interests which was calculated to impair that of the body generally.

The professional and social intercourse of medical men, in this city especially, is on a wrong and improper footing; there is to as great, if not to a greater extent here than elsewhere, a degree of jealousy and unkind feeling which ought nowhere to exist.

It would appear that many of our body fall into the gross error of considering that their individual success depends on decrying their professional rivals and indirectly leading patients to conclude that they alone, of all others, are able and capable of rendering effectual assistance. This has been everywhere noted as a common and general fault of the faculty, and those who indulge in the practice are most woefully mistaken in the result which they hope it may produce. I have yet to learn that a single instance can be found in our annals, in which eventual or lasting success has attended the exertions of individuals who have endeavored to gain a position by so unfair and dishonorable a course. The public is generally sufficiently versed in these matters to be able to distinguish between genuine merit and boastful pretension, and it rarely or ever accords confidence to those whom it cannot esteem. All who are in the habit of indulging in this very censurable and disloyal course would do well to bear in mind the established truism, "that every physician who decries another, injures himself by depreciating the general estimation in which his profession should be held." Or in the words of Mr. Percival: "A physician should (from motives of interest) cautiously guard against whatever may injure the general respectability of his profession; and should avoid all contumelious representations of the faculty at large, or of individuals; all general charges against their selfishness or probity; and the indulgence of an affected jocularity or scepticism concerning the efficacy and utility of the healing art."

That this evil exists to a deplorable extent amongst us cannot be denied; and it is the more to be regretted, because it is so generally unjust, from the circumstance of its being almost impossible to ascertain the real qualifications of medical men (after graduation), and from depreciating language being frequently used in reference to individuals with whom the party has no personal acquaintance, and whose impressions are often formed from hearsay, or are the result of some pique or supposed cause of complaint, for real or imaginary injuries, and rivalry.

A part of this evil results from the fact that social meetings of medical men are not of sufficiently frequent occurrence amongst us.* The advantages of this kind of intercourse are most manifest, and it should be heartily encouraged, as it always serves the purpose, by bringing individuals together in a friendly way, of engendering kindly sentiments and exciting mutual regard and esteem which will ever be accompanied by courteousness of demeanor and general respect. . . .

By our charges we sometimes excite in the public mind a feeling of doubt and distrust; in some instances by demanding more for our services than they are really worth, and in other instances so far undervaluing them, or rather allowing them to be undervalued, as to lead people to think that, when thus tacitly

---

*It is, I am sorry to say, a very rare circumstance for the physicians of New York to meet together sociably at each other's houses, or indulge in an interchange of friendly civilities. Here, there are no convival assemblings of those whose tastes and occupation should draw them frequently together; and although some laudable efforts have been made to break through the icy circle that surrounds us, they have not been responded to in a proper manner, and consequently have failed to accomplish the desired end.

acknowledged to be worth so little, they may in reality be worth nothing. This is one of the great difficulties with which we have to contend, and unfortunately it would scarcely seem capable of being remedied. No fixed and satisfactory tariff, applicable to all cases, can be established, and it is a matter which had probably better be left to the judgment and discretion of each individual. A just medium in charges, however, should always be observed, and we should never be so unreasonable as to ask $100 for a single and inactive consultation visit in the city, nor yet condescend to allow our services to be estimated at the value of ten cents a visit, or one shilling for vaccination or venesection. When persons are really able to do so, they are, for the most part, both ready and willing to grant a fair and adequate remuneration for professional services, and when too poor to pay more than the paltry sums last indicated, we should refer them to the public charitable institutions provided for them, or, at all events, a feeling of pride should lead us to reject all compensation and find our reward in the conscious pleasure of doing a good action.

Feuds amongst ourselves are of too frequent occurrence; they should always be condemned and avoided, as they are the means of retarding the progress of the profession and frequently throw impediments in the way of science. These, however, when strictly confined within professional limits, cannot produce the great and serious evils which must ever result from their being made public. All of our faults and errors should be kept within our own bounds, and on no account should medical men allow their feelings to get the better of their judgments, so far as to lead them to commit a positive and irreparable injury on the profession, the evil consequences of which they are sure to experience themselves, in the depreciation of public respect and confidence in their profession. They should recollect the advice given by the venerable Hufeland and bear in mind his declarations on this subject, to the effect that:

> In proportion as the public is made acquainted with the faults and defects of physicians, and as they are made to appear suspected and contemptible in its eyes, so is the estimation in which medicine is held, lowered; and as this diminished confidence is extended from the science to those who practise it, the censurer soon experiences the consequences of it himself. Public malice against physicians would certainly be less indulged in, and their faults would much less frequently furnish food for general conversation, if they never themselves set the example. . . .

Of the influence of quackery as operating to the injury of our profession here, I shall have but little to say. That it occasions a large pecuniary loss to us cannot be denied; but when practiced openly, and by persons not *bonâ fide* members of the faculty, I do not conceive that it acts in manner otherwise hurtful to our interests or reputation.

It is only when degenerate members of our own body condescend, from the desire of pecuniary gain, to embrace the trade of the charlatan, that they are capable for a time of influencing public opinion, and may, until found out, which they invariably have been and always will be, sooner or later, produce an impression injurious to our general character and interests.

I consider it bad policy, as well as bad taste, to indulge in abusive language against this class of persons, who should always be left to the upbraidings of their own consciences, and that severe and most keenly felt punishment which consists in an entire exclusion from their society, and from any association with their professional contemporaries. They may succeed for a time, and accumulate money, but what shall repay them for loss of caste and that inward feeling of shame and degradation which they must experience on finding themselves despised and rejected by their fellows, and eventually sinking to an oblivion from which they may never again hope to emerge—leaving behind them when they die, as an inheritance to their children, a patrimony which, though it may be rich in the blessings of the world, can never be disconnected from the recollection of the manner in which it was obtained?

These persons are most truly to be pitied; and their bowed head and downcast look, evincing shame and inward suffering, should rather excite in our breasts feelings of commiseration than of ire; and although we can never permit ourselves to regard them in the light of fit associates, we should charitably hope that they have been led astray, and that their minds are so constituted as to render them incapable of experiencing, in its full force, that acute sense of degradation which would be so severely felt by honorable men of cultivated intellect.

That some few of them honestly believe in the virtues and superior advantages of a system that they may have adopted, is most certain; but that numbers of them profess what they cannot believe and do not practice, is equally certain, and may be easily proved; it is the latter class to whom I would have these remarks apply—those who make use of a novelty as a stepping stone to success and cheat the public by promising to pursue a course which they know to be wrong and which they rarely, if ever, in reality follow.

There can be no harm in it, nor can a physician be justly blamed for practicing according to any method that he may conclude, after proper study and inquiry, to be best; it is his duty to follow the course that he conscientiously believes will prove most conducive to the interests of his patients; but, then, he should do so quietly and unostentatiously—as a man who is entitled to the privilege of judging and acting independently—and scorn to call himself, or allow others to call him, the blind follower of a master, or of a particular and exclusive system, for the purpose of attracting attention and gaining notoriety; thus acting the part of an imposter whose province and aim is to deceive. The answer of a friend of mine to a lady, when questioned by her as to what "*class* of doctors" he belonged, will illustrate what I desire to say better, probably, than I have explained. "Madam," said he, "I am a physician who has studied his profession in all its branches and departments; I have examined, and continue to examine, every new theory and everything proposed as useful, and I practice in all instances for the good of my patients."

I would congratulate the Society upon the gradual declension from public favor and sympathy which animal magnetism, homeopathy, and similar delusions are now daily experiencing, as it evinces a return of the sound common sense of the people, which has been for a time diverted by plausible theories and amusing practical exhibitions.

All that might in any way be gleaned as useful or interesting, from these innovations, has long since been adopted by the regular profession and incorporated into our system of treatment. As was our duty, we have examined and studied thoroughly, as it has ever been our interest to do, everything that has been supposed to be calculated to extend our field of knowledge, or enable us to render ourselves more useful to our fellow creatures; what little wheat has been met with, has been most cautiously and industriously separated from the mass of chaff with which it was encumbered, and although the grains are found to be both small and imperfect, they may possibly produce, if properly cultivated, some little fruit.

No sooner, however, is one method of imposture on the wane than we find another brought forward to supply its place; so it has ever been, and so it must and will be always. Homeopathy, lately so fashionable amongst us, finding no resting place in Europe, at least out of Germany—scouted in France, where its absurdities were fully demonstrated by positive and actual experiment—rejected in Italy—discountenanced in England—some few years since took its flight across the Atlantic and implanted itself in our soil. Here it took root, and after supplanting Thomsonianism, and making sad inroads in the fertile fields of the "Herb Doctors," it flourished for a time. Its day, however, is now nearly at an end, and it is rapidly retiring before the enterprising and successful rivalry of hydrosudopathy, and the crono-thermal system, which, likewise, will have their turn and flourish until novelties of more recent date, such as the Russian "mud baths," or perhaps a revival of the old "water casting," come to usurp their places and their profits.

All the endeavors of the profession can never accomplish much against new and plausible medical theories, and by far the most prudent and the wisest course is to abstain from all abuse against them. When asked his opinion of their merits, it is the duty of the upright and conscientious physician to express it frankly, and if in disapprobation, let it be done in courteous language devoid of all abusive epithets. By such a course we are sure to obtain a fair hearing, and our friends will be ever ready to acknowledge the force of remarks and reasoning directed to their understanding, and which shall be unaccompanied by evidences of personal pique or the expression of feelings of dislike and hatred evincing undue prejudice or a desire to condemn unheard.

Having indicated, in a very imperfect manner, however, some few of the many evils that exist in our profession, and endeavored to convey a just impression of its present condition and of some of the causes which operate to injure it, I shall not trespass longer on your time by offering suggestions as to the best and most proper means for remedying them. The most important, and perhaps the only subject entirely within the control of the profession is that of education. But I leave this very difficult and embarrassing question to the united wisdom of the gentlemen who will, I hope, shortly assemble in our city for the special purpose of investigating it. Amongst them there will doubtless be found competent and able representatives of this Society.

EDWIN L. GODKIN

ORTHOPATHY AND HETEROPATHY

Editor's Note

Edwin Lawrence Godkin (1831–1902), an Irish-born lawyer, came to New York in 1856. Here he continued to play the role into which he naturally gravitated even before he left Great Britain, that of publicist. When a new liberal weekly journal, *The Nation*, was founded in 1865, Godkin became its editor. His interests were those of the magazine's subtitle: "A Weekly Journal devoted to Politics, Literature, Science, and Art." Godkin soon took up the cause of Negro rights, he constantly stressed popular education, filled his pages with discussions of current affairs and literary criticism, and led *The Nation*, along with the *Times* and others, in the fight against the Tweed Ring and Tammany domination of New York City.[1]

Its broad editorial policy frequently permitted *The Nation* to comment on medical affairs, particularly the public health. As is evident from this article, Godkin was much more impressed by sanitary science, or the methods of preventing disease, than he was by the doctor's ability to cure.

Godkin defended homeopathy, much to the disgust of his correspondent from Kentucky, mainly on grounds of "scientific" freedom. He believed that the case for or against homeopathy was no better or no worse than that for regular medicine if one applied fairly rigid criteria in judging the results.[2]

The fight between the regular or allopathic physicians and the sectarians continued throughout the century. In New York, in the 1880's, it caused dissent in the regular profession. Many members of the Medical Society of the State of New York left that group in 1882, when a change in the code of ethics, contrary to the AMA Code, allowed consultation with homeopaths and other practitioners. The dissident group formed the New York Medical Association, which held separate meetings and did not merge again with the older group until 1905.

Although much of what the reader "S" from Louisville, presumably a physician, had to say in the letter quoted in this article was true and is what most physicians would have said, Godkin's argument seems more attractive.

The Nation 5 (1867): 335–36, 439–40.

[1] See Frank L. Mott, *A History of American Magazines*, 5 vols. (Cambridge: Harvard University Press, 1957–68) 3: 331–56.

[2] The so-called irregular physicians, homeopaths, eclectics, botanical doctors, phrenologists, water-cure men, and the like, played a substantial role in the dispensation of medical care to nineteenth-century Americans. A large number of flourishing journals were edited and written by members of one sect or another. Because they are not represented in this book, one should not conclude that they were unimportant.

The recent expulsion of a member from the New York Academy of Medicine for having met a homeopathic practitioner in consultation, coupled with the observations made by Dr. Stone in support of the motion, in which, if correctly reported, he strongly insinuated that even the maintenance of intimate personal relations with a homeopathist was an ethical offence in a regular physician of the old school, helps to confirm us in doubts which we have long entertained whether doctors rightly understand their own philosophical position. We are far from denying their right to prescribe to the members of their own profession the terms on which they shall be received as brethren and met in friendly professional intercourse. Any number of men are perfectly justified, if they believe the interests of either science or good manners or good morals will be advanced, or even their social enjoyment promoted thereby, to form themselves into a club or academy, or any other kind of corporation, and lay down certain rules for the guidance of even the professional conduct of those who wish to be of their number, and to make the observance of these rules a condition of business intercourse.

In all professions in which the result of labor is uncertain, and of such a nature that the public cannot at once judge of its quality, a professional tribunal which undertakes to sift the members, and by its recognition to furnish a kind of certificate of character, is of the highest use. The surveillance which the medical profession exercises over its own members undoubtedly goes a great way to protect laymen of ordinary intelligence from quacks and impostors; the ignorant or credulous of course no machinery can protect. We say all this by way of explaining that whatever objections we may make to the allopathic treatment of homeopathists are not due to any general dislike of corporate feeling or corporate interference with freedom of trade. What we say is that this treatment seems to us to rest on a total forgetfulness or total misapprehension on the part of the regular practitioners of their position as scientific men.

The class of men against whom regular practitioners are bound to protect the public by refusing to meet them or treat them with ordinary professional courtesy are quacks and charlatans and cheats—that is, persons who practice medicine without being able to furnish evidence of having undergone any regular training for it or having in any way acquired a fair knowledge of the art; persons who pretend to possess a panacea; persons who, being professionally qualified as far as knowledge goes, have shown a want of moral fitness for it, and other such people. But the homeopathic doctors do not come under any of these heads. They are regularly trained for their calling. As regards character, we presume the average is as high as amongst their allopathic bretheran. They have a code of professional ethics, and enforce it, and they command the confidence of a large and highly respectable portion of the community. In fact, the objection, and the only one, if we are not mistaken, made against professional intercourse with them or even ordinary courtesy towards them, is based on the assumption that, their system being false and absurd, those who practice it must be either fools or knaves. But this notion of the character of the homeopathic system, though it may be true, is in the first place incapable of proof; and in the second place, if it were capable of proof, the demonstration would also destroy the claims of the allopathic system to either our confidence or respect.

The theory of many allopathic doctors seems to be that they have means of verifying their conclusions which the homeopathists do not possess, and that while the latter are empirics, the former are men of science. But the truth is that medicine is not a science in the strict sense of the term, or anything approaching to a science. It is, rather, an immense body of facts out of which a host of able and acute and disciplined observers are endeavoring to construct a science, but hitherto with very indifferent success. The only thing a doctor can predict with any approach to certainty is a portion of the action of certain remedies on the human frame. The *whole of the* action of any of them no doctor can foretell; and therefore what effect any drug will have on disease, no doctor can say with certainty. When the doctor gives a sick man a blue pill, he can tell with an approach to certainty what one result of it will be, but it may and does produce a dozen other results of which he knows nothing. What kills one man cures another; and the treatment of every case is, in reality, a series of experiments conducted under conditions which deprive them almost altogether of the right to be called experiments at all in any scientific sense. The reports of cases which are read at medical meetings are not reports of scientific processes such as a chemist may make. They are records of a series of phenomena of which nobody knows the relation or connection, and the repetition of which in the same order of succession nobody can predict or produce.

The fact is that the art of *curing*, except in its mechanical branch, surgery, has made but little progress from the earliest times. The improvement which we see in it has consisted rather in the abandonment of old processes than the discovery of new ones. There has been an immense change in medical practice within two hundred years, for instance; but, if examined minutely, it will be found that it is due mainly to doctors giving up remedies they once believed in, rather than in their devising new ones. There have been two or three remarkable and valuable discoveries, such as vaccination and quinine, but they have been the result of accident rather than of research or experiment, and the tendency amongst all the best class of practitioners is in the direction of distrust of all "active treatment," as it is called. The older doctors grow—as everybody must have remarked—the less medicine they give; and the practitioners of our day do not give a gill where their predecessors in the last century gave a gallon. They are falling back, as if in despair about medicine, more and more on the plan of simply placing the patient in the most favorable natural conditions, giving him good food and drink and plenty of fresh air when he is weak, prescribing abstinence when he is overfed, exercise when he is too sedentary, rest when he is jaded. For those, and they are unhappily the great bulk of mankind, by whom these remedies are unattainable, there is little hope in the medical art, except in a few acute diseases. In fact, the main value of physicians is now to be found in diagnosis—in plain English, in their ability to tell people what is the matter with them, or whether anything is the matter, and what to eat, drink, and avoid, and to raise the patient's *morale* and that of his friends.

It is in the art of *prevention* and not that of curing that medical men have made real progress. There may be said to be now a sanitary science, and experiments of considerable value in this science are possible and are made every day. Given certain conditions of food, clothing, ventilation, and drainage and exposure, and doctors can tell with a fair amount of accuracy what the effect on the health of masses of people will be; and it is to the progress of this science that we owe the rise in the average duration of life which within the last two hundred years has been witnessed all over the civilized world. And we venture to predict that it is in the cultivation of this science that the medical profession will hereafter win its principal victories, though we certainly do not relinquish the hope that it will yet hit upon something which will enable it to make headway against the ravages of consumption as effectually as vaccination has against small-pox and quinine against certain forms of fever.

The bearing of all this on the professional standing of homeopathists is obvious. One does not need to claim for their system any greater curative power than the allopathic system in order to show the title of its practitioners to respect and recognition. They are—though professing to act on a theory—largely empirics, we grant; but so are the allopathists. The action of their remedies is uncertain; it is even uncertain whether in any given case their medicines will produce any effect on disease whatever; but the same thing may be said of allopathic treatment. The smallness of their doses may seem "absurd," but nothing can in science be called absurd which cannot be demonstrated to be so, and there is no process whatever in the possession of the medical faculty by which it could be shown that an ounce is more likely to cure than the twentieth part of a grain except a simple enumeration of observed cases, which in this matter is of no value whatever, because the homeopathists will produce as many "cases" in proportion to their numbers as their older brethren. As to the novelty of their practice we shall say nothing, because no doctor laying claim to the character of a scientific man will, with the history of his own art before his eyes, consider this an objection to it. The main thing, therefore, for consideration, it seems to us, in fixing the relations which the allopathic profession ought to occupy to the homeopathists, is the personal character of the latter. If they are well-educated men, gentlemen, men of honor and courage and delicacy, to refuse to associate or compare views with them because they use a different class of drugs or use drugs in different quantities, is a course worthier of trades-unionists or of young army officers than a body of grave students of science. So far from condemning them, real philosophers ought to encourage them. In a field in which so little is known there cannot be too many explorers, provided they are governed in their explorations by the laws of honor and by a great or even average devotion to truth. When Napoleon was at the Red Sea he rode over the strand with his staff, and was caught at nightfall by the rising tide and lost his bearings. He therefore disposed his officers round him in a circle and ordered each man to ride out from him, as a center, in a straight line. Those who found the water growing shallower were, of course, in the right track, and were speedily followed by the rest. Academies of medicine might well take a hint from this ingenious but simple contrivance of the great master of the art of war. We would not have them exact one guarantee the less as to character or education, but there is nothing in the present condition or past history of their art to warrant them in concluding with certainty that any school of practitioners is working in the wrong direction, and they owe it to the human race to give all honest and properly qualified explorers a fair chance. We suppose few people care under what system they are cured, whether through a bolus, a globule, or simply through the imagination. The medical profession is not an end but a means. It exists not that a certain number of gentlemen may preserve a good social standing and good emoluments, but that the sum of human misery may be abated. It seems to us that this is forgotten by those who outlaw the homeopathists.

ORTHOPATHY AND HETEROPATHY

To the Editor of The Nation:

In quite an elaborate and very well written article in *The Nation* for October 24, you take to task the allopathic school of doctors for their persistent determination to ignore the disciples of Hahnemann. Presuming, of course, that you lay no stress upon the exceptional case of Dr. Stone, who would forbid social relations as well, let us look for a moment at the real point made by the article referred to.

You admit frankly enough the necessity of organization, association—out of which grows a system of ethics—but claim that the rule which forbids the allopathist meeting in consultation the homeopathic practitioner suggests "a doubt whether the doctors rightly understand their own philosophical position." You assert that doctors are bound to protect the public against charlatans and cheats, but that homeopathic doctors do not come under these heads; "they are regularly trained for their calling." Suppose that this regular training starts from a point which, in the judgment of the old-school doctors, leads to imposture and is, to the public which doctors are bound to protect, simply a cheat; suppose these doctors, in the exercise of their best judgment, believe that the facts out of which Hahnemann claims the growth of "similia similibus curantur" are themselves a cheat—as, for instance, that the millionth part of a grain of sulphur tells upon human organization for a hundred days, and that during these hundred days all the *symptoms felt* are due to the action of sulphur and that whenever these symptoms are found in the sick-room the remedy is sulphur, for "similia similibus curantur." *This is* their system—that is their mode of arriving at the facts upon which the practice is based. You, as a representative man, a standard of health, swallow oyster-shells or opium or charcoal or sulphur, and, with an eye turned inward for ten or twenty or fifty days, note down in a book properly ruled and headed all the sensations you may experience during these days of trial, and thus secure in the fact that oyster-shells or opium produce certain symptoms in the well man, *you know*—"similia similibus curantur"—that oyster-shells or opium will remove these symptoms in the sick man. In order, however, to this removal, you must have your dose of opium homeopathically prepared, and you get that just as readily as you get at the fact of its action. To one grain of opium you add ninety-nine grains of sugar of milk, and triturate for a certain specified number of minutes, turning the mass over with a spatula a certain specified number of times; then of this mass you take out one grain (the one-hundredth part of a grain of opium) and add ninety-nine fresh grains of sugar of milk, triturate and manipulate as before, and one grain of this has the ten-thousandth part of a grain of opium—this is the 2d potency. Carry on this process till you have reached the 30th potency, and you have the ordinary dose of this country, the 30th dynamization being about as much as Americans can stand. They take it stronger on the other side of the water; even as potential as the two-thousandth "attenuation." If you don't want an infinitesimal globule but prefer a fluid, the process is precisely the same—one drop to ninety-nine of alcohol, and one drop of this to ninety-nine fresh drops (you have the ten-thousandth part of a drop already). You may make it a great deal stronger by adding a great deal more alcohol; for a principle of the system is "the greater the dilution, the greater the strength."

Now, without attempting to controvert their foundation principle, "similia similibus curantur," may not those who are "bound to protect the public" insist upon the utter absurdity—demonstrable absurdity—of this mode of arriving at facts, and this *hocus-pocus* manipulatory mode of preparing globules and tinctures?—for any practice of homeopathy without these infinitesimals is a fraud, a sailing under false colors. It is the play of "Hamlet" with *Hamlet* left out. Take their own books from Hahnemann down, passing no judgment upon their philosophy, and looking only at their claimed facts and their *materia medica*, and tell your readers whether the world's common sense does not revolt at the possibility of professional consultation between a practitioner of the old school and a follower of such teaching as this, and tell them whether these old-school men do not show some right understanding of their position as guardians of the public when they repudiate all such tampering with human credulity.

Your statement that the allopathists justify their opposition to this professional intercourse by assuming that those who practice such an absurd and false system are either knaves or fools is rather startling coming from one who knows so well how to use words with meaning in them. I think the course of *The Nation* for two years past justifies me in saying that you lean a little toward Radicalism in politics—so do I; not that you are *very* radical, but conservatively radical—so am I. From the reading of some other papers you and I have both learned that a good many of your neighbors and a great many of mine drift strongly in an opposite direction. We think their teachings are false—very false. They think ours false—very false. Of course there can be no political affinity, association, consultation, or whatever else saves antagonism between such elements; but are we all knaves or fools? You and I are bound to "protect the public," so far as in us lies, against the teachings of those who differ from us as the nadir from the zenith; but they are not fools, nor do they so regard us.

You say the "smallness of the homeopathic doses may seem absurd, but this cannot be proven." That may be so. But if the trituration and spatulation of a grain of sulphur with successive additions of sugar of milk till you have reached the millionth part of a grain, and then claiming for this an influence upon human organization for a hundred days, is not "absurd," the world's common sense and all science hitherto has been wonderfully befooled. It strikes that common sense and that hitherto science as being a little "absurd," also, to claim that these infinitesimals have power to remove morbid action when they have no recognized effect upon any healthy stomach taken either by the globule or the bottleful; and then to get rid of this absurdity by claiming that they act only upon morbid conditions, diseased parts, while all the facts of their action are derived from standards of health, looks more like another absurdity than a rational explanation.

The upshot of your view of the whole matter is, that there is a very unimportant difference of opinion between two sets of men pursuing the same vocation, the one believing in the necessity of large doses, the other in small doses—in either case the object being *to cure*, and the public caring not one whit whether the dose which does it is large or small. Now, to the public I confess this view of the matter is very plausible and lies palpably *on the surface*. But the old school of doctors claim that while the homeopathist is professing to cure, he is doing absolutely nothing, is in fact playing the charlatan—educated charlatan he may be, but still the charlatan—giving minute directions about the taking of minute particles of charcoal, modifying in no possible degree the morbid state with which he professes to deal. But you say the patient gets well—so he does; and this brings us to the standpoint from which we may fairly look at the *successes* of homeopathy.

The fact, which is growing more and more rapidly upon the profession all over the world, that *disease has a history*, goes far toward an explanation of the recoveries under every conceivable form of medication. In the hands of the most enlightened medical men of the day much disease is conducted to a favorable termination without an atom of physic; but then the enlightened medical men *don't pretend to give physic*, allopathic or homeopathic—indeed, stoutly deny that you need physic, only need to be cured—that is, taken care of—and frankly tell you that nature is doing for you infinitely more and better than they can do.

What possible community of thought can exist between two men who start off in such opposite directions: the one recognizing a history in disease and trusting largely to "vis medicatrix naturae"—*taking care* of his patient and thus *curing* him; the other claiming to war with almost unerring certainty against a tangible malady, and feeding his patient upon thin air and a drop of water? Let your medication be much or little, but don't delude your patient, don't deceive "the public you are bound to protect," and don't play falsely with your own soul.

Louisville, Ky.   S.

[We do not profess to be able to decide whether allopathy or homeopathy is the right system; all we know is that scientifically there is as much to be said for one as for the other. The description "S." gives of the way in which homeopathic doses are prepared seems funny to us; but it does not seem "absurd," from a scientific point of view, to suppose that such doses affect the human frame, either in health or disease, because we do not *know* anything accurately about the effects of any dose on the human frame. "S." may give the most "sensible" dose in the world, and yet will be entirely unable to say what the result will be . "Common sense" is no guide in such matters, as everybody knows who has the slightest knowledge of the history of science. "Common sense" said for a long time that the sun moved round the earth; but common sense was wrong. Therefore, we say allopathic doctors may *not* insist on "the demonstrable absurdity" of the homeopathic practice, for the simple reason that they cannot "demonstrate" it; and it is because we find that they sometimes labor under the delusion that they can, that we have expressed the doubt whether they understand their own scientific position. Nor is the reproach that they practice on a theory, or in other words, *à priori*, one which allopathic doctors can fairly cast at the homeopathists, for the simple reason that they themselves do the same thing and have always done it; and some of their theories have been, as the world now believes, as absurd as could be desired by their worse enemies. Take, for instance, the celebrated medical "Doctrine of Signatures," which maintained that a substance possessing medicinal value had some outward mark indicating the disease for which it was a remedy. Under this sytem the lungs of a fox were good for asthma, because a fox is long-winded; tumeric was good for jaundice, because it is yellow; the bloodstone was good for bleeding at the nose; and so on through scores of substances. One school of regular practitioners at one time ascribed the operation of mercury and iron in the human system to their specific gravity. Moreover, there is, we presume, no doctor at the present day who does not practice on a theory which he thinks diseases in our day are of the "low" type; others never give any alcohol, because they think alcohol poisonous. As to which is right we are certainly incompetent to decide or even offer an opinion. All we say is that gentlemen in this position must not ask us to believe that homeopaths are quacks because their doses seem absurd. Of course, we would not expect a doctor who did not believe in homeopathy to consult with one who did; but we do maintain that if any doctor thinks he can get light thrown on one of his cases by taking counsel with a homeopathist, science as well as humanity demands that his brother doctors shall not interfere with him. "S." accounts for the success of homeopathists by the growing recognition of the fact that "diseases have a history." This may have much to do with it; but we confess we think people's growing indifference to the mode of their cure, provided they get well, has more; and this indifference we ascribe to the growing disbelief in the existence of a science of medicine. The public feeling in the matter is, in fact, well expressed by Lisette in Molière's "Amour Médicin." She tells M. Tomès, the doctor, that the coachman is dead. "Impossible," says M. Tomès; "a fact," says she; "he can't be dead," says he; "he is, and buried too," says she; "you're mistaken," says he; "I have seen him," says she; "impossible," says he; "Hippocrates declares that these diseases do not terminate till the fourteenth or twenty-first day, and it is only six days since the coachman fell sick;" "Hippocrates may say what he pleases," replies Lisette, "the coachman is dead."—Ed. Nation.]

PART IV
MEDICAL PRACTICE

INTRODUCTION

The title "Medical Practice" for this section is inadequate and perhaps misleading. "Therapeutics" would be too restrictive, but that is the focus of most of the following papers. Four of the writers (Bigelow, Bartlett, Davis, and Flint) address themselves to general questions of therapy, to treat or not to treat, as it were. Rush, Chapman, and Delafield are concerned with more specific problems. They describe and discuss some of the commonest illnesses to which nineteenth-century Americans fell prey. Only Seguin focuses on a diagnostic approach to illness, and surgery is relegated to another section entirely.

One of the leaders in the movement for a rational medicine, utilizing less heroic remedies, was the Connecticut physician Worthington Hooker, who throughout his career made a number of perceptive remarks about the character of the profession and the society in which it practiced. The healing art would make progress in America, Hooker assumed, because people here were characterized by a great fondness for novelty and experimentation. But Americans were activists too, and this could explain why active dosing was not met with great resistance by the public.

> Perhaps the disposition to demand of the physician an active medication in all cases exists to a greater degree in this than other countries. We are preeminently an energetic and enterprising people, and therefore the bold "heroic" practitioner is apt to meet with favor from the public.[1]

Despite Hooker's pessimism about Americans resisting bleeding and purging, many of them did turn to the various medical sectarians flourishing at mid-century.[2]

---

[1] "Nature of evidence in practical medicine," *New Englander* 11 (1853): 549–70; 559. This article was unsigned, but from editorial comments it is safe to assume Hooker was probably its author. Austin Flint (see introduction to paper by Seguin) a decade later believed that Americans had too little fondness for novelty.

[2] The declining popularity and acceptance of the sectarians in the latter nineteenth century, on the other hand, was one indication of the increasing effectiveness of regular medicine. As Professor Shryock has remarked, "The gradual shift in the status of homeopathy, from the dignity of a system to the heresy of a sect, may be viewed as a turning point in medical thought." *Medicine and Society in America; 1660–1860* (New York: New

As late as 1900 some clinicians were still very sparing in their use of drugs. William Osler, in 1901, told an audience at the Johns Hopkins Medical History Club that,

> A new school of practitioners has arisen which cares nothing for homeopathy and less for so-called allopathy. It seeks to study, rationally and scientifically, the action of drugs, old and new. It is more concerned that a physician shall know how to apply the few great medicines which all have to use, such as quinine, iron, mercury, iodide of potassium, opium, and digitalis, than that he should employ a multiplicity of remedies the action of which is extremely doubtful.[3]

Bibliographical Note

Little has been said so far in our discussion about the actual conditions of medical practice. Nor do the papers of this section deal with this in any general way. The topic is of such magnitude that probably the best way to deal with it in a brief introduction is to guide the reader to a number of very useful secondary sources.

As a first source of information, as well as of references, one should turn to the many writings of Professor Richard H. Shryock. See especially his *Medicine and Society in America: 1660-1860*, New York: New York University Press, 1960; and the recently reprinted essays *Medicine in America*, Baltimore: The Johns Hopkins Press, 1966. Charles E. Rosenberg has used an approach that should be more widely incorporated in the writing of medical history in his "The practice of medicine in New York a century ago," *Bull. Hist. Med.* 41 (1967): 223-53.

Many of the state histories of medicine contain much information about conditions and types of medical practice. See especially John Duffy's *The Rudolph Matas History of Medicine in Louisiana*, 2 vols., Baton Rouge: Louisiana State University Press, 1958; Thomas N. Bonner, *The Kansas Doctor, A Century of Pioneering*, Lawrence: University of Kansas Press, 1959; and his *Medicine in Chicago 1850-1950*, Madison: American History Research Center, 1957.

David J. Davis, ed., *History of Medical Practice in Illinois*, vol. 2, Chicago: Illinois State Medical Society, 1955; James J. Walsh, *History of Medicine in New York*, 5 vols., New York: National Americana Society, 1919; and Wyndham B. Blanton's three books: *Medicine in Virginia in the Seventeenth Century*, Richmond: The William Byrd Press, 1930; *Medicine in Virginia in the Eighteenth*

York University Press, 1960), p. 144. For recent discussions of homeopathy in America see chapter 5 of Joseph F. Kett's, *The Formation of the American Medical Profession* (New Haven: Yale University Press, 1968), and Martin Kaufman's, *Homeopathy in America: The Rise and Fall of a Medical Heresy* (Baltimore: The Johns Hopkins Press, 1971). One of the best known contemporary discussions was Oliver Wendell Holmes's "Homeopathy and its kindred delusions," in his *Medical Essays, 1842-1882* (Boston: Houghton, Mifflin, 1895), pp. 1-102, first delivered as two lectures in 1842. For extensive discussion of the botanical sect see Alex Berman's articles, "The Thomsonian movement and its relation to American pharmacy and medicine," *Bull. Hist. Med.* 25 (1951): 405-28; 519-38; and "Neo-Thomsonianism in the United States," *J. Hist. Med.* 11 (1956): 133-55.

[3] "Medicine in the Nineteenth Century," in *Aequanimitas* (3rd ed.; New York: McGraw-Hill, 1932), pp. 219-61; 255.

Century, Richmond: Garrett & Massie, 1931; and *Medicine in Virginia in the Nineteenth Century*, Richmond: Garrett & Massie, 1933.

The medical problems of special groups, such as slaves and pioneers has also received attention. Shryock has an essay on the former in *Medicine in America*. See also John Duffy, "Medical practice in the ante-bellum South," *J. Southern Hist*. 25 (1959): 53–72. For frontier medicine see R. Carlyle Buley, "Pioneer health and medical practices in the old Northwest prior to 1840," *Miss. Valley Hist. Rev.* 20 (1933–34): 497–520; and Madge E. Pickard and R. Carlyle Buley, *The Midwest Pioneer, His Ills, Cures, and Doctors*, Crawfordsville, Ind.: Banta, 1945.

One of the widespread medical practices of the first half of the century was blood-letting. Under the influence of Benjamin Rush, a great deal of blood was taken from patients for a variety of ills. Leon S. Bryan has shown that the practice began to decline by mid-century, but that much of the discussion of pros and cons found in American literature had European origins. "Blood-letting in American medicine, 1830–1892," *Bull. Hist. Med.* 38 (1964): 516–29. Another extremely important paper, one of much broader scope, is Alex Berman's, "The heroic approach in 19th century therapeutics," *Bull. Am. Soc. Hosp. Pharmacists* (1954, Sept.–Oct.): 320–27. One cannot stress too often that the history of American medicine cannot be studied without fully recognizing that, more often than not, it took its problems and answers from Europe.

For information regarding the economics of medicine see George Rosen, *Fees and Fee Bills: Some Economic Aspects of Medical Practice in Nineteenth Century America*, Baltimore: The Johns Hopkins Press, 1946, published as Supplement No. 6 to the *Bulletin of the History of Medicine*.

The numerous biographies and autobiographies that have been published are rich sources of information about how individual doctors lived and practiced. For conditions early in the century, see the *Autobiography* of Charles Caldwell, Philadelphia: Lippincott, Grambo, 1855; reprinted with a long introduction by Lloyd G. Stevenson, New York: (Plenum Publishing Co.), Da Capo Press, 1968. The two-volume memoir of Samuel D. Gross, *Autobiography*, Philadelphia: George Barrie, 1887; and J. Marion Sims' *The Story of My life*, New York: D. Appleton Co., 1884 (also reprinted by Da Capo Press) are useful. For an account of medical practice in the latter nineteenth century see William Allen Pusey, *A Doctor of the 1870's and 80's*, Springfield: Thomas, 1932.

BENJAMIN RUSH

ON THE CAUSES OF DEATH IN DISEASES THAT ARE NOT INCURABLE

Editor's Note

Benjamin Rush (1745–1813), one of America's most famous physicians, signer of the Declaration of Independence, medical writer and teacher, needs no introduction. His influence during the first decades of the nineteenth century was widely felt. Although the lancet and calomel purge that he favored so much doubtless caused much harm, his work for education, temperance, and the care of the mentally ill more than balanced the ledger.

Rush, who was active in various religious causes, sometimes sounded more as if he were delivering a sermon than a medical school lecture. The sermonizing is apparent in the following essay, which also nicely illustrates his opinion of the efficacy of active treatment and his contemptuous dismissal of the "ill directed operations of nature." It was partly against views such as Rush's that some of the writers of a later generation reacted. The school of therapy that relied more on nature than on art received a considerable hearing just after the middle of the century.[1]

Bibliographical Note

Rush's monistic theory of disease causation is not well expressed in the essay which follows. It has been described by Professor Shryock in *Medicine and Society in America, 1660–1860*, New York: New York University Press, 1960, available in paperback reprint; and in his article "Benjamin Rush from the perspective of the twentieth century," *Trans. Studies Coll. Phys. Phila.* 14 (1946): 113–20, reprinted in *Medicine in America*, Baltimore: The Johns Hopkins Press, 1966, pp. 233–51. See also Nathan G. Goodman, *Benjamin Rush, Physician and Citizen, 1746–1813*, Philadelphia: University of Pennsylvania Press, 1934; *Letters of Benjamin Rush*, L. H. Butterfield, ed., 2 vols., Princeton: Princeton University Press, 1951; and George W. Corner, ed., *The Autobiography of Benjamin Rush*, Princeton: Princeton University Press, 1948.

Sixteen Introductory Lectures (Philadelphia, 1811), pp. 65–87. This is Lecture III, delivered November 26, 1793.

[1] As Professor Shryock has pointed out, the condemnation of Rush at mid-century also reflected the influence of the Paris school on American medical thought.

Our city has again been afflicted by a malignant bilious fever. Its mortality has been much greater, in a given number of sick people, than in former years. In meditating upon the causes of this extraordinary mortality, I was led to contemplate the causes of death, not only in our late epidemic, but in other diseases which are not incurable, for the malignant bilious or yellow fever is not necessarily a mortal disease. In considering this subject, the first thing that occurred to my mind was the small proportion of people who die of diseases that are acknowledged to be incurable. In examining the bills of mortality, of all countries, how few people do we find die of aneurysms, epilepsy, internal cancers, and casualties, compared with the number of people who perish from fevers and other diseases which are admitted to be under the power of medicine. Perhaps the proportion of deaths from the former, compared with the deaths from the latter diseases, does not amount to more than one in a hundred. Ninety-nine persons, of course, die who might be cured by the proper application of remedies which are within the reach of reason and power of man. The business of the present lecture shall be to point out the various causes which render the means of saving life, that are known or attainable by us, thus abortive. The discovery of these causes will open a wide field for speculative truth, as well as practical virtue and happiness.

In considering the causes of death in diseases which are not incurable, I shall mention:

I. those which are derived from physicians;

II. those which arise from the conduct of sick people; and

III. those which arise from the conduct of their attendants and visitors.

1st. Under the first general head, I shall first mention *ignorance* in a physician, arising from original incapacity or a want of proper instruction in medicine. But where there have been both capacity and instruction, there is sometimes an obliquity in the human understanding which renders it incapable of perceiving truth upon medical subjects. A mind thus formed, may acquire learning without knowledge, and it may even acquire knowledge upon all subjects except in medicine. But where there are talents that are in every respect equal to the profession (and these are by no means so rare as has been commonly supposed), there is often a deficiency in their application. This deficiency extends to reading and observation. Few physicians read after they enter into business, and still fewer profit by their observations. It is from the neglect of these two sources of medical knowledge, that we consider so many cases as new, that have existed a hundred times before, and that we prescribe the same remedies in all countries and seasons for diseases of the same name. No epidemic has the same symptoms or will bear the same treatment in a warm and cold climate. The muslin dresses of the East and West Indies would not be more unsuitable for the citizens of Philadelphia in the autumnal months, than the remedies of a tropical climate are for the diseases of those months in the middle states of America.

But again, epidemics often differ so much in their character in the same climate in different years as to require a difference of treatment. The yellow fevers of 1793, 1794, and 1797 in our city yielded, in most cases, to copious bleeding. They were, moreover, aggravated in those years in every case by bark and laudanum. In the yellow fever of the present year, the lancet was used more sparingly, and bark and laudanum were administered in some cases with success. Lastly, the same epidemic differs in the *same* season in different kinds of weather. This remark was obvious in our late fever. Copious bleeding was forbidden, in almost every case, in the month of August. Emetics at this time had a much happier effect. After the 20th of September, and during the whole month of October, copious bleeding, in many instances, supplied the place of emetics, and produced, when properly used, a safe and easy termination of the disease.

2d. A cause of death in diseases that are not incurable arises from the *negligence* of physicians. This negligence extends to their delays in not obeying immediately the first call to a patient, to their inattention to all the symptoms and circumstances of a disease in a sick room, and to the time of their visits not being accommodated to those changes in a disease in which remedies of a certain character can be applied with effect. Negligence from the first of those three causes has occasioned the death of many patients. A conduct, the reverse of that which has been mentioned, is happily commended by Dr. Johnson in his friend and physician, Dr. Levet, in an elegant ode to his memory. The talents of this physician were said to be moderate, but his success was considerable in his extensive practice among the poor, owing chiefly to his early and immediate compliance with the calls of his patients.*

3d. Physicians render curable diseases mortal, in many instances, by their connecting the measure of their services to the sick with pecuniary considerations. This is one reason why more of the poor than of the rich die of mortal epidemics. They are in general either deserted by physicians altogether or attended in such a desultory manner that medicine has but a slender chance of doing them any service. Extravagant charges for medical advice and attendance have, in several cases that have come to my knowledge, produced such delays in sending for a physician as have given a curable disease time to advance to its incurable stage. These delays, though apparently originating with patients, should be traced wholly to the conduct of physicians.

4th. Forgetfulness in a physician to visit his patients or to send them medicines at regular and critical hours has occasioned the death of many persons in diseases that might, under other circumstances, have been cured.

5th. A preference of reputation to the life of a patient has often led physicians to permit a curable disease to terminate in death. This disposition is more

*"No summons mock'd by *chill* delay,
No petty gain disdain'd by pride,
The modest wants of every day,
The toil of every day supply'd."

general than is known or supposed by the public. The death of a patient, under the ill-directed operations of nature, or of what are called lenient and safe medicines, seldom injures the reputation or business of a physician. For this reason many people are permitted to die who might have been recovered by the use of efficient remedies.

6th. A *sudden indisposition* attacking a physician, so as to prevent his regular and habitual visits to his patients, has often been the cause of death, where a favorable issue of a disease would otherwise have taken place. This source of mortality is most obvious in general epidemics, when the disease is dangerous, the patients numerous, and the time of brother physicians so completely occupied as to prevent their affording the persons who have been deserted the least substituted aid.

7th. Where none of the causes of mortality which have been enumerated have occurred, patients are sometimes lost in curable diseases by fraud and uncertainty in the composition and doses of medicines, by which means they produce greater or less effects than were intended. Many persons have died from an excess in the operation, or from the inertness of a dose of James's powder. The tartarized antimony has as often deceived the hopes of a physician. It was to obviate these evils that Mr. Chaptal expressed a wish that "Those heroic remedies which operate in small doses, should produce constant and invariable effects through all Europe," and wisely proposed that "Governments, which do not apply their stamp of approbation to objects of luxury, until they have passed a rigid inspection, should prohibit traders from circulating, with impunity, products upon which the health of the citizen so essentially depends."*

8th. The prescriptions of physicians, written in a careless and illegible hand, have sometimes produced mistakes in the exhibition of medicines which have been the means of destroying life in diseases that had no tendency to death. Verbal prescriptions have occasionally been followed by the same unfortunate issue. The bare recital of these facts should render perspicuity in writing and speaking an essential part, not only of the learning but of the morality of every physician.

We proceed, in the second place, to mention those causes of death in curable diseases which originate with sick people; and here we must begin, as under our former head, by mentioning *ignorance*. Medicine has, unhappily for mankind, been made so much a mystery that few patients are judges of the talents or qualifications of physicians; hence the bold and the artful are often preferred to the modest and the skilful. The desire of health, like the love of money, it has been said, levels all ranks and capacities; and, however much what is called a liberal education may enable men to form correct opinions upon certain subjects, it gives them no preeminence in medicine. In this science the rich and the poor, the learned and the illiterate are actuated, in common, by the same vulgar

---

*Vol. ii, p. 261, 262.

prejudices. Our late epidemic furnished many proofs of the truth of these re-marks. An opinion had become current and popular that the disease was aggra-vated by harsh remedies and that it was to be cured by the operations of nature, aided by the most simple medicines. To the influence of this opinion must be ascribed, in part, its greater mortality than in former years. Patients who suf-fered by this species of ignorance, not only renounced all knowledge upon other subjects where innumerable analogies suggested the reasonableness of accom-modating means to ends, but they rejected the analogy of a practice in diseases which habit had long made familiar to them. What patient is so ignorant as not to use more powerful remedies in a pleurisy than in a common cold? and yet the same patient cannot comprehend that a yellow fever is to a mild remittent, what a violent inflammation of the lungs in a pleurisy is to a moderate affection of the same parts in a catarrh.

2d. *Prejudice* in patients in the choice of a physician has sometimes rendered diseases mortal which are not incurable. This prejudice is either of a religious or a political nature. The former leads men to prefer physicians of their own sect; the latter, of their own party, without any regard to talents or knowledge. It is because our profession is a degraded one, that gentlemen of other professions usurp the right of thinking for us upon political questions. The world does not treat the profession of the law with so much disrespect. Eminent talents at the bar command business from men of all parties. The reason for this difference in the conduct of mankind towards the two professions is that the value and danger of property is better known and more sensibly felt than the value and danger of health and life.

3d. *Fashion* has a powerful influence in determining sick people in the choice of a physician; and as the leaders in it are generally as ignorant as those who follow them of the true characters of physicians, men are preferred who add by their ignorance to the mortality of curable diseases. In Europe the common people follow the example of the privileged orders in their choice of a physician. In this country, wealth gives the tone to medical reputation. It is remarkable that the effects of patronage, whether it be derived from titles or money, are as little influenced by success in the treatment of diseases as they are by talents, for it has frequently been observed that the most fashionable physicians are the least successful in their practice. Nor does a general knowledge of this fact affect the business of such physicians while they retain the favor of the great. This imita-tive disposition in human nature extends to other things as well as to the preser-vation of health. It discovers itself in acts the most opposite to the common feelings and principles of action in man. It leads man, in some instances, to delight in deformity. The humpback of Alexander was aped by all his officers. It does even more. It leads men to covet diseases and pain. Dionis tells us in his surgery, that after he had cut Lewis XIV, for a fistula in ano, he was called upon by a great number of the nobility of France to examine whether they had not the same loathsome disorder, and he adds that they always appeared to be offended when he informed them they were not affected with it.

4th. Many patients die of curable diseases by neglecting to apply in *due time* for medical air. Cancers and consumptions have been called incurable diseases. This is far from being true. If the tumors which precede nearly all cancers were extirpated immediately after they were discovered, and if the premonitory symptoms of consumption were met by proper remedies we should seldom hear of persons dying of either of those diseases. Our newspapers frequently told the public that our late epidemic baffled the skill of our physicians. This assertion was not well founded. Most of our physicians declared that the disease, after the *first* day, was incurable. In this they discovered a just knowledge of it; and in this knowledge skill consists. It should rather have been said that the disease baffled the hopes of patients who supposed their indisposition was occasioned by a trifling cold and neglected to send for a physician at the only time in which it was under the power of medicine. Few cases proved fatal under any mode of practice where physicians were called in the *forming* state of the disease.

5th. The *neglect* in patients to comply with the prescriptions of their physicians has, in many instances, rendered diseases fatal that might have been cured. It is from disobedience to our prescriptions, whether it be founded in ignorance of the danger of the disease under which sick people labor, or upon the calls of business or pleasure predominating over sickness and pain, or upon the unpalatable nature of certain medicines, or upon a dread of the pain of others that we sometimes discover, after the death of our patients, medicines that would probably have saved them upon a mantlepiece or in the drawers of a dressing table. Patients, who recover sometimes humorously insult their physicians by telling them of the improper and even prostituted use to which they have applied their medicines. Sir Richard Nash was once asked by his physician if he had followed his prescription "If I had," said Sir Richard, "I should certainly have broken my neck, for I threw it out of my window." Fear has prevented, in many instances, the successful application of bloodletting in the cure of diseases. False delicacy, by restraining the use of clysters, has sometimes been attended with the same fatal consequences. The former weakness is the more mischievous, from its disguising itself under the apparent dictates of judgment.

6th. The neglect in patients to make use of the remedies of their physicians at the *time* and in the *manner* in which they were prescribed is a frequent cause of death in curable diseases. In acute indispositions, the cure often turns upon a remedy being used, not only on a certain day, but at a certain hour. Purges, vomits, bleeding, blisters, sweats, and laudanum have all their precise days, hours, and perhaps less divisions in time, of being useful; before or after which they are either ineffectual, or do harm. Our late epidemic furnished many proofs of the truth of this remark, more especially in the use of blood-letting. Few persons died of it where the prescription of the lancet was complied with in the early part of the first day of the fever; and few recovered where it was used for the first time on the second or on any other of its subsequent days. Its efficacy was most observable in its paroxysms. In its remissions, bleeding was less proper, and sometimes hurtful. But patients not only injure themselves by neglecting to use remedies at the *time*, but by using them in a *different manner* from that in which they are prescribed. They take more or less of their medicines, or they lose more or less blood than was intended, and often at a time when life and death are perched upon the same beam and when the smallest particle of error gives it a preponderance in favor of the grave. . . .

Thus have I pointed out the principal causes of death in diseases that are not incurable. If the operation of any one of those causes has been attended with fatal consequences, what must be the combined effects of them all?

Here gentlemen let us make a pause. Many useful reflections are suggested by the observations which have been delivered. I shall briefly mention such as are obviously connected with the subject of our lecture.

1. In the first place, let us do homage to the divine goodness. From what has been said, it is evident that our Creator has provided us in the most ample manner with the means of health and life; and if they fail of producing their intended effects it is only because they are rendered ineffectual by the ignorance, folly, and wickedness of man.

2. Let us duly appreciate the difficulties of a physician's studies and labors. He must embrace and control as many objects in contending with a disease, more especially if it be of a dangerous nature, as a general does in arranging his troops and fighting a battle. Death presses upon him from numerous quarters; and nothing but the most accumulated vigor of every sense and faculty, exerted with a vigilance that precludes the abstraction of a single thought or the repose of a moment, can ensure him success in his arduous conflict. It is possible for a patient to reward the mechanical parts of the labor and knowledge of a physician, but no compensation can ever be an equivalent for such paroxysms of solicitude and mental excitement as have been described and which occur at all times, and more especially during the prevalence of great and mortal epidemics.

3. From what has been said we may learn that medicine is a more certain and perfect science than is commonly supposed. To judge of its certainty by the limited nature of its usefulness is to exclude from our calculations all the circumstances which have been mentioned that militate against successful practice. As well might we deny the fertility of a soil because the owner of it neglected the proper seasons and ways of cultivating it, as deny the certainty of medicine because it does not produce salutary effects in spite of the combination of voluntary ignorance, error, and vice against them.

4. In contemplating our present want of success in curing diseases that are not necessarily mortal let us apply ourselves with fresh ardour to remove the obstacles which are opposed to the perfection of our science. It was often and well said by the late Dr. Jebb, "that no good effort was lost." The seeds of improvement and certainty in medicine, which are now sown and seem to perish, shall revive at a future day and appear in a large increase in the health and lives of our fellow creatures. Let this reflection console us under the disappointments we meet with in our attempts to extend the usefulness of our profession. The distance occasioned by time between the different generations of mankind will

soon be destroyed, and we shall find, with inexpressible comfort, in the final settlement of our account of the good and evil we have done in this life that our abortive labors of love to our contemporaries have not been lost in the total amount of human benevolence.

5. I have said that the ignorance, folly, and wickedness of man have hitherto defeated the purposes of the divine benevolence to his creatures. The force of human reason has long been tried without effect as a remedy for folly and vice. The true character of this operation of the mind has been discovered, in an eminent degree, in the absurd principles and criminal pursuits which have lately actuated the greatest part of mankind. To remove the folly and vice which obstruct the progress of medical knowledge and assist in rendering curable diseases mortal, the influence of religion must be added to the operations of reason. I once conversed with an ingenious traveller in this city upon the subject of language. He remarked that it would never be perfect while morals continued in their present imperfect state, for words could never have a just and appropriate meaning until a sacred regard to truth regulated their application to qualities and actions. This connection between morals and philology, thus pointed out, is not more intimate and necessary than the connection of morals and medicine. I admit in this place of no mortality but that which is derived from religion. It is this divine principle alone that can subdue all the folly and wickedness which concur in rendering curable diseases incurable. Physical and moral evil begin together. They have constantly kept pace with each other, and they must decline and cease at the same time. It is the business of reason to remove physical evil; moral evil can only be removed by religion; but to ensure the success of the former it must be combined with the latter, for reason without religion is like the clay-formed image of our first parent, before his Creator infused into him the breath of life. It is true, the dictates of right reason and religion are the same, for they both hold out truth and virtue as our supreme good; but they differ in this particular—reason furnishes the feeble and transitory motives to pursue them, while religion, by its powerful and durable impressions upon the will, disposes us to choose them as the only means of regulating our conduct and ensuring our happiness.

I shall conclude this lecture by remarking that I have many reasons of a personal nature for being thankful to God for my preservation from death during our late mortal epidemic, but none of them operate with more force upon my mind than the privilege I this day enjoy of again meeting my beloved pupils, in order once more to disseminate among them principles in medicine which I believe to be true and which I know to be useful.

JACOB BIGELOW

ON SELF-LIMITED DISEASES

Editor's Note

Jacob Bigelow (1787–1879) after receiving his medical degree in Philadelphia spent his professional career in Boston. Known as one of America's foremost early botanists, Bigelow was Harvard's first professor of materia medica and played an important role in bringing her medical school and the Massachusetts General Hospital to the forefront of medical education.

Henry Nash Smith has described the American love for oratory as one of the most conspicuous features of American culture in the decades before the Civil War.[1] In medicine this judgment is readily borne out if one looks at the tremendous numbers of printed orations, discourses, and dissertations stemming from medical schools and societies throughout the land. Although their prose is usually florid and their sentiment lofty, these speeches provide a useful source of information for the historian. The selection by Bigelow fits the category of orations. Delivered before the august Massachusetts Medical Society in 1835, when its author was forty-eight years old, it soon became a classic, widely referred to. It was Bigelow's central theme, that nature not art should more often be relied upon, and not his words themselves that received the most attention.

Bibliographical Note

George E. Ellis, *Memoir of Jacob Bigelow, M.D., LL.D.*, Cambridge: Wilson, 1880.

The death of medical men is an occurrence which eminently demands our attention, for it speaks to us of our science and of ourselves. It reminds us that we, in turn, are to become victims of the incompetency of our own art. It admonishes us that the sphere of our professional exertions is limited, at last, by

---

Med. Communications Mass. Med. Soc. 5 (1836): 319–58. Reprinted from *Nature in Disease* (Boston: Ticknor & Fields, 1854), pp. 1–58. This is a paper delivered before the Massachusetts Medical Society, May 27, 1835.

[1] *Popular Culture and Industrialism, 1865–1890* (New York: Anchor, 1967), p. 428.

insurmountable barriers. It brings with it the humiliating conclusion that while other sciences have been carried forward within our own time and almost under our own eyes to a degree of unprecedented advancement, medicine, in regard to some of its professed and most important objects, is still an ineffectual speculation. Observations are multiplied, but the observers disappear and leave their task unfinished. We have seen the maturity of age and the ardent purpose of youth called off from the half-cultivated field of their labors, expectations, and promise. It becomes us to look upon this deeply interesting subject with unprejudiced eyes and to endeavor to elicit useful truth from the great lesson that surrounds us.

In comparing the advances which have been made during the present age in different departments of medical science, we are brought to the conclusion that they have not all been cultivated with equally satisfactory success. Some of them have received new and important illustrations from scientific inquiry, but others are still surrounded with their original difficulties. The structure and functions of the human body, the laws which govern the progress of its diseases, and more especially the diagnosis of its morbid conditions are better understood now than they were at the beginning of the present century. But the science of therapeutics, or the branch of knowledge by the application of which physicians are expected to remove diseases, has not, seemingly, attained to a much more elevated standing than it formerly possessed. The records of mortality attest its frequent failures, and the inability to control the event of diseases, which at times is felt by the most gifted and experienced practitioners, give evidence that in many cases disease is more easily understood than cured.

This deficiency of the healing art is not justly attributable to any want of sagacity or diligence on the part of the medical profession. It belongs rather to the inherent difficulties of the case and is, after abating the effect of errors and accidents, to be ascribed to the apparent fact that certain morbid processes in the human body have a definite and necessary career from which they are not to be diverted by any known agents with which it is in our power to oppose them. To these morbid affections, the duration of which, and frequently the event also, are beyond the control of our present remedial means, I have on the present occasion applied the name of *self-limited diseases*, and it will be the object of this discourse to endeavor to show the existence of such a class and to inquire how far certain individual diseases may be considered as belonging to it.

By a self-limited disease, I would be understood to express one which receives limits from its own nature and not from foreign influences; one which, after it has obtained foothold in the system, cannot, in the present state of our knowledge, be eradicated or abridged by art, but to which there is due a certain succession of processes to be completed in a certain time; which time and processes may vary with the constitution and condition of the patient, and may tend to death or to recovery, but are not known to be shortened or greatly changed by medical treatment.

These expressions are not intended to apply to the palliation of diseases, for he who turns a pillow or administers a seasonable draught of water to a patient palliates his sufferings, but they apply to the more important consideration of removing diseases themselves through medical means.

The existence of a class of diseases like those under consideration is, to a certain extent, already admitted, both by the profession and the public, and this admission is evinced by the use of certain familiar terms of expression. Thus, when people speak of a "settled disease," or of the time of "the run of a disease," it implies on their part a recognition of the law that certain diseases regulate their own limits and period of continuance.

It is difficult to select a perfectly satisfactory or convincing example of a self-limited disease from among the graver morbid affections, because in these affections the solicitude of the practitioner usually leads him to the employment of remedies, in consequence of which the effect of remedies is mixed up with the phenomena of disease, so that the mind has difficulty in separating them. We must therefore seek for our most striking or decisive examples among those diseases which are sufficiently mild not to be thought to require ordinarily the use of remedies, and in which the natural history of the disease may be observed divested of foreign influences. Such examples are found in the vaccine disease, the chicken pox, and the salivation produced by mercury. These are strictly self-limited diseases, having their own rise, climax, and decline, and I know of no *medical* practice which is able, were it deemed necessary, to divert them from their appropriate course or hasten their termination.

It may appear to some that the distinction of these diseases from others is the old distinction of acute and chronic. Yet on due inquiry, such an identification is not found to be sustained, for there are some acute diseases which, we have reason to believe, are shortened by the employment of remedies; while, on the other hand, certain chronic cases of disease are known to get well spontaneously after years of continuance.

If the inquiry be made, why one disease has necessary limits while another is without them? the reply is not uniform nor always easy to be made. Sometimes the law of the disease may be traced to the nature of the exciting cause. Thus the morbid poison of measles, or of small pox, when received into the body, produces a self-limited disease; but the morbid poisons of psora and syphilis may give rise to others which are not limited, except by medical treatment. Sometimes, also, the cause being the same the result will depend on the part, organ, or texture which is affected. Thus if we divide with a cutting instrument the cellular or muscular substance, we produce a self-limited disease which, although it cannot by any art be healed within a certain number of days or weeks, yet in the end gets well spontaneously, by one process, if the lips are in contact, and by another and slower process, if they are separated.* But if, on the other hand, we

_____

*In one case, the disease is a solution of continuity; in the other, a solution of continuity and contact.

divide a considerable artery, we have then an unlimited disease, and the hemor-rhage or the aneurysm which follows does not get well, except through the interposition of art.

The class of diseases under consideration comprehends morbid affections differing greatly from each other in the time, place, and nature of their spon-taneous developments, so that they may admit of at least three general sub-divisions. These may be called, 1st. The *simple*: in which the disease observes a continuous time and mostly a definite seat; 2d. The *paroxysmal*: in which the disease, having apparently disappeared, returns at its own periods; and 3d. The *metastatic*: in which the disease undergoes metastasis or spontaneous change of place. In the present state of our knowledge, we have no difficulty in finding examples of each of these subdivisions. There are also other examples in which the disease, although capable of being in part influenced by medical treatment, still retains a portion of its original intractability and has strong relations to the class in question.

As a mode of directing our inquiries toward these diseases, we may suspect those complaints to be self-limited in which it is observed that the unwary and the sceptical, who neglect to resort to remedies, recover their health without them. We may also suspect diseases to be of this character when we find op-posite modes of treatment recommended and their success vouched for by prac-titioners of authority and veracity. We may moreover attach the same suspicion to cases in which the supposed cure takes place under chance applications or inconsiderable remedies; as in the empirical modes of practice, on the one hand, and the minute doses of the homeopathic method on the other. Lastly, we may apprehend that cases are fatally self-limited* when enlightened physicians die themselves of the diseases which they had labored to illustrate—as in the case of Corvisart, Laennec, Armstrong, and others.

In proceeding to enumerate more precisely some of the diseases which appear to me to be self-limited in their character, I approach the subject with diffi-dence. I am aware that the works of medical writers, and especially of medical compilers, teem with remedies and modes of treatment for all diseases; and that in the morbid affections of which we speak, remedies are often urged with zeal and confidence, even though sometimes of an opposite character. Moreover, in many places, at the present day, a charm is popularly attached to what is called an active, bold, or heroic practice; and a corresponding reproach awaits the opposite course, which is cautious, palliative, and expectant. In regard to the diseases which have been called self-limited, I would not be understood to deny that remedies capable of removing them may exist; I would only assert, that they have not yet been proved to exist.

Under the simple self-limited diseases, we may class *whooping cough*. This disease has its regular increase, height, and decline, occupying ordinarily from

---

*In the following article on the Treatment of Disease, it has been found convenient to divide diseases into the curable, the self-limited, and the incurable. In a general sense, however, the last term falls within the second.

one to six months, but in some mild cases only two or three weeks. During this period, medical treatment is for the most part of no avail. Narcotic appliances may diminish the paroxysm, but without abridging the disease. After whooping cough has reached its climax, change of air sometimes appears to hasten convalescence. Also, if inflammatory or other morbid affections supervene upon the pure disease they may become subjects for medical treatment. With these exceptions, whooping cough appears to be a self-limited disease.

Most of the class of diseases usually denominated eruptive fevers are self-limited. *Measles*, for example, is never known to be cut short by art or abridged of its natural career; neither can this career be extended or the disease kept in the system beyond its natural duration by the power of medicine. *Scarlet fever*, a disease of which we have had much and fatal experience during the last three years, is eminently of the same character. The reasons which induce me thus to regard it are the following. The writings of medical observers agree in assigning to it a common or average period of duration, and this is confirmed by the observations of practitioners at the present day. From this average duration and character there are great natural deviations, the disease being sometimes so slight as to attract the notice of none but medical eyes, and sometimes so malignant that treatment is admitted to be hopeless. The modes of treatment which have had most testimony in their favor are various and opposite. By Dr. Fothergill, stimulants were relied on; by Dr. Currie, cold water; by Dr. Southwood Smith, and others, blood-letting. But it is not satisfactorily shown that either of these modes of practice has been particularly successful, for where the writers have furnished us anything like definite or numerical results, it does not appear that the mortality was less in their hands than it is among those who pursue a more expectant practice. The post mortuary appearances, which in many diseases furnish useful lessons for practice, are in scarlet fever extremely various and uncertain, and sometimes no morbid changes, sufficient to account for death can be discovered in any of the vital organs or great cavities.

Small Pox is another example of the class of affections under consideration, its approach and disappearance being irrespective of medical practice. It may, at first view, appear, that inoculation has placed artificial limits on this disease. But it must be recollected, that inoculated small pox is itself only a milder variety of the same disease, having its own customary limits of extent and duration, which are fixed, quite as much as those of the distinct and confluent forms of the natural disease. . . .

But that the usefulness of our profession may extend, our knowledge must go on to increase, and the foundation of all knowledge is truth. For truth then we must earnestly seek, even when its developments do not flatter our professional pride nor attest the infallibility of our art. To discover truth in science is often extremely difficult; in no science is it more difficult than in medicine. Independently of the common defects of medical evidence, our self-interest, our self-esteem, and sometimes even our feelings of humanity may be arrayed against

the truth. It is difficult to view the operations of nature divested of the inter-
ferences of art, so much do our habits and partialities incline us to neglect the
former and to exaggerate the importance of the latter. The mass of medical
testimony is always on the side of art. Medical books are prompt to point out
the cure of diseases. Medical journals are filled with the crude productions of
aspirants to the cure of diseases. Medical schools find it incumbent on them to
teach the cure of diseases. The young student goes forth into the world believing
that if he does not cure diseases it is his own fault. Yet, when a score or two of
years have passed over his head, he will come at length to the conviction that
some diseases are controlled by nature alone. He will often pause at the end of a
long and anxious attendance and ask himself how far the result of the case is
different from what it would have been under less officious treatment than that
which he has pursued; how many in the accumulated array of remedies which
have supplanted each other in the patient's chamber have actually been instrumental in doing him any good. He will also ask himself whether in the course of
his life he has not had occasion to change his opinion, perhaps more than once,
in regard to the management of the disease in question, and whether he does
not, even now, feel the want of additional light.

Medicine has been rightly called a conjectural art, because in many of its
deductions, and especially in those which relate to the cure of diseases, positive
evidence is denied to us. We are seldom justified in concluding that our remedies
have promoted the cure of a disease, until we know that cases exactly similar in
time, place, and circumstances have failed to do equally well under the omission
of those remedies; and such cases, moreover, must exist in sufficient numbers to
justify the admission of a general law on their basis. Nothing can be more
illogical than to draw our general conclusions, as we are sometimes too apt to
do, from the results of insulated and remarkable cases, for such cases may be
found in support of any extravagance in medicine, and if there is any point in
which the vulgar differ from the judicious part of the profession it is in drawing
premature and sweeping conclusions from scanty premises of this kind. Moreover, it is in many cases not less illogical to attribute the removal of diseases, or
even of their troublesome symptoms, to the means which have been most recently employed. It is a common error to infer that things which are consecutive
in the order of time have necessarily the relation to cause and effect. It often
happens that the last remedy used bears off the credit of having removed an
obstruction or cured a disease, whereas in fact the result may have been owing to
the first remedy employed, and to the joint effect of all the remedies, or to the
act of nature, uninfluenced by any of the remedies. We see this remarkably
exemplified in recoveries from amenorrhea and from various irregularities of the
alimentary canal.

An inherent difficulty, which every medical man finds to stand in the way of
an unbiased and satisfactory judgment, is the heavy responsibility which rests
upon the issue of his cases. When a friend or valuable patient is committed to

our charge, we cannot stand by as curious spectators to study the natural history of his disease. We feel that we are called on to attempt his rescue by vigorous means, so that at least the fault of omission shall not lie upon our charge. We proceed to put in practice those measures which on the whole have appeared to us to do most good, and if these fail us, we resort to other measures which we have read of or heard of. And at the end of our attendance we may be left in uncertainty, whether the duration of sickness has been shortened or lengthened by our practice, and whether the patient is really indebted to us for good or evil. In the study of experimental philosophy, we rarely admit a conclusion to be true until its opposite has been proved to be untrue. But in medicine we are often obliged to be content to accept as evidence the results of cases which have been finished under treatment, because we have not the opportunity to know how far these results would have been different, had the cases been left to themselves. And it too frequently happens that medical books do not relieve our difficulties on this score, for a great deal of our practical literature consists in reports of interesting, extraordinary, and successful results, published by men who have a doctrine to establish or a reputation to build. "Few authors," says Andral, "have published all the cases they have observed, and the greater part have only taken the trouble to present to us those facts which favor their own views."* A prevailing error among writers on therapeutics, proceeds from their professional or personal reluctance to admit that the healing art, as practiced by them, is not, or may not be, all sufficient in all cases; so that on this subject they suffer themselves, as well as their readers, to be deceived. Hence we have no disease, however intractable or fatal, for which the press has not poured forth its asserted remedies. Even of late, we have seen unfailing cures of cholera successively announced in almost every city in which that pestilence unchecked has completed its work of devastation!

It is only when, in connection with these flattering exhibitions, we have a full and faithful report of the failures of medical practice in similar and in common cases, setting forth not only the truth but the whole truth, that we have a basis sufficiently broad to erect a superstructure in therapeutics on which dependence may be placed. Such, it must give the friends of science gratification to observe, is a part of the rigid method which characterizes the best examples of the modern French school; and such, it is not difficult to foresee, must ultimately be the only species of evidence on this subject to which the medical profession will pay deference.

It appears to me to be one of the most important desiderata in practical medicine to ascertain in regard to each doubtful disease, how far its cases are really self-limited and how far they are controllable by any treatment. This question can be satisfactorily settled only by instituting, in a large number of

---

*Bien peu d'auteurs ont publié tous les cas qu'ils ont observès, et la plupart ne se sont empressés de nous transmettre que les faits que caressaient leurs idées.—*Clinique* III. 618.

cases which are well identified and nearly similar, a fair experimental comparison of the different active and expectant modes of practice, with their varieties in regard to time, order, and degree. This experiment is vast, considering the number of combinations which it must involve, and even much more extensive than a corresponding series of pathological observations; yet every honest and intelligent observer may contribute to it his mite. Opportunities for such observations, and especially for monographs of diseases, are found in the practice of most physicians, yet hospitals and other public charities afford the most appropriate field for instituting them upon a large scale. The aggregate of results, successful and unsuccessful, circumstantially and impartially reported by competent observers, will give us a near approximation to truth in regard to the diseases of the time and place in which the experiments are instituted. The *numerical* method employed by Louis in his extensive pathological researches, and now adopted by his most distinguished contemporaries in France, affords the means of as near an approach to certainty on this head as the subject itself admits. And I may add that no previous medical inquirer has apparently submitted to the profession any species of evidence so broad in its foundations, and so convincing in its results, as that which characterizes the great works of this author on Phthisis and Typhoid fever.

In regard to acknowledged self-limited diseases, the question will naturally arise, whether the practitioner is called on to do nothing for the benefit of his patient; whether he shall fold his hands and look passively on the progress of a disease which he cannot interrupt. To this I would answer—by no means. The opportunities of doing good may be as great in these diseases as in any others; for in treating every disease there is a right method and a wrong. In the first place, we may save the patient from much harm, not only by forbearing ourselves to afflict him with unnecessary practice but also by preventing the ill-judged activity of others. For the same reason that we would not suffer him to be shaken in his bed when rest was considered necessary to him, we should not allow him to be tormented with useless and annoying applications in a disease of settled destiny. It should be remembered that all cases are susceptible of errors of commission, as well as of omission, and that by an excessive application of the means of art, we may frustrate the intentions of nature, when they are salutary, or embitter the approach of death when it is inevitable. What practitioner, I would ask, ever rendered a greater service to mankind, than Ambrose Paré, and his subsequent coadjutors, who introduced into modern surgery the art of healing by the first intention? These men with vast difficulty succeeded in convincing the profession that instead of the old method of treating incised wounds by keeping them open with forcible and painful applications, it was better simply to place the parts securely in their natural situation and then to let them alone. In the second place, we may do much good by a palliative and preventive course, by alleviating pain, procuring sleep, guarding the diet, regulating the alimentary canal—in fine, by obviating such sufferings as admit of mitigation and preventing or removing the causes of others which are incidental, but not necessary, to the state of disease. In doing this, we must distinguish between the disease itself and the accidents of the disease, for the latter often admit of relief, when the former do not. We should also inquire whether the original cause of the disease, or any accessory cause, is still operating and, if so, whether it can in any measure be prevented or removed; as, for example, when it exists in the habits of life of the patient, in the local atmosphere, or in the presence of any other deleterious agent. Lastly, by a just prognosis, founded on a correct view of the case, we may sustain the patient and his friends during the inevitable course of the disease and may save them from the pangs of disappointed hope on the one side or of unnecessary despondency on the other.

It will be seen that in the foregoing remarks a low estimate has been placed on the resources of art, when compared with those of nature. But I may be excused for doing this in the presence of an audience of educated men and the members of a society whose motto is *Naturá duce*. The longer and the more philosophically we contemplate this subject, the more obvious it will appear that the physician is but the minister and servant of nature; that in cases like those which have been engaging our consideration, we can do little more than follow in the train of disease and endeavor to aid nature in her salutary intentions, or to remove obstacles out of her path. How little, indeed, could we accomplish without her aid!—It has been wisely observed by Sir Gilbert Blane, that "the benefit derivable to mankind at large, from artificial remedies, is so limited, that if a spontaneous principle of restoration had not existed, the human species would long ago have been extinct."*

The importance and usefulness of the medical profession, instead of being diminished will always be elevated exactly in proportion as it understands itself, weighs justly its own powers, and professes simply what it can accomplish. It is no derogation from the importance of our art that we cannot always control the events of life and death, or even of health and sickness. The incompetency which we feel in this respect is shared by almost every man upon whom the great responsibilities of society are devolved. The statesman cannot control the destinies of nations, nor the military commander the event of battles. The most eloquent pleader may fail to convince the judgment of his hearers, and the most skilful pilot may not be able to weather the storm. Yet it is not the less necessary that responsible men should study deeply and understandingly the science of their respective vocations. It is not the less important, for the sake of those whose safety is, and always will be, committed to their charge, that they should look with unbiased judgment upon the necessary results of inevitable causes. And while an earnest and inquiring solicitude should always be kept alive in regard to the improvement of professional knowledge, it should never be forgotten that knowledge has for its only just and lasting foundation a rigid, impartial, and inflexible requisition of the truth.

Medical Logic, p. 49.

NATHANIEL CHAPMAN

REMARKS ON THE CHRONIC FLUXES OF THE BOWELS

Editor's Note

Nathaniel Chapman, 1780–1853, was a Philadelphia physician of wide influence and repute. He founded and edited the *Philadelphia Journal of the Medical and Physical Sciences* in 1820. Its name was changed to the *American Journal of the Medical Sciences* in 1827 by its new editor, Isaac Hays. In 1816 Chapman was elected to fill the prestigious Chair of the Theory and Practice of Medicine at the University of Pennsylvania, thereby following in the footsteps of Benjamin Rush. In 1847 Chapman was elected as first president of the American Medical Association.[1]

The paper by Chapman, somewhat difficult to read through, illustrates, nevertheless, a number of important points. It is one of the few examples in this book of a purely medical paper. Chapman describes the symptoms, causes, geographical distribution, prognosis, pathological findings, and treatment of the nonspecific but very common disorder of chronic diarrhea. The reader can readily see how a leading practitioner of the early nineteenth century approached his work. Chapman's language seems almost foreign to us. The present-day physician who has difficulty with such terms as gleety, lientery, pediluvium, and cubeb, will appreciate how his patients feel when he speaks in medical language to them.[2]

Not a little diversified are the symptoms of this pathological condition, though in nearly all instances the bowels are very irritable and consequently excited by the slightest causes. The stools may be small and of mucus, sometimes tinged with blood or containing fragments of lymph, or are glairy or

Am. J. Med. Sci. 19 (1836): 86–98.

[1] There have been numerous articles about Chapman and his various activities. A recent biography tells the whole story: Irwin Richman, *The Brightest Ornament, A Biography of Nathaniel Chapman, M.D.* (Bellefonte, Pa.: Pennsylvania Heritage, 1967).

[2] Gleet referred to gonorrhea, but as used here meant a chronic discharge from a mucous membrane. Lientery meant diarrhea, or frequent liquid fecal discharges. A pediluvium was a foot bath. And cubeb referred to a drug derived from the dried berries of *Piper cubeba*, used as an anti-inflammatory agent. Drugs and medical terms can be easily looked up in a nineteenth-century medical dictionary, such as the one compiled by Robley Dunglison. For more detailed information about drugs, their origin, history, and use, see any of the books on materia medica. A very useful one is Alfred Stillé's *Therapeutics and Materia Medica*, 2 vols. (Philadelphia: Blanchard & Lea, 1864).

gleety—or exceedingly copious and of a light clay color—or dark and granulated like coffee grounds, or resembling greasy water, and of a cadaverous odour—or are seemingly of putrid chyme, or pulpy, mixed with ingesta, very frothy, and of divers hues, though usually of an ashy or slaty aspect, and are attended by more or less tormina and tenesmus or straining, or come away at once in a gush, or by a sudden ejection or squirting without any uneasiness.

The mode of evacuation depends much on the character of the stools—slow and difficult when they are small and tenacious, and the reverse if large and watery. Little appetite exists, or it is very capricious, and the food taken is seldom thoroughly digested. The tongue is heavily furred in the center and at the root, with florid tip and edges, or red and raw throughout, as if scalded—or with scattered superficial ulcers on it, and the inside of the cheeks and lips, or down into the fauces—or it is pallid, attenuated, and flaccid. The skin is dry, furrowed, and of a dingy white or sallow or leaden hue—the eyes sunken, with a shrivelled and meagre expression of countenance. Tenderness of the abdomen is felt on pressure, though not uniformly, and it is tumid or the contrary, lank, relaxed, or even collapsed. Borborigmus is very troublesome. The pulse is often contracted, hard, and accelerated, with an irregular febrile movement, especially in the evening—but it may be natural, or very diminutive and feeble, with low temperature of the surface, or while the extremities are cold, the belly is preternaturally hot. Emaciation advances rapidly, with corresponding debility, till finally the individual sinks from absolute exhaustion, death being preceded by edema of the lower limbs, apthae of the throat and mouth, redness and ulceration around or within the verge of the anus, and the Facies Hippocratica strongly marked. The duration of an attack is very various, from a few weeks to months or years, subject, when long continued, to alternate remissions and exacerbations.

Chronic fluxes may be an original affection or the consequence of an acute attack protracted by neglect or ill-management—and when of the former or primary nature, are assignable to many of the causes of the latter operating less actively.

They are undoubtedly induced by malaria, whether the vitiation of the atmosphere be owing to the effluvia of vegetable or animal decomposition, or other offensive impregnations—scarcely less so by the excesses or variations of temperature, particularly moist, austere weather, and by the occupany of cellars and other damp confined places.

As much, perhaps, may be ascribed to the direct irritation of the *primae viae* from aliments or drinks, such as tainted or tough indigestible meats, sour or mouldy bread, or crude or decayed vegetables or fruits, the intemperate use of ardent liquors or bad water, putrid or charged with adventitious matters.

They result, too, from the long persistence in purging with drastic articles, as is practiced by some for the removal of diseases, and above all dropsy, of which I have seen repeated instances, and by whatever indeed is calculated thus to worry the bowels into a state of exasperation, or to destroy their tone, or otherwise throw them into derangement. It is in this way, I have little doubt, that the horrible abuse of mercury throughout a considerable extent of our country concurs in the production of similar mischief. Nothing is more irritating to the alimentary tube, the liver, and to the whole of the abdominal viscera, than this very article, unless cautiously regulated—and when we advert to the indiscriminate and exorbitant employment of it by confessedly too many of the practitioners in the region to which I have alluded, the conjecture advanced seems scarcely to require any confirmation.

Nor must the exanthemata be omitted in the enumeration of causes. These have their origin in the mucous membrane of the alimentary canal—and the translation to the skin not perfectly taking place leaves behind an irritation productive of this effect, as is strikingly exemplified in scarlatina, measles, etc. Chronic eruptions of different kinds receding from the cutaneous surface occasionally operate also in the same mode, two instances of which I have seen.

Certain sections of our country are singularly liable to the disease, and it prevails to a great extent especially at or near Richmond and New Orleans. Cases of it I have annually from each of these cities and am assured that it is one of the most terrible of their maladies: no age, sex, or condition of life is entirely exempt from it, though it rarely occurs before puberty. What occasions it is not ascertained: nothing peculiar about Richmond exists to which its production can be referred, but at New Orleans the popular notion connects it with the use of the turbid waters of the Mississippi. Never having seen a case in the early stage, I am not able to describe it from any knowledge of my own, but I learn that it usually commences with the symptoms of dyspepsia. As it has come before me, the disease was far advanced and only distinguishable from more common diarrhea by less emaciation, the flesh and integuments being rather flaccid than wasted, and by a peculiar sallowness of skin, more of the light lemon than the orange hue, and by the number and copiousness of the discharges, which invariably resemble pale clay or Fuller's earth dissolved in a quantity of water.*

Chronic fluxes are moreover of a secondary nature, from the extension of irritation to the bowels of other diseased organs, as the stomach, liver, spleen, pancreas, kidneys, uterus, the lungs—and I have seen it occasioned by hemorrhoidal tumors or ulcerations at the termination of the rectum.

No perplexity can prevail in the recognition of diarrhea. It were highly important, however, in a therapeutic and practical view, could we discriminate the several states of the bowels on which the discharge depends—but I am apprehensive we cannot do this with any uniformity or precision. Neither the symptoms

---

*Diarrhea of a somewhat different kind appears to be hardly less frequent among our Eastern population, especially that of Boston, the source of which is as little intelligible. But the individuals whom I have attended with it, in their passage through this city to the South, all concurred in stating that the attacks were ushered in as dyspepsia, followed after a long interval by the bowel affection, then cough and other pectoral symptoms, marasmus, hectic fever, etc.

nor the appearance of the stools may be relied on under all circumstances. Generally, however, inflammation is denoted by pain in the abdomen, hot skin, corded, frequent pulse, and by slimy, membraniform or bloody dejections. But on the contrary, how often is there pain without phlogosis, and ulcerations and other lesions are to be met with where no expression had been given by this or any more distinctive sign of their existence?

Genuine mucous or serous discharges, though ordinarily indicative of simple irritation or phlogosis, are occasionally found in every variety of case—and even the most copious effusions of blood, the common product of phlogosis, may be owing to merely a turgescence or perhaps relaxation of vessels.

Gleety stools usually denote a subdued state of previous inflammation—though not always, they sometimes proceed from an ulcerative condition. Chymous dejections are more uniformly significant of an imperfection in the digestive powers of the colon or, in other words, the process of fecation.

Evacuations thin, greasy, and of a cadaverous odor, mixed with sanious, purulent, or fibrinous matter are to be deemed, in my opinion, the least unerring criterion of organic mischief. But this test is also fallible, having seen extensive lesions of the same kind with stools of the earth-like solution I have just mentioned.

In a disease so various in its character, and occasioned by such diversity of causes or conditions, the grounds of prognostication must necessarily be vague and uncertain. Not much more can be determined, than that in proportion to the duration and severity of the attack, the degree of constitutional disturbance, emaciation, and debility is the prospect of a cure or otherwise. What is to be deduced from the aspect of the stools I have previously stated. Cases with mucous or gleety discharges are usually the most curable, and those earthy or watery, and of cadaverous smell, the least so.

From autopsic inspections, evidence is afforded of inflammation in its several gradations, in the mucous coat especially, confined to a part or embracing a considerable extent, and sometimes every variety of organic injury, from the simplest to an entire change of structure, the most common of which, however, is ulceration. This consists of a single ulcer, or a few only, though often innumerable. Cases have repeatedly been examined by me where it was as impossible to count them as the stars in the firmament. Large portions of the bowels are, indeed, sometimes found cellulated like a honey-comb. The ulcers are of various sizes, from that of the head of a pin to an inch or more, and have a close similitude to the venereal chancre. Connected with these, or independent of them, mere vegetation or fungous excrescences are occasionally to be met with. I once opened a subject who died of the disease, where a fungoid growth in the colon was discovered nine inches in length, two in breadth, and half an inch in thickness. But in other instances, the mucous surface seems to be scalded, as it were, here and there a vesicle or superficial sore, or more decidedly apthous, in the whole, analogous to the state of the tongue, mouth, and fauces, which I have noticed. . . .

To determine, however, the exact pathology of the case we have seen is very difficult, and so long as it remains in such obscurity the practice must be some-what tentative and empirical. Nevertheless, in the want of more perfect informa-tion we may be guided, in part, by the character of the stools and, still more, by the general state of the system.

The pulse being tense or corded, with pain and tenderness of the abdomen, aggravated by pressure, florid tongue, and not extreme weakness, we can scarcely err by a resort to venesection, the propriety of which, indeed, is attested by ample experience. To Sydenham, in his account of the diarrhea of measles, we are indebted for this great practical improvement, which is not the least of his valuable contributions. Claimed recently as a discovery, it may have been overlooked or disregarded by others, though not by the practitioners of this city. From the time of my connection with the profession, such, at least, has been the plan of treatment of every description of inflammatory bowel affection, chronic or acute. Nor will a single bleeding, however copious it may be, always or even generally suffice. Chronic inflammations, though not so immediately dangerous, has a much stronger hold of a part than recent, and accordingly proves more difficult to dislodge or subdue. Not discouraged, then, if no very striking advan-tage accrues from the first bleeding, in such cases, let it be repeated every two or three days, while the pulse and strength warrant the continuance, and we cannot fail ultimately to be well satisfied with the consequences. Certainly, in some instances, I have bled from ten to fifteen times, taking away four, six, or eight ounces of blood each operation and found it essential to the cure. Topical bleeding is a very important auxiliary to venesection, sometimes superseding altogether the necessity of it where the means of accomplishment, which is seldom the case in country practice, can be conveniently obtained.

The inflammatory state having been overcome, gentle emetics of ipecacuanha, exhibited occasionally, may be useful. They are not prescribed here as evacuants, though not always without advantage in this respect, as to renovate by insti-tuting a series of new actions the condition of the whole alimentary canal. Nor in their immediate operation, by arresting the peristaltic motion, are they with-out good effect, and perhaps not less so by inducing a determination to the dermoid surface. In the management of this disease it is of the last importance to restore to the skin its healthy functions, for till this is accomplished no decided and permanent impression will be made. Great benefit accrues from the frequent use of the warm bath with this view. To command, however, its full effect, where the skin is dry and the capillary circulation torpid, some stimulating article should be added to the water, as salt, and, on the patient entering his bed, he is to be rubbed with a flesh-brush till a universal glow is diffused over his body. The bath being not readily commanded, a stimulating pediluvium or fric-tion with fine warm salt may be employed as a succedaneum—and further to promote the effect, a small dose of Dover's powder will prove serviceable. During the day, a pill may be given every two or three hours, composed of a small portion of torrefied rhubarb, ipecacuanha, and opium. The ipecacuanha, on every account, is singularly valuable in this disease, though there are some who prefer the antimonials, and especially the cerated glass of antimony, with opium—a preference, I suspect, without any just foundation.

These medicines having been tried unavailingly, we may next resort to alum, which is much prescribed in the form of whey. My mode of directing it, however, is in the dose of two, three, or four grains to a quarter of a grain of opium, several times in the twenty-four hours. In some instances, a small portion of ipecacuanha may be added, and especially if the skin continues dry and the bowels harassed by griping or other uneasiness. By Mosely, a combination of alum and white vitriol, called by him the vitriolic solution, has been greatly extolled in chronic dysentery and diarrhea. Of this, I cannot say a great deal from my own experience, having been discouraged from any extensive use of it by its very disagreeable taste and nauseating effects. Entitled to greater regard, is a union of alum and the sulphate of iron in equal portions, say a grain or two of each, occasionally repeated, with or without opium, as the indication may be.

The acetate of lead, with opium and ipecacuanha, has strong claims to attention, and the camphorated mixture, with nitrous acid and laudanum, is of late strongly commended, though, I think, undeservedly.* In some instances, particularly where the liver is concerned, the nitro-muriatic acid internally or as a pediluvium or by frictions has certainly proved of service. It ought, however, to be cautiously used and its effects carefully watched. Even when endermically applied I have known it, in several instances, to bring on the most distressing dysenteric affections.

Contrary to common opinion, by which they are forbidden, I have seen the vegetable acids eminently beneficial. Diluted vinegar I allude to especially, though lemon juice sometimes also answers.

Much the most, on the whole, however, may be expected from the use of mercury. This is an indispensable remedy when the case is associated with hepatic derangement, and even if such do not exist it proves serviceable. Calomel or the blue pill is given in minute doses with opium, and sometimes ipecaeuanha and prepared chalk, to attain the alterative and not the salivant effect.

By the unanimous voice of practitioners, blisters are declared to be of the greatest utility at this conjuncture, which are applied to the abdomen or the extremities and may be alternately put on the ankles and wrists. The principle on which they act, in the latter instance, is that of revulsion.

Chronic fluxes, with such discharges as to constitute merely a gleet of the bowels, are most successfully managed by the balsamic and terebinthinate preparations. The copaivae I have often used advantageously; also the spirit of turpentine, and sometimes, even more so, common rosin, in the dose of four or five

---

*This is called Hope's mixture, from the author of it, and is prepared as follows,—the dose of which is a tablespoonful, several times a day: R. Mist. camph. ℥viij., acid. nitrous. ℨj., tinct. T. heb. gtt. xl.

grains several times a day. Cubebs, repeated in the same dose and manner, I have known to be serviceable. . . .

We come now to the consideration of regimen, on the due regulation of which everything depends.

As to diet, it is usual to select those articles supposed from their astringency to bind the bowels, which I think is a mistaken notion derived from the false doctrine that the discharge constitutes the disease—the great purpose in the cure is to restrain it. The indication, on the contrary, is to soothe irritation by the blandest nutriment, thus making it harmonize with the other parts of the treatment. It is customary, as having this property and by which they are so well adapted, to commence with the mucilaginous or farrinacious matters—that of gum arabic, the slippery elm or the benne, and tapioca, sago, sallop, arrow root, rice, flour, etc. Gruel and thin broths, though usually proscribed, from an apprehension of their running through the bowels, I have found, on the same principle of allaying irritation, very appropriate. We direct them in cholera morbus, and why not in the present case? Milk, on some occasions where the stomach is not sour, answers very well—and perhaps no article more uniformly agrees with the patient than buttermilk.*

Digestible solids, as mutton, or fowl, or game, or oysters, raw or slightly roasted, may subsequently, on the abatement of irritation, be allowed—and I have seen benefit from an occasional indulgence in a small portion of ham or salt fish under similar circumstances.

Crackers or stale leaven bread are only proper. Fruit I have sometimes known to be appropriate, particularly peaches. The dew or blackberry has a large share of popular confidence in this respect, to which it is not more entitled than strawberries. These, and I may add oranges, habitually and almost exclusively used, have cured the disease. Mentioning on a former occasion some cases to this purport as regards the latter, the physician-general of the British forces in Canada, who happened to be present, informed me that his wife, having suffered from diarrhea for a long period, during which she had visited Europe and received there the best medical advice without avail, was finally cured by living entirely on oranges, to which she was prompted by an irresistible instinctive desire. Yet generally fruits disagree, or prove as injurious as the common vegetables. The best drink at first is rice or barley-water, or some·similar article, and brandy and water or port wine in the advanced atonic stages. Neither much food nor drink should be permitted at a time, it being very apt at once to run though the bowels, nor the latter be very cold for the same reason.

Many of the cases of diarrhea, and especially of long standing, may be considered as materially dependent on dyspepsia, and hence all the dietetic rules in

---

*Milk may be given alone or thickened with some of the farinaceous matters mentioned above, the best of which is wheat flour, thus prepared:—Enclose in several folds of linen half a pound or more of it, drawn tight into a ball, and then boil it for several hours in a pot of water. On cooling it becomes hard and must be grated into a powder.

relation to that affection are to be observed, together with a recurrence to the ordinary remedies for its removal.

No one questions the necessity of preserving an equable temperature on the surface in the intestinal affections, and among the best means of securing it is a flannel roller, while at the same time by its compression, further and more decided efforts are attained. Equally important is it carefully to protect the feet—these, when cold, hardly ever failing to revive or exasperate the affection.

Exercise has been greatly insisted on as a curative measure: but whether it operates for good or evil will depend on its being properly timed. During the continuance of any activity of phlogosis it must be avoided—absolute rest, even in the recumbent posture, having the most beneficial influence under such circumstances. It is indeed, in many instances, the *sine qua non*, or without which everything else will prove nugatory—while, in an opposite or atonic condition, taken in any mode it is eminently serviceable, though more so on horseback, and particularly if it be extended to a long journey. More than one of our watering places, the White Sulphur and Warm Springs of Virginia especially, are deemed very efficacious and hence may be worthy of trial.

Even, however, if all these expedients fail, we are not to abandon the patient. As a last resort a sea voyage to some temperate climate should be recommended. This is a very important measure and will sometimes succeed when all others have proved unavailing.

It is matter of great moment to remove these fluxes. Exhausting as they may be in their immediate effects, they are connected with pathological conditions which become aggravated by delay, leading too often to the saddest catastrophe. Looking at some of the results only, "the bowels," says a late writer rather quaintly, "being unfaithful to the stomach, and, instead of playing fair, let go their hold of the *pabulum vitae* before the lacteals have properly performed the process which that grand organ has prepared for them, nutrition must be deficient, and the consequences of inanition ultimately take place. Nor," continues he, "does the mischief stop here." Locke tells us that people with relaxed bowels have seldom strong thoughts or strong bodies. To a certain extent this may be true, and it is one of the numerous instances illustrative of the ultimate dependence of our moral on our physical condition.

ELISHA BARTLETT

AN INQUIRY INTO THE DEGREE OF CERTAINTY IN MEDICINE; AND INTO THE NATURE AND EXTENT OF ITS POWER OVER DISEASE

Editor's Note

Elisha Bartlett (1804–55) practiced and taught medicine in several states from Kentucky to New England. In 1844 he published his *Essay on the Philosophy of Medical Science*, reflecting the Parisian influence. His reputation, like that of many historical figures before and since, has had its ups and downs at the hands of historians. According to his contemporaries, and many who followed, Bartlett's chief claim to fame rests on his magnificent book, *The History, Diagnosis, and Treatment of Fevers in the United States* (Philadelphia: Lea and Blanchard, 1842), that went through four popular editions.[1]

The "elegant and classical" essay of Pierre Jean George Cabanis, on which Bartlett's *Inquiry* is patterned, was published as *Du Degré de Certitude de la Médecine*, in 1797, with a new edition in 1803. R. LaRoche translated it into English as *An Essay on the Certainty of Medicine* (Philadelphia: Desilver, 1823). By presenting to students and practitioners of medicine a philosophical analysis of its methods, Cabanis believed he would perform a service for all mankind. Himself a physician, Cabanis (1757–1808), was one of the best known members of the group of philosophers known as the *idéologues*. These men sought to bring about a medical revolution at the time of the great political and social upheaval we know as the French Revolution. Based on sensualist doctrines of Condillac and others, this new approach to medicine was to be founded on close observation of patients, both during life and at autopsy.

Cabanis began his essay on certainty by stating the objections against certainty in medicine alleged by cavillers against it. The mysteries of life, of disease, and the action of drugs were held by some to be beyond our grasp, hence uncertainty prevailed. This opinion, Cabanis argued, was contrary to the facts and was a product of bad reasoning, as was, unfortunately, much of the thinking applied to medicine.

As one example, he cited: "A cure follows the application of a remedy; the remedy therefore has produced the cure; *post hoc, ergo propter hoc.* This is,

---

Philadelphia: Lea and Blanchard, 1848.

[1] Lester King has recently characterized him as a shortsighted, arrogant, and "empirical" writer. "Medical philosophy, 1836–1844," in *Medicine, Science, and Culture, Historical Essays in Honor of Owsei Temkin*, Lloyd G. Stevenson and Robert P. Multhauf, eds. (Baltimore: The Johns Hopkins Press, 1968), pp. 143–59. To an earlier generation, such as William Osler's, Bartlett was a very appealing figure. See Osler's "Elisha Bartlett, A Rhode Island Philosopher," in *An Alabama Student and other Biographical Essays* (New York: Oxford University Press, 1908), pp. 108–58. See also Erwin H. Ackerknecht's important appraisal of Bartlett in "Elisha Bartlett and the philosophy of the Paris clinical school," *Bull. Hist. Med.* 24 (1950): 43–60.

undoubtedly, a specimen of very bad reasoning, yet by this fallacious rule have all the articles of the materia medica been arranged, and the mode of administering them reduced to a system. Assuredly nothing demands a more enlightened mind, more sagacity, and circumspection than the discovery of truths of this kind."[2]

While the problems were real, they were not insurmountable. "I dare make bold to predict," concluded Cabanis, "that together with the true method of observation, the spirit of philosophy which should always predominate in it will soon revive in medicine, and that the science will assume a different aspect."[3]

John Forbes (1787–1861), a distinguished British physician and medical editor, to whom Bartlett refers in rather unfriendly terms, wrote a great deal on the subject of "nature and art." The particular piece that offended Bartlett, and many others, was a long review essay Forbes published in the journal he edited. Forbes entitled his piece "Homeopathy, allopathy, and 'young physic.' "[4] Although purporting to be a collective review of nine books on homeopathy, including an 1819 edition of Hahnemann's *Organon der Heilkunst*, Forbes really examined the whole problem of therapeutics. He provided his readers with a concise history and theory of homeopathy and then inquired into that system's ability to cure disease and in the power of allopathy, or regular medicine, to achieve the same goal.

Forbes was duly impressed by some of the results reported by followers of Hahnemann. About one case of dyspepsia treated by a highly diluted preparation of strychnine, Forbes waxed lyrical, much to the disgust of many later commentators on his article: "Can anything in therapeutics," Forbes asked, "surpass the evidence of the marvelous effects produced in this case by the 1,000,000 part of a grain of *nux vomica*."[5] Forbes also boldly ventured further: "What, then, it will naturally be asked, is the explanation of the momentous fact we have announced, that a considerable number of diseases have been, and perhaps continue to be, treated as successfully by homeopathists as by allopathists? *Is it that the one kind of treatment is as good as the other*? IS IT THAT HOMEOPATHY IS TRUE?"[6] Forbes answered his question in the negative in regard to the theory of homeopathy. But, perhaps in practice, he surmised, it may not be false. By comparing the results of homeopaths with those of regular physicians, one could readily see the lamentable condition of medicine. It was to this point that Bartlett addressed himself in the essay that follows.

PREFACE

The main title of my inquiry is the same as that of the very elegant and classical essay of Cabanis, published half a century ago. I adopt it for the simple reason that there is no other at all appropriate. Since writing my own essay I

---

[2] Cabanis, *On the Certainty of Medicine*, p. 32.

[3] Ibid., p. 110. Bartlett fifty years later had a similar goal in mind. As Ackerknecht has pointed out, however, the *Inquiry*, unlike its model by Cabanis, was predominantly non-philosophical in nature.

[4] *British & Foreign Medical Review* 21 (1846): 225–65.

[5] Ibid., p. 248.

[6] Ibid., p. 250. Italics and capitals by Forbes.

have read, for the first time for nearly twenty years, the work of Cabanis. Besides the differences that must almost unavoidably exist in the conception and treatment of a complex and difficult question by different minds, I may be permitted to say that the leading and principal design and purpose of the two works are not exactly identical. The essay of Cabanis is more elementary than my Inquiry is; it deals more systematically with the fundamental nature and philosophy of medicine than my Inquiry does. The latter may be said to take up the subject where it is left by Cabanis. I have no pretensions to supplant or to rival the finished and beautiful essay of the French philosopher and physician; and the unlikeness of the two works is at least sufficient to save me from the imputation of having merely repeated my forerunner or of having merely gone over the same ground.

Some of my readers, especially the more staid and older ones—my esteemed and venerable seniors and contemporaries—may think, perhaps, that I have now and then suffered myself to be seduced into dangerous proximity to the boundary line which separates good taste and simplicity from their opposite qualities. If I have done so, it has been from yielding to an impulse excited and kindled by the task in which I have been engaged and which I found it difficult to resist. If the drapery of our philosophic muse wears a somewhat warmer and livelier hue than the sober coloring which more appropriately belongs to it, it has been caught from the sunny fields through which her pathway has lain. If the axle of our car has now and then waxed fervid, and if an occasional gleam of light has flashed from its flying wheels, let us at least plead, in extenuation of the weakness, that it is not from the careless rein, or any perilous speed with which our coursers have been driven, but from the glowing and radiant atmosphere through which we have been carried along.

There may, possibly, be others who will say that my advocacy of the claims of medicine is more zealous and earnest than is becoming in one of its practitioners and teachers. I can only answer that I do not think so. I speak for the art and the science, not for myself. This art and science have been violently and, I think, blindly and unjustly assailed by parties who understand neither their own strength and position nor ours. I have endeavored to make fair and manly stand against them, and I have done nothing more. When crowds of epauletted and bedizened coxcombs, who have never smelt gunpowder, make the air clamorous with their noisy boastings, the war-worn and scar-covered veteran may, at least, point to the trophies that he has brought from a hundred battlefields.

I am stating only what everybody knows to be true when I say that the general confidence which has heretofore existed in the science and art of medicine, as this science has been studied and as this art has been practiced, has within the last few years been violently shaken and disturbed and is now greatly lessened and impaired. The hold which medicine has so long had upon the popular mind is loosened; there is a widespread skepticism as to its power of curing diseases, and men are everywhere to be found who deny its pretensions as a science and reject the benefits and blessings which it proffers them as an art.

It is not necessary for my present purpose to point out the causes and influences which have led to this state of things. I will merely say, in this connection, that however trifling and inconsiderable may have been the effects upon the feeling to which I have alluded, of the famous article of Dr. Forbes, first published in the *British and Foreign Medical Review*, I give utterance, I suppose, to the almost universal sentiment of the profession when I express regret that the author of that article did not accompany his official and voluntary confession of medical delinquency, incompetency, and uncertainty with the qualifications and conditions absolutely essential to the truth of the confession itself. This, Dr. Forbes has almost wholly neglected to do. Without entering into any elaborate criticism of his paper, it is quite safe to say that he has taken, if not a distorted, at least a partial, view of his subject; he has looked at one side only of the shield; one hemisphere only of his world of truth has been turned to the sun. Now this partial view is necessarily a false view: it is false because it is partial,—if for no other reason. Dr. Forbes has drawn, in strong and exaggerated colors, the manifold imperfections of medical science and the discouraging uncertainties of medical art; but he has neglected to show the limits of these uncertainties and to circumscribe the boundaries within which these imperfections are confined. This he should have done, and not only would his second picture have constituted, on the principle of contrast often followed by artists in such matters, an appropriate companion to his first—the clearer and more radiant sky, the steadier and serener light, the erect figures with hopeful and forward-looking faces of the former, brought into striking and beautiful relief by the cloudy and uncertain horizon, the murky and dim atmosphere, and the constrained and groping shapes of the latter—but more than this: his first delineation is a true one only when the second hangs by its side; the harmony of the lights and shadows and the truthfulness of the objects in each picture are dependent upon the presence of the other.

The canvas which now stands upon my easel is placed there to receive at least the outlines and some of the leading and more prominent features of this second picture. I have waited, I think, long enough for Dr. Forbes, or for some one else better qualified than myself, to do the work which I have here undertaken. If Ulysses is not present in the field to bend his own bow, some weaker arm from the camp must essay the enterprise. It seems to me high time that a clear and earnest word should be spoken for the science which we study and teach and for the art which we inculcate and practice. The interests of truth of our profession and of humanity alike demand that the legitimate claims of medicine to the regard and confidence of mankind should be vindicated and maintained. And this is the task I have set myself. I wish to show as clearly and as positively as I can, the nature and the degree of the certainty that belongs to medicine as a science and as an art. In doing this, I shall deal but little in general assertions, unsustained by positive proofs, and not at all in empty and vague declamation; I shall state the reasons of the faith that I profess, and I shall exhibit the evidence upon which it rests. . . .

I do not mean to say by these remarks, that the sciences of anatomy and physiology are by any means finished and complete; this can hardly be said of any subject of human inquiry. I mean merely to say that this degree of completeness is as satisfactory as it is in any of the natural sciences and that it is daily advancing. There are impassable barriers to our investigations into the secrets of nature, whatever may be their character or direction; and here, as elsewhere, we are surrounded on all sides by a ring of darkness which no power of ours can ever penetrate or dispel. But we may rest assured that here, too, as elsewhere, all that is knowable will be known. Every passing month furnishes its contribution to the work; some new discovery is made or some old truth is strengthened and illustrated, or some error or delusion is corrected or dispelled; a thousand microscopes are prying into the deepest and darkest recesses of organization; a thousand laboratories are busy with the chemistry of life; myriads of patient scalpels are plying their careful and laborious dissections, and so these, like all other branches of human knowledge, are carried slowly but steadily forward in their interminable career.

It is not, however, against these departments of our science that the accusations to which I have alluded have been brought, so that there is no occasion for my giving to them anything more than this general and passing notice. It is unnecessary to make a formal defence of a point which is never attacked. The charges of which I have spoken refer particularly and almost exclusively to that department of medical science designated by the terms *pathology*, and *therapeutics*. This department is constituted by the phenomena and relations of disease; it embraces all these phenomena and all these relations. It professes, and claims to consist of, a knowledge of the causes of disease, of the seat and phenomena of disease, and of the means of preventing, mitigating, and removing disease. The charges against our science are that it deceives itself in this matter—that its pretensions are either altogether false or greatly exaggerated—that its knowledge of disease is vastly less than it professes to be—and, especially, that its power of curing and of mitigating disease has been immensely over-estimated and over-stated. These charges sometimes deny altogether the existence of this power, although, in most instances, they content themselves with the allegation that it is very limited in extent and very uncertain in its application.

These are grave charges and I think they should be gravely met; they strike at the very foundations of our science as a power and means for removing and diminishing the physical ills of life; they rob it of its chiefest grace and glory; they take away its highest claim to the regard and gratitude of men; they deserve, I think, an honest and thorough investigation; and this investigation, subject to the conditions of the space within which I wish to work, and the ability with which I may be enabled to work, I now proceed to undertake. I shall endeavor to show the nature of our knowledge of disease—its extent, and its degree of positiveness; I shall endeavor to show how far and with what measure of certainty and of constancy we are able to control, to mitigate, and to remove disease.

The best way and, indeed, the only way within the limited sense which I have assigned myself, in which I can do this is to rely principally upon the evidence and illustrations which may be derived from the study and examination of some individual disease. This disease, in order to answer my purpose, should be of frequent occurrence, not confined to any particular localities, susceptible of being clearly marked in its characteristic features, and sufficiently severe, more or less seriously, to endanger life. I do not know any acute affection that so nearly fulfils all these conditions, as *pneumonia*, or inflammation of the substance of the lungs; and I shall accordingly make use of this disease in the further prosecution of my subject. It is only important for me to add here, in order to remove any suspicion that may arise in the minds of my skeptical readers, that I have chosen a one-sided and an unfair subject for the illustration of my inquiry, that after having gone through with this detailed and special illustration, I intend to point out the differences which exist between this disease and others, whether these differences are in my favor or against me. I shall strive not only to tell the truth, but to tell the whole truth.

There are several forms or varieties of pneumonia; it is necessary for me to state here that in the use which I propose to make of this disease I shall confine myself to its ordinary sporadic form, occurring in persons after the age of puberty and, at the period of attack, in the enjoyment of, at least, an average degree of health and free from any other obvious disease.

The first inquiry that presents itself relates to the local lesion which constitutes, anatomically, the disease. What, and how much do we know of this lesion?—of its seat, its phenomena, its nature? What are the foundations, the nature, the extent, and the degree of certainty, of our knowledge of these things? The answer to these questions is at hand; it is definite, and it is sufficiently satisfactory. We know that with the commencement of the inflammation, the portion of lung which is the seat of this morbid action becomes of a deeper red color than it has in health, with a livid or violet tinge; that its specific gravity is increased from an undue accumulation of blood in its vessels and a corresponding diminution of air in its air-cells; that it has lost, in a great degree, its spongy and elastic feel and is more doughy and solid to the touch; that it is less tough and more friable; and that when cut or torn, a large quantity of reddish, turbid, and frothy fluid flows from the surfaces. We know that, except in a very small number of cases in which this stage of engorgement continues until the subsidence of the disease, in the course, generally, of from two to five or six days the diseased lung undergoes other and still more striking changes. Its specific gravity is still further increased, so that it is as heavy and solid as liver; it contains no air and does not crepitate; its air-cells are obliterated; its surfaces, when cut or torn, are of a deep red color, often mottled or marbled; a reddish, thick, opaque, and semipurulent fluid flows from them in moderate quantity, and they are crowded with a multitude of small, red, slightly flattened, granulations. When the disease does not destroy life, this condition of the lung, after having persisted for a few days, gradually disappears, and the lung as gradually returns to its former state. In a few fatal cases, death takes place while the lung is still in the condition just described; but in a large proportion of these cases it becomes soft and still more friable, and from violet-red, it becomes of a grayish or yellowish color. Such are the characteristic anatomical phenomena of this local lesion. They are very constant, with the conditions that have been stated, and they have been ascertained with entire and absolute positiveness. A certain class of physicians—I mean the homeopathists—deny the value and usefulness of this knowledge, but no one doubts the certainty of the knowledge itself. . . .

I cannot see why our knowledge of the pathological anatomy of pneumonia, thus briefly indicated, should not be considered, in a good degree, satisfactory. I do not pretend that this knowledge is perfect and complete. It is at least exceedingly difficult, it may be, in the nature of things, altogether impossible, for instance, to ascertain in what precise tissue the inflammatory process commences and in what minute molecular changes and perversions it consists. But this kind of imperfection belongs to all natural science; as much, for instance, to the science of chemistry as to that of life. I will only add that the other elements of the pathology of pneumonia—the accompanying inflammation of the pleura; the change in the composition of the blood; the striking and singular accumulation of solid masses of fibrine in the cavities of the heart, in a certain proportion of fatal cases; the occasional, but very rare, formation of a distinct abscess in the lungs; the varieties of the lesions at different periods of life, and under other circumstances—have all been ascertained as carefully and as positively as the more essential and characteristic phenomena that I have described.

In the second place, the symptoms of pneumonia, the general and local signs by which it manifests itself and reveals its presence, are not less accurately and positively known. In about one-quarter of the cases, the formal access of the disease is preceded for a few days by various disturbances of the system, usually of moderate severity; in the other three-quarters, the disease commences suddenly, without any premonition. The initiatory symptom in most cases is a chill, accompanied or immediately followed by pain in the side, more or less acute; cough; dyspnea; a feeling of general uneasiness; headache; febrile excitement; and the expectoration of viscid, tenacious, frothy sputa of a uniform brick-dust color. The duration of these and of all the other symptoms, their constancy, their varieties in degree and in kind, their importance and value as diagnostic and as prognostic indications, their differences and peculiarities in different forms of the disease, have all been very carefully studied and very accurately determined. To give the results and details of all these researches would be, so far, to write an elaborate monograph upon pneumonia; but this is not my purpose, and I must content myself with the foregoing general but distinct and unqualified assertion. Besides these rational symptoms, as they are called, there is another class of phenomena of a peculiar character, constituting evidences of the existence, the seat, and the stage of the disease still more conclusive. These are the *physical signs*, as they are called, of pneumonia. They consist in certain modifications of the resonance of the walls of the chest corresponding to the diseased lung on percussion; of the natural sounds of the respiration and the voice, heard when the ear is applied to the chest, and the presence of other sounds of a new and unusual character. By the aid of these acoustic phenomena we can fix upon the exact portion of the lung which is the seat of disease; we can mark out its boundaries; we can follow these boundaries inch by inch as they advance and invade new parts of the lung; we can follow the natural progress of the inflammation from its first, to its second period, and back again in its retrograde march towards health. We know the precise moment of time when the air-vesicles are so blocked up that no air passes into them, and the precise moment, also, when they are again opened to admit it. The roar of conflagration does not mark more clearly the passage of the raging element from chamber to chamber of a burning house, than does the fine dry crackle of the crepitant rhonchus, the presence and march of inflammatory engorgement of the lungs. It cannot be necessary for me to pursue this branch of my subject any further; certainly, I have said enough to convince the most skeptical of my readers, if they believe what I say, that there is no lack of certainty and positiveness in the signs by which pneumonia is revealed to us during life. . . .

The most important and interesting part of our inquiry still remains to be considered, and the space that I have already occupied admonishes me to desist from any further illustrations of the state of our knowledge of the natural history of pneumonia. It can hardly be necessary for me to do so, although nothing would be easier if the subject before me required it. I apprehend that some even of my professional readers would be surprised by a full exposition of the extent and the positiveness of this knowledge. The different forms and varieties of the disease, its various complications, and especially its most important and numerous relations to other diseases, might all of them furnish us with instances and evidences of this knowledge not less striking than those I have already given. But I have said enough, I think, to convince the most skeptical and to satisfy the most incredulous that the science of medicine, so far at least as pneumonia is concerned, in no degree deserves the charges of incompleteness and uncertainty which have been laid at its door.

The value of medical science depends wholly upon its connection with medical art. It might, to be sure, be cultivated as an interesting subject of inquiry, independent of this connection; but it derives most of its interest and all of its importance and practical utility from its agency in the prevention, mitigation, and removal of disease. These are its great ends and objects, and so far only as it attains them or ministers to them can it lay claim to our veneration and regard as a blessing and a benefit to our race. It happens, however, that less confidence is felt in medicine as an art than as a science. It is precisely here, in its chief end and purpose, that it is said to fail. Physicians, it is admitted, may indeed understand the seat and nature of disease, but it is denied that they can, with any certainty or uniformity, control or cure it. Practical medicine, it is asserted, is altogether a haphazard affair of guess and conjecture, doing good when this happens, more by accident than according to any constant and fixed principles and as often doing harm as good. It is my purpose now to inquire honestly and carefully into this matter. I wish to show, and I intend to do so according to the extent of my means and ability, the nature, the degree, and the certainty of our power over disease. For the purpose of illustration, I shall continue to make use of the disease which has already, thus far, furnished me with materials for my investigation.

Considering the very wide differences in the forms and character of pneumonia, there has been for a long time a pretty general agreement amongst medical men in regard to what has been considered as the best method of treating it. General blood-letting during the early periods of the disease has been principally relied upon by the immense majority of careful observers and experienced practitioners. With only occasional and temporary exceptions, this has been the leading and prominent remedy. So strong and so universal was the confidence in this remedy that the feeling became very general that it was essential to the cure of the disease; or, at least, that it would not be omitted without the most imminent hazard to the patient. It was a very common, if not a general, belief not only that the chances of recovery were almost indefinitely increased by the operation, but that the disease was very much shortened in its duration and in many cases wholly and at once arrested. This conviction—the growth of centuries—was the gradual result of the aggregate, common, everyday experience of the profession during this long period of time. And it was never stronger, perhaps, or more firmly fixed in the general medical mind than at the period of the publication, in 1828, of Louis's researches upon this subject—the effects of blood-letting in pneumonia. This is a very remarkable work, and its conclusions have a direct and very important bearing upon the inquiry in which I am engaged. Louis's researches constituted the commencement of a more rigorous and searching investigation than had hitherto been instituted into the actual extent of our power over disease. The time for such an investigation had now fully come. It could not have been made before the great discovery of Laennec had prepared the way for it by giving us more accurate and positive means of diagnosis than we had hitherto possessed. The general belief of which I have spoken, derived from the traditions of general experience, did not satisfy the positive and exacting mind of Louis. He said, in effect, if not in so many words—I know very well that this belief is almost universal; I know that it comes to us sanctioned by the wisdom and sustained by the experience of ages; but other beliefs, not less universal and not less firmly settled, have been proved at last to be partly or wholly false; there have been many and wide-spread medical delusions which time and a sufficiently thorough investigation have at length dissipated; this may be one of the same class; at any rate, it is due to the cause of science and the interests of humanity that the subject should be more closely studied than heretofore. I do not deny that the conviction is well founded—I deny nothing—I only say that the evidences of its truth do not exist or, at least, that they have not been furnished to us—I cannot find them.

Between the years 1821 and 1827, Louis studied carefully, and from day to day at La Charité, the effects of blood-letting in fifty cases of pneumonia terminating favorably, and in twenty-eight cases which terminated in death. The patients were bled from one to four times, according to the indications in each case; from ten to fifteen ounces of blood being taken at each operation. Of the fifty cases terminating in health, twenty-three were bled for the first time within the first four days from the commencement of the disease, and the average duration of the disease in these cases was seventeen days; twenty-seven were bled for the first time between the fifth and the ninth days, inclusive, and the average duration of the disease in these cases was twenty days. Every possible precaution was taken that the two groups of cases, thus compared with each other should be essentially alike in all the circumstances that could in any way affect the danger of the disease. Louis studied, further, the effects of the same remedy upon the leading symptoms of pneumonia. He found that the pain in the side was never wholly and at once removed by an early blood-letting; but that, on the contrary, it was generally more severe for twelve or twenty-four hours after the first bleeding, if this was practiced early in the disease. He found, however, that the average duration of the pain in the first group of cases was six days and a little over eight days in the second group. He found that most of the other symptoms were moderately influenced by the bleedings. Between the years 1830 and 1833, Louis studied in the same manner at La Pitié the effects of blood-letting in twenty-nine cases of pneumonia, four of which terminated fatally. Of the twenty-five cases terminating favorably, thirteen were bled between the second and fourth days of the disease, inclusive; and the average duration of these cases was fifteen days and a half; the other twelve cases were bled from the fifth to the fourteenth day, inclusive, and their average duration was eighteen days and a-quarter. No one of these cases was bled on the first day of the disease. The first bleedings were a little more copious than in the cases at La Charité. The effects of the remedy upon the individual symptoms did not differ from those in the latter cases.

So far as this limited investigation could settle the question, Louis considered himself justified in coming to this conclusion—that blood-letting has a favorable effect upon the march of pneumonia; that it abridges its duration; but that this effect is much less than had generally been supposed, patients who are bled during the first four days of the disease, all other things being equal, recovering four or five days sooner than those who are bled later. And as far as this particular investigation is concerned, the conclusion is perfectly justifiable and legitimate. It results with a slight qualification, necessarily and inevitably, from the facts; and Louis never pretended to carry the conclusion beyond this. He says, expressly, that these facts are neither sufficiently numerous nor sufficiently various finally to settle the question at issue; and that he publishes them principally for the purpose of calling anew the attention of observers to the subject. It is important to bear in mind that these investigations show directly, not so much the absolute effects of blood-letting as the difference in its effects when performed early or late in the disease. His conclusions so far as his own facts are concerned would have been more truly stated if he had confined it to early, compared with late, blood-letting.* . . .

So far as the two principal objects of our inquiry are concerned, we may embody the results of the preceding investigation in the two following brief propositions:

First:—The science of medicine, so far as pneumonia is concerned—although like other natural sciences, still unfinished and progressive—is, to a very satisfactory extent, settled and positive; the principal phenomena and relations to this disease have been well and accurately ascertained; its natural history is, in a good degree and to a considerable extent, complete.

Second:—Medical art, so far as pneumonia is concerned—although not endowed with absolute and unqualified power—is still of great and unquestionable utility. Through the agency, principally, of blood-letting and antimonials, as its most active means, it lessens the severity of the disease, shortens its duration, and in many instances prevents its termination in death.

Such, then, I believe to be a fair and true statement of the nature and the extent of the power of art over this form of disease. It may seem to some that this power is circumscribed within very narrow limits—that it is so *"cabin'd, cribb'd, confined,"* so qualified and contingent as to be of little worth. I do not think so. Its power seems to me to be very great and its value beyond all estimate. Such is the constitution of nature, that some cases of the disease are

---

*There is one other important conclusion of Louis's which is not kept strictly within the limits of his facts. It results from his investigations, he says, that pneumonia is not *arrested* by early blood-letting. It would have been more exact to have said that, according to these investigations, pneumonia is not arrested by bleedings *practiced after the first day of the disease.* I do not mean to say that this conclusion is a false one; I say, merely, that it does not follow directly and necessarily from the facts from which it is derived. The somewhat moderate difference between the effects of early, and late blood-letting, might justify the *probable* conclusion, that blood-letting at the very onset of the disease, would still fail to arrest it; but this question could be positively settled, only by this particular application of the remedy. The effects of blood-letting might be very different within the first few hours, and after the first day of the disease.

beyond its reach; others would struggle through their successive stages without its formal and active aid; but the hard rigor of the former is often softened by its ministry; the latter are almost always benefitted by its interference; while in many other cases it determines the momentous issue of life or of death and turns the trembling balance in the sufferer's favor.

As I have already said, I am not laying down rules for the treatment of pneumonia; but before leaving this subject it may be proper for me to remark, for the information of my nonprofessional readers, that in addition to the heroic remedies which are chiefly relied upon there are numerous other means of secondary and subordinate value, but the utility and importance of which are not less certain than those of the former. . . .

Surgery has escaped almost entirely the charges of incompetence and uncertainty which have been so liberally bestowed upon practical medicine. The reasons of this are simple and obvious enough. Its processes are not only more showy than those of practical medicine, but they are more easily seen and apprehended; they appeal immediately and strongly to the senses; they are so manifest that they can be neither doubted nor mistaken. The restoration of a dislocated bone to its socket; the removal of a calculus from the bladder, either by the lithontriptor or by the knife and forceps; the closure of an aneurysm by a ligature on the diseased vessel; the instantaneous arrest of the spouting torrent of blood from a cut artery; the re-admission of the long-excluded light to the retina by the withdrawal, or the dropping down, of the darkened curtain of the crystalline lens are achievements so brilliant in their execution and so striking and positive in their results as not merely to leave no room for cavilling or for skepticism, but to excite in us at once, emotions both of wonder and delight. And we may now add that surgery does its most formidable work—sundering the large limbs with its bold and free incisions, rending by main force the ligamentous fastenings and the strong adhesions of anchylosed joints, and carrying its exploring probes amongst the exquisitely sensitive filaments of exposed and irritated nerves whose every slightest touch has heretofore been intolerable agony—doing all this, I say, and more, after having steeped the senses and the mind in total unconsciousness or lapped them in positive elysium. But there is no essential difference, after all, between the certainty of surgical and the certainty of medical art. The processes and operations of the surgeon, like the medicines of the physician, are his means for the removal or mitigation of disease and, like the latter, their efficacy and success are always more or less contingent and uncertain. I mean to say by this, simply, that great and unequivocal as is the power of surgical art over disease, that of medical art is none the less so; they are both subject to similar conditions and their degree of certainty is much the same. . . .

NATHAN S. DAVIS

NATURE AND ART. THEIR RELATIVE INFLUENCE IN THE MANAGEMENT OF DISEASES. ARE THEY ANTAGONISTIC OR CO-OPERATIVE?

Editor's Note

Nathan Smith Davis (1817–1904) is best known for his efforts to reform medical education. He was one of the principal founders of the A.M.A. and in 1859 helped to establish the three year curriculum at the medical department of Lind University (later Northwestern). Davis was also an energetic medical editor. He founded the *Chicago Medical Examiner* in 1860. With the establishment of the *Journal of the American Medical Association*, in 1883, he became its first editor, resigning in 1889.

In the early 1860's two conflicts in regard to therapeutics exemplified the stresses within the profession. Both were part of a larger discussion about the role of nature in the cure of disease. This latter, a subject going back at least to the Hippocratic writers, was also prominent in contemporary European thought, where therapeutic nihilism was becoming widespread among the academic centers. While Americans usually did not adopt a posture of actual nihilism, the discussions regarding "rational medicine," or reliance on less active bleeding and purging did fill many pages of American medical journals.

The first of the two conflicts alluded to above was over statements made by Oliver Wendell Holmes in his oration to the Massachusetts Medical Society in 1860. Since the paper by Davis was, in part, an answer to Holmes, the latter's remarks deserve our attention.[1]

Holmes's speech "Currents and Counter-Currents in Medical Science," greatly disturbed a large number of America's doctors. Indeed, the society that had invited him to deliver the annual oration publicly disavowed itself from what he said, an unusual step, to say the least. "The object of Dr. Holmes," the reviewer in the *American Journal of the Medical Sciences* pointed out, "in his address is to favor a general current which has manifestly been setting in during the past twenty-five or thirty years in favor of assisting nature in the treatment of disease, and in opposition to a predominant dependence on art."[2]

Holmes in his oration took to task many aspects of his profession's practices, its journalism and therapeutics coming in for the most scorn. The passage most

---

Chicago Med. Examiner 2 (1861): 129–39. An essay read to the Chicago Medical Society, October 19, 1860.

[1] I have elsewhere dealt with the other therapeutic discussion, the banning of calomel and tartar emetic by Surgeon-General Hammond. "Therapeutic conflicts and the American medical profession in the 1860's," *Bull. Hist. Med.* 41 (1967): 215–22.

[2] *Am. J. Med. Sci.* 40 (1860): 462–74; 463. This was one of the most thoughtful reviews; it was also friendly to Holmes. The reviewer was Worthington Hooker, a kindred spirit in the quest for a "rational medicine."

often quoted and that which doubtless gave most offense to his colleagues and the greatest satisfaction to the medical sectarians had to do with the materia medica:

> Throw out opium [meaning retain for use], which the Creator himself seems to prescribe . . . ; throw out a few specifics which our art did not discover, and is hardly needed to apply; throw out wine, which is a food, and the vapors which produce the miracle of anesthesia, and I firmly believe that if the whole materia medica, *as now used*, could be sunk to the bottom of the sea, it would be all the better for mankind—and all the worse for the fishes."[3]

Although a medical man believes he treats his patients on principles founded in his experience, this is not always the case. Much is really belief or fashion of the time. There are in every calling, Holmes pointed out, those who go about their daily tasks according to the rules of their craft, without questioning past or future. These he called the practical men; "They pull the oars of society." Holmes wanted to awaken his audience to the intellectual currents of the time, such as positivism. And awaken them he did—to the point where many became enraged. Nathan Smith Davis was one who felt compelled to answer some of Holmes's charges.

Bibliographical Note

Thomas N. Bonner, "Dr. Nathan Smith Davis and the growth of Chicago medicine, 1850–1900," *Bull. Hist. Med.* 26 (1952): 360–74.

An extensive discussion of works by Jacob Bigelow, Worthington Hooker, and John Forbes appeared as an essay review, "Nature and art in the cure of disease," *North Am. Rev.* 89 (1859): 165–208.

A general history of the role of nature in the treatment of disease is Max Neuburger's *Die Lehre von der Heilkraft der Natur im Wandel der Zeiten*, Stuttgart: Enke, 1926. It has been translated into English as *The Doctrine of the Healing Power of Nature*, New York, 1933.

During the last ten or fifteen years much has been said and written concerning the curative powers of Nature; as though she was an actual *entity*—a fair Goddess of health, ruling over the animal economy with the ubiquitous power to meet disease at every point.

And while nature has been thus personified and exalted as an active curative power, *Art* has been caricatured as little else than an indiscriminate exhibition of harsh and deleterious drugs. Drs. Forbes and Bigelow took the lead in this modern effort to deify nature, and it has been followed up, both in and out of the profession, until we can hardly take up a popular address, an introductory

---

[3] "Currents and Counter-Currents," in *Medical Essays, 1842–1882* (Boston: Houghton, Mifflin, 1895), pp. 173–208; 202–3. The italics were Holmes's.

lecture, or an essay in the pages of a medical journal without finding the curative powers of *nature* extolled and the assumed *over-drugging* of the human race, under the direction of art, soundly berated.

One of the latest and most noted productions of this kind is the annual address, delivered before the Massachusetts Medical Society, by Dr. Oliver Wendell Holmes, of Boston; entitled, "Currents and Counter Currents in Medical Science." In perusing this kind of literature, two questions always arise in the mind, namely: 1st, what is meant by *Nature* as used in medical language; and 2d, what are the true relations between nature and art? Most of that class of writers who extoll nature and depreciate art use the two words as though they were necessarily antagonistic, but make no attempt to define either of them. Dr. Holmes, however, has so far deviated from the beaten path as to define both terms as follows: "*Nature*, in medical language, as opposed to Art, means trust in the reactions of the living system against ordinary normal impressions."

"*Art*, in the same language, as opposed to Nature, means an intentional resort to extraordinary abnormal impressions for the relief of disease."

"*Disease*, dis-ease—disturbed quiet, uncomfortableness, means imperfect or abnormal reaction of the living system and its more or less permanent results."

"*Food*, in its largest sense, is whatever helps to build up the normal structures or to maintain their natural actions."

"*Medicine*, in distinction from food, is every unnatural or noxious agent applied for the relief of disease."

These definitions, emanating from a high literary source and directly from what is claimed as the headquarters of conservatism in medicine, may reasonably claim a little examination. It will be seen by the first paragraph quoted that *nature*, in medical language, "means *trust*," that is, reliance, faith; therefore, according to Dr. Holmes, *nature* is merely a *mental* act, capable of being exercised either by the patient or the physician, or by both. "*Trust* in the reactions of the living system against ordinary normal impressions" constitutes *nature*. Surely, the definition if sufficiently simple, but can anything be more manifestly absurd? It is probable, however, that Dr. Holmes meant to convey the idea that *nature* is the reaction of the living system against ordinary normal impressions, instead of *faith* or *trust* in such reaction. But while his language makes nature consist in a mere mental act of faith, *Art* consists in the production of "extraordinary abnormal impressions;" and disease simply "means imperfect or abnormal reaction of the living system," etc. Surely, the author of definitions so lucid and so comprehensive should have a monument erected to his memory!

Nature is the normal *reaction* of the living system.

Disease is imperfect or abnormal *reaction* of the living system.

Art is the production of abnormal *impressions* on the living system. But what is meant by the words "*reaction*" and the "*living system*"? According to lexicographers, *re-action*, means action restored, renewed, re-established; and necessarily presupposes a previous diminution or suspension of action.

But can "ordinary normal impressions" produce anything more than simply, *action*? If not, how can *nature* be synonymous with *re-actions*? It was no part of our intention, however, to waste time in criticising the absurd definitions of Dr. Holmes. On the contrary we quoted them for the purpose of exhibiting more clearly, certain fundamental errors that are common to the whole class of writers, represented by Holmes, Bigelow, Forbes, etc. The first and most important of these errors is the assumption that *nature* and *art*, as used in reference to the treatment of disease, are antagonistic or opposed to each other.

The second, is the assumption that all medicines are "unnatural or noxious agents" producing "extraordinary abnormal impressions" on the living system.

The third, is the assumption that whatever is injurious or debilitating to the human system in health, is equally so to the same system affected by disease.

These three assumptions constitute the foundation on which is based all the reasonings and deductions of "Young Physic"—"Nature and Art in the cure of Disease"—and a host of minor productions in the form of addresses, essays, etc. To expose the fallacy of these assumptions and point out, what we deem to be, the true relations of *nature* and *art* in the cure of disease are the special objects of this paper.

Nature is a word which occurs so frequently in the medical writings of all ages that its import, or the ideas sought to be conveyed by it, ought to be clearly understood. It is generally used in such a manner as to indicate not only an active but a more or less intelligent power. . . .

We thus see clearly that *nature* in medical language, when not used merely as a cloak for ignorance, means simply the ordinary processes that take place in the living animal body; and the *curative efforts* or *powers of nature*, the *vis medicatrix naturae*, are the performance of one or more of these processes in such a manner as either to remove the causes or overcome the effects of disease. Having thus defined nature and her efforts, we will next inquire into the nature of *art* and her real relations to nature.

Dr. Holmes has defined Art, to consist in the use of medicine for the production of extraordinary abnormal impressions to relieve disease. And medicines he defines to be *unnatural noxious* agents. These definitions, however, are only equalled in absurdity by his declaration that nature means a mental act of faith or *trust*. We should say that *disease* consisted in extraordinary and abnormal impressions and actions; and that *art*, as used in medical language, meant the use of such agents as would diminish or *remove* such "extraordinary and abnormal impressions" and their results. In the illustrations already given we have seen that nature has three methods of resisting disease; first, by expelling the cause, as when offending matter is ejected by gastric or intestinal discharges or by increased secretions from the skin, kidneys, etc. Second, by increasing the action of one secretory organ sufficient to compensate for the diminished action of another. Third, by allowing the accumulation of such material in the blood, as by its narcotic or sedative qualities is capable of overcoming morbid excitement and favoring critical evacuations.

So the enlightened physician, the practitioner of the true medical art, instead of using noxious agents to produce abnormal impressions, acts in strict imitation of nature's own processes by endeavoring first of all to remove the noxious causes—second, to use one organ when necessary for the temporary relief of another, which may be disabled by disease—and third, to bring into requisition such agents as will allay irritation or excitement when in excess or prop up and sustain the properties and functions when too much depressed.

We thus see that the operations of nature herself or, in other words, the processes that take place in the human system when embarrassed by morbid impressions or disease, plainly indicate the use of agents to remove offending matter, either by evacuants, such as cathartics, diuretics, diaphoretics, etc., or by antidotes to destroy its noxious qualities. And when the morbid actions do not cease with a removal of the causes from which they originated, nature points with equal clearness to the employment of sedatives, anodynes, or tonics, according to the nature of the morbid action.

The very existence of disease is a confession on the part of nature that she has been unable to resist the action of those noxious influences to which she has been exposed. And the true object of art is to interpose timely and well directed assistance in her behalf, either by removing the evil influences or lessening their effects on the organized structures, or by both. Hence the skill of the physician in the practice of his art will be in direct proportion to the clearness with which he sees the exact nature and tendency of the morbid actions constituting disease, and the precision with which he adapts the application of remedial agents to the accomplishment of the special change indicated by the nature of the morbid action. If there is any truth in the foregoing observations, they show clearly that the physician is what his name imports, namely, a student of nature in its most comprehensive sense. For he studies nature, not only in her healthy manifestations but also in her embarrassments, her deformities, and morbid conditions. And his *art*, instead of being antagonistic or opposed to nature, is in the truest sense of the word her ally, her assistant, exerted only when she is embarrassed and in a direction to relieve such embarrassment.

Hence, the assumption of Dr. Holmes, and the school he represents, that nature and art stand in opposition to each other is a fundamental error that vitiates all their reasoning. Equally faulty is the definition of medicines given by the same class of writers, and the distinction between food and medicine. The assertion that food embraces all substances capable of nourishing the tissues or supporting the functions of the organs; and that medicines are simply "unnatural or noxious agents," is neither explicit nor truthful. Will any respectable physiologist deny that calorie, electricity, oxygen, etc., are capable of supporting the various functions of the system, and yet will he pretend that these agents are food? Again, it is perfectly well known that under certain circumstances strychnine, the preparations of iron, or peruvian bark, etc., are capable of aiding very much in supporting the various functions of the system; but will any one pretend that these agents are food! Neither is it true that all medicines are "unnatural or noxious agents." Are not the gentian, the poppy, and the rhubarb just as *natural* as the potatoe, the corn, or the wheat? And, when properly used, are they any more noxious? If improperly used, they may produce injurious or noxious effects, and so may a loaf of bread. The truth is that the human system is capable of being acted upon by three distinct classes of agents. The first embraces all such substances, whether solids, liquids, or gases, as are capable of being assimilated and converted into any part of the natural structures of the body. These constitute *food*.

The second embraces those agents which though not constituting a part of the living structures are yet essential to the healthy performance of the various functional and organic actions, such as atmospheric oxygen, caloric, light, and electricity. These are the natural *stimuli* or *excitors* of action, and are essentially distinct from food.

The third class embraces all such agents as are capable of modifying the properties and actions of the system, without being themselves assimilated. These are *medicines*.

Another fundamental error, that vitiates the reasoning of all that class of writers who delight to deify nature and caricature art, consists in the assumption that all medicines or substances capable of affecting a well man injuriously, must also affect a sick man in the same direction. Thus, if a bleeding, a purge, or a blister debilitates a person in health, the same effect must necessarily follow their administration to one affected with disease. To the observing and experienced practitioner, the fallacy of such a statement is abundantly obvious; and yet it is well calculated to deceive the inexperienced and the nonprofessional. Those who assert such a doctrine forget that the intense engorgement of the capillaries of an important organ like the lungs or brain may so interfere with the performance of its function as to threaten a speedy and fatal exhaustion, while a timely bleeding, sufficient to make a well man faint, would, by relieving the oppressed organ and restoring its function, positively add to the strength of the sick one. They seem to forget that all disease or morbid action is accompanied by abnormal susceptibilities and diminished strength; and consequently that agents which might act positively injurious on organs with their normal susceptibility and action, might be exactly adapted to remove abnormal susceptibility and action and thereby restore strength and health. Without pursuing these strictures further we will briefly state a few rules which we think should govern the physician in the investigation and treatment of disease.

First, he should regard the living body as a complex organization composed of various delicately organized structures and organs, each designed to perform its own proper function and all endowed with elementary properties that distinguish them from inorganic or dead matter.

Second, he should remember that the body so organized and endowed is constantly surrounded by agents, ponderable and imponderable, so numerous and so changeable that they are capable of influencing the properties and functions of its several structures in every possible direction. Thus, some are capable of exalting the properties and inducing excited action; others of depressing the properties and inducing diminished action; while others still pervert the properties and functions, instead of simply exalting or depressing them.

Third, the physician should aim to make himself so familiar with the physiology and pathology of every structure and organ, that he is capable of analyzing the complex phenomena of disease and of tracing accurately its location, its grade of action, its stage of progress, its tendencies, and its influence on other organs more or less remote from its own location.

Having done this, he should have such a knowledge of the materia medica as will enable him to apply such remedies as are exactly adapted to the existing grade of morbid action. In doing this he will find use for depletives, sedatives, and anodynes to soothe pain and diminish excited action; for tonics and restoratives to prop up and sustain functions already impaired; and for alteratives and antidotes to correct perverted action and neutralize noxious ingredients.

Following these rules and objects, the enlightened physician will neither become a skeptical advocate of expectancy, nor an indiscriminate administrator of heroic remedies, nor yet a dreamy advocate of some vague theory by which he attempts to reduce all disease to a unit and all remedies to one principle of action, whether such theory be the *asthenia* of Brown and Todd or the similia similiabus curantur of Hahnemann. But he will become a true observer of nature in health and disease and will be ever ready to aid her when embarrassed by disease or morbid action, strictly in accordance with the dictates of an enlightened *common sense.*

AUSTIN FLINT

CONSERVATIVE MEDICINE

Editor's Note

Austin Flint (1812–86), who taught in six schools in his forty-year teaching career, was a prolific writer of books, articles, and editorials. His text of 1866, *A Treatise on the Principles and Practice of Medicine* (Philadelphia: Henry C. Lea), was one of the most popular American medical books of its time. His case records alone are said to fill nearly 17,000 folio pages. His writings reflect careful observation and recording of clinical cases, a procedure he urged his many students to follow. The work of Louis and Laennec in Paris impressed him greatly, although he did not go abroad to study. Samuel D. Gross called Flint the Sydenham of his time.[1]

This paper on "Conservative Medicine" followed in the tradition of rational therapeutics, although Flint was not as staunch a believer in nature as were Worthington Hooker or Jacob Bigelow, for instance. Flint's paper, as he explained, was inspired by the surgeons and their interest in conservative operations.

Bibliographical Note

Flint wrote two other essays dealing with a similar theme: "Conservative medicine as applied to therapeutics," *Am. J. Med. Sci.* 45 (1863): 22–43; and "Conservative medicine as applied to hygiene," ibid. 46 (1863): 361–77. These essays are collected and published as *Essays on Conservative Medicine and Kindred Topics*, Philadelphia: Lea, 1874.

For biographical information on Flint see A. S. Evans, "Austin Flint and his contributions to medicine," *Bull. Hist. Med.* 32 (1958): 224–41; and Norman Shaftel, "Austin Flint, Sr. (1812–1886): educator of physicians," *J. Med. Educ.* 35 (1960): 1122–35.

"What does the writer mean by *conservative medicine*?" This will be the mental inquiry of the reader when the caption of this article meets his eye. It is

---

Am. Med. Monthly 18 (1862): 1–24.

[1] S. D. Gross, *Autobiography*, 2 vols. (Philadelphia: Barrie, 1887) 2: 161.

desirable, first of all, for the writer to explain the subject which he ventures to hope will appear to possess interest enough to lead to a perusal of the pages which are to follow.

The meaning of *conservative surgery* is well understood. This phrase has been sufficiently common of late years. The conservative surgeon aims to preserve the integrity of the body. He spares diseased or wounded members whenever there are good grounds for believing that by skillful management they may be saved. He resorts to mutilations only when they are clearly necessary. He weighs carefully the dangers of operations, so as not to incur too much risk of shortening life by resorting to the scalpel. By conservative medicine, I mean an analogous line of conduct in the management of maladies which are not surgical. The conservative physician shrinks from employing potential remedies whenever there are good grounds for believing that diseases will pursue a favorable course without active interference. He resorts to therapeutical measures which must be hurtful if not useful only when they are clearly indicated. He appreciates injurious medication, and hence does not run a risk of shortening life by adding dangers of treatment to those of disease. Such, in brief, is an explanation of the subject of this article. For the phrase *conservative medicine* I am indebted to a distinguished friend and colleague, well known as eminently a conservative surgeon.

During the last quarter of a century a change has taken place in medical sentiment as regards surgical operations. New and grand achievements in surgery seemed formerly to be the leading objects of personal ambition. To borrow a fashionable expression, they were decidedly the rage. Boldness in the use of the knife was the trait in the character of the surgeon which was most highly admired. The history of surgery during the first third of the present century is characterized by the introduction and frequent performance of numerous formidable operations. It was customary to speak of them as brilliant, and the daring surgeon enjoyed somewhat of the *eclat* which belongs to the hero of the battlefield. This analogy was implied when one of the greatest of our American surgeons wishing to distinguish his most brilliant exploit styled it his Waterloo operation. The change that has taken place is marked. We hear now comparatively little of terrible operations and of that sort of heroism which is associated with bloody deeds. What would once have been considered as a degree of courage to be admired is now stigmatized as rashness. It is an equivocal compliment to say of a practitioner that he is a bold surgeon. The change, it may be said, is in a measure due to the fact that the great number of new operations which have been introduced since the beginning of the present century leaves but a limited range for further explorations in that direction; but this explanation will go only a little way. The change is one of sentiment. The desire is to preserve the integrity of the body, to avoid mutilations, to incur the dangers of capital operations only when they are imperatively called for—in a word, conservatism has become the ruling principle in surgery. The most important of the most recent improvements in surgery exemplify the influence of this principle on the medical mind.

An analogous change, within the same period, has taken place in medical practice. Formerly, boldness was a distinction coveted by the medical as well as by the surgical practitioner. "Heroic practice" was a favorite expression, consisting in the employment of powerful remedies or in pushing them to an enormous extent. The physician emulated the surgeon in daring. The change is not less marked in medicine than in surgery. We hear now oftener of diseases managed with little or no medication than of cases illustrating the abuse of remedies. In the treatment of many affections it is not considered necessary to employ measures which but a few years ago it would have been considered culpable to withhold. The change, too, is here one of sentiment. We desire to preserve the vital forces, to avoid the perturbations and damaging effects of potential therapeutic agencies—in short, conservatism has become a leading principle in medicine as well as in surgery. The improved method of managing a host of affections will be found to illustrate this fact.

Before proceeding further, let us inquire how the contrast between medical practice at the present moment and a quarter of a century ago should affect our estimation of medicine. Is medicine disparaged by the changes which have actually taken place? It is not enough to answer this question in the negative. Mutations, when they denote progress, are, of course, desirable. In so far as the contrast shows improvement, medicine at the present moment is deserving of esteem, the more, as the changes are great. It redounds to the glory of medicine that it admits of illimitable progressive changes. In this fact lies the distinctive feature of legitimate medicine as contrasted with illegitimate systems of practice. But, some one may say, is there to be no stability in medicine, no traditional authority, and is reverence for the past to have no influence? If not, where is our ground of confidence in the practice of the present day? And is it not probable that at the end of another quarter of a century mutations will have occurred twice as great as those which have taken place during the last twenty-five years? These questions are to be met fairly and squarely; let us endeavor so to meet them. . . .

All that society can claim of medicine in any generation is the capabilities of the medical science in that generation. All that society can claim of physicians is that these capabilities shall be understood and judiciously applied. But we are opening up trains of thought which will lead us a long way from our subject, and we must abruptly return to the consideration of conservative medicine.

It is an interesting point of inquiry, whence came the influences leading to conservatism as a principle of medical practice? The answer to this inquiry would not be the same in all countries and sections. It must be admitted that in our country the earliest and fullest development of the principle was in New England. Our New England brethren are fond of dating a new order of medical ideas from the publication of an address more than twenty years ago, by Jacob

Bigelow, on the self-limited character of certain diseases. Not underrating the importance of that publication, the spirit of the oral teachings of James Jackson and John Ware has exerted on the medical mind of New England an influence which can only be appreciated by those who have experienced it. To those who have known experimentally the value of their teachings, it is a source of deep regret that the influence of these admirable professors has not been more widely diffused by means of larger contributions to medical literature. British conservatists attribute much to the writings of Dr. Forbes. Among the nonmedical observers of the change in practice which has taken place, some have been persuaded that it is due to the disciples of Hahnemann, an idea too preposterous to need refutation. The truth is, we are not to look for the causes of the change exclusively in the views emanating from particular persons. It is rather a legitimate result of scientific researches in different directions. If we were to specify circumstances which have more especially been instrumental in leading to the principle of conservatism, we would mention, *first*, the abandonment of the attempt to found a system or theory of medicine after the decline and fall of Brunonianism and Broussaisism; and *second*, the study of diseases after the numerical method with reference to their natural history and laws.

Strange as it appears, the importance of determining by clinical observation the intrinsic tendencies of different diseases at the basis of therapeutics seems to have been heretofore overlooked. Physicians have acted on the presumption that most diseases do not pursue a favorable course without treatment more or less efficient. This has been, to a still greater extent, the popular belief. The apparent proof of the success of the Hahnemannic treatment rests on this belief. What are the facts already ascertained with respect to the intrinsic tendencies of different diseases? We know that diseases in the management of which but a few years ago the physician would not dare to omit potent therapeutical measures, almost invariably end in recovery without any active treatment. Take, as examples, pneumonia, limited to a single lobe, and acute pleurisy. It is sufficiently settled that these diseases involve very little danger in themselves, proving fatal only in consequences of complications. The practitioner, therefore, no longer feels obliged to employ blood-letting, mercurialization, cathartics, blisters, etc., in these diseases, with reference to the saving of life. The only question is, do patients pass through these diseases as well without as with such measures of treatment? Clinical observation following up this inquiry arrives at results which exemplify conservative medicine.

Our acquaintance with the natural history of the great majority of diseases is, as yet, very incomplete. Knowledge of the tendencies of diseases allowed to pursue their course without active treatment is not readily acquired. We cannot conscientiously withhold remedies which we have reason to believe may prove useful. Cases are therefore to be slowly accumulated in which, from circumstances not under our control, diseases have been uninfluenced by therapeutic interference. This knowledge, it is evident, is the true point of departure for the

study of the effects of remedies as regards the termination and duration of
diseases. The information already obtained has rendered the use of powerful
therapeutic agencies far less common than they were but a few years since. It
remains to be seen hereafter what will be the further effect on medical practice
of continued researches in this direction.

Conservative medicine assumes that remedial measures, according to their
potency, must either do harm or good; that they can never be neither hurtful
nor useful. Prior to the advent of conservatism, this important fact was not duly
appreciated. Blows were leveled at diseases, but the patient was not enough
considered. It did not enter sufficiently into the calculations of practitioners
that if successive blows dealt at a disease were misdirected, the effect was not
lost, but injury was inflicted in proportion to their force. Hence, it must needs
follow that the sick man sometimes encountered, in addition to his malady,
assaults not less real because well meant. In this respect, certainly, we have
evidence of progress. We are satisfied that we do not err in saying that the most
judicious practitioners of the present day accept the following maxims of that
eminently conservative physician, Chomel: *first*, that we are not so much to
treat diseases, as patients affected with disease; and *second*, that not to do harm
is no less an object of treatment than to do good.

In defining conservative medicine, we have seen that it expresses a characteristic of the improvements in medical practice during the last twenty-five years. Let
us now direct our attention to illustrations afforded by some of the different
classes of remedial measures. And, first of all, blood-letting suggests itself. How
great the change as regards this remedy! Twenty-five years ago it was employed
as if it were an innocuous remedy. Practitioners thought much more of the risk
of not resorting to it when it was needed than of the evils of its being needlessly
resorted to. Hence, they often acted on the rule inculcated by a medical writer,
viz., when in doubt use the lancet. How different the rule of treatment now!
Few practitioners of the present day would resort to this remedy in any case in
which its appropriateness seemed to them questionable. Why not? Because it has
been ascertained to be a spoliative remedy. It causes a disproportionate loss of
the corpuscular elements of the blood, which are slowly regenerated. These
corpuscular elements are already deficient in many diseases. In short, anemia and
its pathological relations were very imperfectly understood a quarter of a century ago. It is clear now to everyone, that if not indicated, blood-letting should
never be employed. This simple statement explains, in a great measure, the
comparative disuse of blood-letting. The great question now is, whether it is a
remedy called for more or less frequently in the management of certain diseases,
chiefly the acute inflammations. I do not propose to enter here into a discussion
of this question. This much may be said: Clinical observation, which is alone
competent to settle the question, has shown that it is a remedy not called for so
often or to so great an extent in acute inflammations as was supposed but a few
years ago. A single incidental remark with respect to blood-letting, and it is one

which will apply to other remedies: In determining its influence for good or evil by means of clinical observation, it is not enough to take into account the ratio of recoveries and the duration of cases of disease. Blood-letting may not increase the mortality from a disease, nor protract its continuance, and yet prove injurious. The injury may be manifest only in the slowness of convalescence and the impaired condition of the system after recovery.

Cathartics were prescribed a quarter of a century ago much more generally and to a much greater extent that at the present time. In fact, purgation was considered as rarely out of place, whatever might be the nature or seat of the disease. This harmonized with the notion that very many diseases originated in, and nearly all were liable to be perpetuated by, causes acting within the alimentary canal. . . .

It is needless to remind the reader familiar with the practice current twenty-five years ago, of the frequency with which emetics were employed. Of morbid causes referred to the alimentary canal, a large share were supposed to exist in the *prima viae*—an expression then often used by writers and in common parlance. The same notion taken up by the public was conveyed by the homely expression "foulness of the stomach." Emetics were prescribed by physicians to remove saburral matters and vomiting desired by patients as a cleansing operation. Severe and prolonged vomiting by lobelia, in conjunction with the vapor bath, constituted the Thomsonian practice, which, in certain parts of our country, for several years was considerably patronized. At the present time, emesis, irrespective of cases of poisoning and over-repletion, is rarely produced, excepting as incidental to the use of remedies not prescribed for that purpose, such as the nauseant sedatives, colchicum, veratrum viride, etc. What would be thought of a practitioner now who treated cases of phthisis with emetics repeated almost daily! Yet, within the memories of physicians of twenty-five years' standing, this practice has been advocated and to some extent adopted. The progress of medical conservatism has led to the abandonment of emetics as perturbatory and debilitating agents, excepting in the rare instances in which they subserve an explicit purpose.

The practice of the present time presents a striking contrast with that twenty-five years ago, as regards the use of counterirritant applications. The physician whose professional career has already extended over that period is sometimes reminded of the severe measures then in vogue by the exhibition of indelible scars on the bodies of his old patients. He is not likely now to contemplate these traces of his former vigorous practice with lively gratification. Blisters, sometimes applied successively over the same space, and not diminutive in size, tartar-emetic ointment and plasters, issues, the moxa, etc., were considered as among the most efficient of the means of influencing the cure of a host of local affections. How much less frequently are they now used and, when counterirritation is deemed advisable, how much milder are the applications chosen! Physicians were strongly impressed with the belief that local affections were often removed by revulsion. They accepted the doctrine of Hunter, that two diseases rarely concur and, hence, that an artificial disease is likely to effect a cure by a process of displacement. Not only has this doctrine been disproved by pathological researches, but these have shown a large number of the local diseases formerly regarded as primary, to be the secondary or tertiary effects of morbid conditions then unknown. Bright's disease had not been discovered, and its multitudinous pathological consequences were, of course, unintelligible. In those days solidism prevailed, and hematology has been since created. Physicians made no account of blood-poisons, and the old humoral notions of coction and fermentation had not been revived under the modern but equally indefinite garb of catalysis. Mr. Farr had not invented the name Zymosis, a name expressive of our ignorance rather than conveying any precise knowledge, but, nevertheless, significant of a wide and most important leap from the doctrine of solidism; or, in other words, of a passage backward, guided by the light of modern science, to humoralism which, as Rokitansky remarks, is simply a requisition of common sense. This change in pathological views, in conjunction with clinical observation, has led physicians to distrust more and more the value of counterirritant applications and, at all events, to conclude that severe revulsive measures are rarely called for; hence, the change in practice is in conformity to the principle of conservatism.

The contrast as regards the use of mercury affords a signal instance of progressive change. The remarkable efficacy of this remedy in certain affections naturally led to the expectation of its utility in many diseases. Mercurialization being a disease, it accorded with the current belief of the incompatibility of different affections, to suppose that it displaced other diseases. It was considered as *par excellence* an *alterative* remedy; and what a latitude for imagined results was afforded by that title! Moreover, its supposed special action on the liver accorded with the notion that the secretion of bile had much to do with morbid phenomena. The relief or prevention of portal congestion was incidental to its hepatic effects. It lessened exudations; it promoted the absorption of morbid products; it altered the secretions; it dispelled local engorgements and, by exciting stomatitis, it acted by way of revulsion. Waiving here, as in the other instances, discussion of the actual value of this remedy, the extravagance of the views formerly entertained is now sufficiently evident. The statements of those who have made war upon this article of the materia medica, and the popular prejudices thereby produced, are equally, or still more, extravagant; but it is a remedy potent for harm when inappropriate, as it is powerful for good when indicated; and, therefore, the great change that has taken place as regards its use exemplifies conservatism.

These examples are sufficient to show how conservative medicine is illustrated by recent improvements as regards the employment of particular therapeutic measures. They furnish evidence of immense progress in practical medicine. Let not this statement be misunderstood. The improvements which have been noticed consist in the restricted use of blood-letting, cathartics, emetics, counterirritants, and mercurials. Does the restricted use of these measures detract from their real therapeutic value? Not at all. Medicine has by no means repudiated them. She employs them with better judgment and discrimination; thus, availing herself of the good they can accomplish, she escapes the evils arising from their injudicious and indiscriminate use.

If we look at the progress of medicine during the last quarter of a century from another point of view, we find additional examples of conservatism. Regarding it exclusively from the point of view already taken, it appears that in proportion as the practice of medicine has improved, reliance on certain active or heroic measures of treatment has diminished. This is true, but it is not the whole truth. Some measures are employed with much more freedom now than a few years ago. The use of opium and alcoholic stimulants, in certain diseases, affords the most striking illustrations of this truth. These instances also exemplify the principle of conservatism. Opium and alcohol, in excessive doses, occasion immediate disorder of more or less gravity and may destroy life. But given so as not to incur any risk of these effects, they do not conflict with conservatism, because their operation is transient, and unless their use be continued they do not leave behind them damaging effects. Given in quantities which are confortably borne, they certainly do not impair the vital forces by perturbation, by loss of fluids, by affecting the constitution of the blood, or by inducing local changes, as do the measures previously noticed. This statement, of course, has nothing to do with the ulterior consequences, moral and physical, of intemperance or opium-eating. Here, too, as in other instances, discussion of the *modus operandi* of remedies is waived. Most physicians will agree in the statement that, when indicated as remedies, opium and alcohol sustain the vital forces. In this respect they are positively conservative. But a point of distinction is, when not indicated, if given within certain limits and not continued, they are neither spoliative, exhausting, disturbing, nor disorganizing, as are various other measures and, therefore, not like the latter even then, antagonistical to conservative medicine. . . .

A comparison of cases of pulmonary tuberculosis now and twenty-five years ago illustrates the importance of the practical views just presented. The management of this disease twenty-five years ago was certainly not in accordance with the principle of conservatism. The measures employed, medicinal and hygienic, were, indeed, directly opposed to this principle. The antiphlogistic system of treatment was often adopted, under the belief that inflammation was the most important element of the local affection. Blood-letting, cathartics, mercurialization, severe counterirritation were considered as remedial, and to these were conjoined low diet and confinement within doors. Now, pulmonary tuberculosis is not cured in the majority of cases, although it is not incurable; and there is reason to believe that the proportion of cures is considerably larger than under the treatment just referred to. But, directing attention to the incurable cases, under the plan of treatment generally pursued at the present time, which is eminently conservative, how striking the contrast! Formerly, the instances of rapid progress of the disease were more numerous, and it almost invariably advanced with a steady march, rarely occupying many months in completing its fatal career. Patients were usually confined to the bed for weeks before death, lingering on the borders of the grave, suffering from extreme debility, bed-sores, aphthae, and colliquative diarrhea. It was difficult to conceive of a picture more distressing and repulsive than that of an unfortunate being in the last stage of consumption. Conservatism has done much towards ameliorating the condition of consumptives, even when it is hopeless as regards recovery. Cases of so-called galloping consumption are less frequent. Life is not infrequently prolonged and made comparatively confortable for years. It is not uncommon to meet with instances of a considerable deposit of tubercle remaining quiescent or progressing very slowly and the patient able to engage in the active occupations and enjoyments of life. Even when the disease is progressing to a fatal termination, the strength is usually so far preserved that a bedridden consumptive is now rarely seen, and it is not uncommon for patients to be out of doors almost up to the hour of their death. I appeal to those whose medical experience has extended over a quarter of a century for the truthfulness of this comparison.

In concluding these fragmentary remarks, let it be borne in mind that important as is conservatism in medical practice it is by no means inconsistent with the employment of efficient therapeutic agencies in the management of diseases. The conservative surgeon does not hesitate to use the knife and dismember the body when convinced that thereby he may save life. So the conservative physician resorts without hesitation to his potential remedies—not less potent for good or evil than the scalpel—whenever he sees clearly that they will contribute to the safety and welfare of the patient.

EDOUARD SEGUIN

CLINICAL THERMOMETRY

Editor's Note

Edouard Seguin (1812–80) was born and educated in France. He came to the United States at mid-century and soon established himself in the field of education for the mentally deficient. His son, Edward C. (1843–98) became a well-known neurologist in New York and, owing to the similarity of the names, is often confused with his father. The elder Seguin published several books on thermometry in the 1870's. The fever chart in the article that follows was one of the earliest to appear in the American medical literature.

Of the medical developments introduced in the mid-nineteenth century, certainly the diagnostic instruments were of the first order of importance. The microscope was successfully used by pathologists studying disease and by biologists studying tissue reactions and phenomena of growth, healing, cell morphology, and reproduction. The ophthalmoscope, laryngoscope, and the binaural stethoscope played an increasingly important role in physical diagnosis after about 1860. At the same time the use of the clinical thermometer, not a new invention, was urged on physicians in Europe and America. As in most things medical and scientific, Europe took the lead—both in development and discovery as well as in introduction for standard use.

Writing just a few months before Edouard Seguin published the article that follows, his fellow New Yorker, Austin Flint, pointed out that, "Hitherto, in this country, the thermometer has been but little used in medical investigations, owing, probably, to a prudential reserve with regard to novelties. Many, however, are now interested in confirming, by personal observation, the correctness of what has been set forth in publications on the other side of the Atlantic."[1]

Bibliographical Note

Charles L. Dana, "The Seguins of New York," *Ann. Med. Hist.* 6 (1924): 475–79.

Ivor Kraft, "Edouard Seguin and 19th century moral treatment of idiots," *Bull. Hist. Med.* 35 (1961): 393–418.

E. Seguin, *Medical Thermometry and Human Temperature*, New York: Wood, 1876. In 1873 Seguin published an earlier version entitled *Family Thermometry*.

Med. Record 1 (1866–67): 516–19.

[1] Austin Flint, "Remarks on the use of the thermometer in diagnosis and prognosis," *New York Med. J.* 4 (1866): 81–93.

For a history of the use of thermometers and measurement of temperature in medicine, see the standard European work by C. A. Wunderlich, *On the Temperature in Diseases: A Manual of Medical Thermometry*, trans. from 2nd German ed., London: New Sydenham Society, 1871.

A few words on vital thermometry will help us to understand the range of clinical thermometry.

John Davy's name will remain intimately connected with the origin of animal and human thermometry. His observations, made upon many men and animals, were carried on in Europe, Asia, and Africa with a small pocket thermometer and a strong passion for his undertaking. The results of his experiments were very imperfect, owing to his applying the instrument under the tongue, where the temperature is constantly changed by the current of air. Nevertheless, Davy's observations determined the difference between warm- and cold-blooded animals; the former whose physiological temperature never falls below 96.5°F.; and the latter, whose heat never rises above 82.5°F. and may fall as low as 74°F., thus putting an impassable barrier of at least 14 degrees between the two classes of animals. This is due to Davy (1803).

Though in common with others he made also many pathological observations with the thermometer, they had no clinical import because they were not based upon a correct physiological standard. It is not out of place in this connection to relate the following anecdote.

The little thermometer of Davy once became famous for having accomplished a miracle, which was as follows: Doctors Beddoes, Coleridge, and Davy had undertaken to cure a desperate case of rheumatism by some new remedy, and previous to giving it, Dr. Davy, according to his irrepressible habit, wanted to ascertain the temperature of the patient. But no sooner was the thermometer between the patient's teeth than he exclaimed "that the instrument was operating," and that he felt better. The physicians, in the presence of such a curious instance of moral action, did not administer their drug, but continued the application of the instrument, with the effect of loosening the stiffened limbs and restoring the cripple to active life in a fortnight.

After John Davy, French physicians seemed to have taken up the question of animal heat. To Brechet, and Drs. Becquerel and Jules Seguin (the last-named submitting himself to tedious and painful experiments) belong the honor of having established with their thermoelectrical apparatus the standard of human physiological temperature (98.5 F.), which external agencies can make to vary but a few tenths of a degree more or less. True, Brechet and his then (1838) young associates left to subsequent observers the task of finding out the second term of the problem, viz.: that any greater deviation above or below that standard, testified to inward anomaly or disease.

After these, further experiments upon human temperature were made by the Germans. Here, Wünderlich appears, with his half-million clinical observations, as the founder of clinical thermometry, with Traube, of Berlin, L. Thomas, Uhle, etc. The German school took the discovery of Brechet as the basis of physiological thermometry.

The normal temperature of the human body at completely sheltered parts of its surface amounts to 98.5° Fahrenheit.

The average variations of a few tenths announced by Brechet, and certified by the numerous observations of Professor Traube, are as follows:

98.24°	Fahr.,	7 A.M.
98.69	Fahr.,	10 A.M.
98.65	Fahr.,	1 P.M.
98.78	Fahr.,	5 P.M.
98.24	Fahr.,	7 P.M.

PATHOLOGICAL THERMOMETRY

What does pathological thermometry teach us?

1st. A rise in the thermometer above 99°F. is an index of the existence of fever.

2d. A fall under 97.3°F. is the index of the presence of a devitalizing agency, such as that at work in cholera.

3d. An elevation of the pathological temperature in the evening is the rule in the period of pyrexia.

(There are febrile states in which, on the contrary, exacerbations occur in the morning.)

4th. A decrease in the temperature in the evening is the rule in the period of *defervescence* and indicates recovery.

5th. An increase of the same precedes, by several hours, the occurrence of fever; that is to say, long before the pulse could tell it.

6th. A sudden increase in the previous uniform or descendent course of the temperature portends some unexpected complication or intercurrent disease.

7th. Each regular disease is thus shown to run in two periods; one of increase, marked by *effervescence* (ebullition of Sydenham) or elevation of temperature; the other of decrease, marked by *defervescence* or abatement of temperature.

8th. When cure is to take place, *effervescence* goes on steadily to what may be termed its pathological height in each disease.

9th. *Defervescence* follows *effervescence* with the same regularity till the temperature of the body has reached the physiological standard, after passing in a more or less marked manner through morning and evening oscillations.

10th. When cure is not to take place, the *effervescence* is more protracted or attains higher degrees; or the *defervescence*, instead of presenting a gradual falling off to the physiological standard, falls suddenly below it and terminal coldness soon closes the record.

If we could deviate from our immediate subject, which refers particularly to the use of the thermometer in diagnosis, we might insist with advantage upon its value as a means of estimating the effects of remedies, and controlling therapeutics. Dr. W. H. Draper says in this respect: "From my own experience in the use of the instrument, I am convinced that it will furnish one of the best tests, perhaps the best that we can have in the administration of alcoholic stimulants in febrile conditions. We have had occasion to observe the utility of the instrument for this purpose at the N. Y. Hospital." Thus are confirmed the early previsions of Davy and his compeers, who lacked only the fundamental point (98.5°, of Brechet and his disciples), to introduce thermometrical positivism as the *mètre* (measurer) of therapeutic action of medicines. Indeed, the thermometer is already a medical power; and, like all powers, nobody knows today to what use it may be adapted tomorrow.

The following are the propositions established lastly by Dr. T. A. Compton, of Dublin, "*Temperature in Acute Disease,*" London, 1860.

1st. That a continued daily temperature of 99° Fah., and upwards, indicates an unhealthy condition and occurs in every case of acute disease. As I have never met with one case in which such a temperature was present under normal conditions in a healthy adult, and as every case of the two hundred taken exhibits this state of temperature, the proposition may be considered to be proved.

2d. That any one observation of a very high temperature (such as 105° Fah.), in any case in which the general symptoms do not appear of any particular severity, should lead to a very attentive re-examination and suggest a very careful watching, especially if occurring in a nondiagnosed case; such a temperature being present only in severe forms of any disease.

3d. That the thermometer is of great use as a means of diagnosis in those cases, which frequently present themselves, of general *malaise*, often accompanied by a history of rigors, loss of sleep, etc.; such symptoms being due either to the commencement of some acute disease or merely to some gastric or uterine disturbance of a temporary character.

4th. That the temperature in every disease has a tendency to run a peculiar course and has a certain range of altitude, a knowledge of which course and range is of great value as an assistance to us in diagnosis and prognosis.

5th. From the last proposition it follows that the same altitude of the thermometer attained at one period of any disease is not of the same importance as the same height reached at another time in the same disease.

6th. That although in all diseases a high range of temperature generally indicates a severe case with a slow convalescence, and a low range usually occurs in a mild case and is followed by a rapid convalescence; yet there is no actual temperature in any disease which necessarily foretells a fatal determination. Thus I have registered 105.6° Fah. in a severe case of typhus ending favorably, 106.3° Fah. in erysipelas, 105.3° in typhoid; and each of these temperatures was the highest I ever took in the respective diseases.

7th. That in the majority of cases a rise of temperature is contemporary with a rise of pulse, but that, on the other hand, there appears generally to be but little connection between temperature and frequency of respirations.

8th. That where the temperature and pulse together do not coincide with the general symptoms, the two former may be generally relied on as to the actual state.

9th. That where the temperature and general symptoms agree together, but do not coincide with the state of the pulse, the two former may generally be relied on as to the actual state.

10th. That in those cases in which the pulse and general symptoms remain the same, a moderate fall of temperature on one occasion is not to be relied on; but should such a fall continue in a moderate and gradual manner for some days and at such a period when a fall was to have been expected, the temperature may then be depended upon. Severe cases of typhus, towards their close, often give examples of this sort.

11th. That in those cases in which the pulse and general symptoms continue the same, being the one frequent and the other severe, a continuous rise of temperature for some days, occurring at a period of disease at which some improvement might generally be expected, is usually the precursor of a fatal termination.

12th. That although it is possible that the state of the temperature alone in acute disease may, perhaps, hereafter prove to be the one safest symptom to rely upon if taken by itself (and I believe it is at present, at least, equal to the state of the pulse and of greater value than this certainly, if only its frequency be taken into account), yet the temperature must be considered merely as an aid, and all other symptoms must be carefully examined, as it is on comparison with these that its greatest value is always to be found.

But the indications of pathological thermometry may be expressed more in accordance with the views of Wünderlich, as follows. Thus we would say, again:

1st. The thermometer gives indications of sudden changes in health, and even permits us to appreciate their imminence.

2d. It detects latent though important diseases.

3d. It corrects—in the course of a settled disease—hasty appreciations and decides doubtful points.

4th. It determines the stage—otherwise inappreciable—of a disease whose previous history is unknown.

5th. It reveals—often timely—complications or changes which may have taken place insidiously or unexpectedly.

6th. It unveils masked fevers* and points earlier than any other sign to a fatal prognosis. Its opposite indications predict recovery.

7th. It enlarges by an entirely new series of facts our circle of pathological phenomena.

8th. In the diagnosis and prognosis of general diseases, the thermometer, whether alone or concurrently with the other vital signs, presents the same character of *positivism* evinced by auscultation, percussion, and mensuration in localized affections.

But clinical thermometry is never practiced alone. On the contrary, it is supported by the study of other symptoms, and its indications are mostly collected with those given by the pulse-beats and the breathing; forming in their ensemble and continuity "the record of the three great vital signs."

This triple observation necessitates the formation of a diagram (in itself an important instrument of diagnosis), upon which the rise and fall of the vital signs are not only recorded daily but connected from morning to night by curves or lines. This triple track of diseases may be seen illustrated in German and English publications, but is in none of them better devised than in the *facsimile* given below.

Of the three component parts of clinical thermometry, we have explained two, the thermometer and the diagram; it remains to speak of the reading. But who can read thermometry on the diagram if he cannot write it? Here the question is merely practical.

Practically, England has contributed the labors of Aitken on thermometry (vulgarization of German doctrines) and thermometrical observations in fevers and pneumonia (clinical records, bearing mostly on the question of *defervescence*), also, of S. Ringer, "on the temperature of the body as a means of diagnosis in phthisis and tuberculosis," accompanied by eight diagrams showing the average heat in these affections to be higher by several degrees than the physiological standard, 98.5°F.

Already the part taken by American physicians in this new movement is not inconsiderable. Thermometry was introduced late in 1865 in the New York, and later in the Bellevue Hospital (and likely in others that we ignore). Dr. William H. Draper had his own diagram of the vital signs appended to the head of the beds of his patients in the first-named institution; and Professor Austin Flint uses in Bellevue the diagram of Dr. Da Costa. Several articles on thermometry have been published by the medical press. One (already referred to), in the *Chicago Medical Journal* of May last; and another, by Dr. Flint, in the New York *Medical Journal* for November. Every sign seems to point to an early generalization of thermometry in hospital and private American practice.

---

*In French, *fièvres larvées*, so specific an expression that it would be very appropriate in English also.

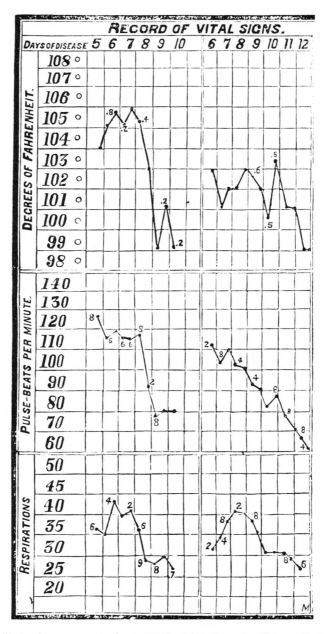

Diagram illustrating two cases of pneumonia, taken from the *Chicago Medical Journal* for May, 1866; article on "The Use of the Thermometer in Clinical Medicine," by Edward C. Seguin, M.D., New York.

It has been said, against the use of the thermometer, that it takes too much time—more time than a practitioner can afford to bestow upon a single case. The objection is grave, but, happily, unfounded. "A sensitive thermometer, placed in the axilla, will, if there is considerable elevation of temperature, rise above the normal degree of heat within the first minute and will exhibit the actual temperature in five; but if it is warmed in the hand before applying, the indication may be obtained in one or two minutes." (Wünderlich, *On the Use of the Thermometer in Private Practice*.) This is the result of the experience of the master with very delicate thermometers. . . .

Where is the physician who cannot give to one patient the five or ten minutes necessary to obtain the full rise of mercury in a thermometer? And who, after reading these few graphic lines, cannot use the thermometer at the bedside?

Thus the thermometer is the instrument of precision by which human heat is measured, as the watch is another with which the pulse-beats are counted. Any physician who can practice without a watch may think that he can diagnosticate without a thermometer. But, like other men, physicians, to do delicate work, need mathematical instruments, meters, compasses, lenses, etc., so as to embrace in the sphere of their judgment phenomena unsuspected by the unaided senses.

Having paid a full tribute to the virtues of the thermometer, we may now refer to what it has not done yet and is expected to do.

It answers very well to measure the general temperature of the body, taken at completely sheltered places; but we must acknowledge that it is not fitted to measure the abnormal temperature of local inflammation upon open surfaces. It would be often desirable that an excess of local heat might be compared, at its different stages, with the normal heat of surrounding healthy parts; and we do not doubt that some mathematical genius will yet devise a kind of thermometer whose broad and yielding bulb shall adapt itself to any surface of the body, at the same time that its superstructure shall be isolated from atmospheric influence. What mankind needs man finds.

And lastly, so far, clinical thermometry has been studied more in its concordance than in its discordance with the other vital signs—pulse-beats and breathing. From this concordance very interesting conclusions have been drawn and even diseases are recognized (read) by German students by simply looking at diagrams. But it may be already affirmed that when the discordances of the vital signs among themselves shall have been studied as well, many new and useful conclusions will be arrived at, and symptoms of diseases already obscure will be evinced.

Let us borrow our last word on the subject from Wünderlich himself:

> The thermometer is indispensable for the exact observation of fever patients. Had we been accustomed to its use, history of diseases, unaccompanied by continuous thermometrical observations, would seem as defective as would reports on diseases of the lungs, heart, spleen, or liver without indications of the physical signs; affections of the brain, unaccom-

panied by accounts of psychical function; and maladies of the intestinal canal, in which no mention is made of the alvine discharges. Perhaps some may complain of the institution of these observations as a new burden, just as was said of the stethoscope and pleximeter. But this must be got over; and the time is not distant when no physician will venture to pronounce upon a febrile disease without the application of the thermometer, etc. (Ib. *On the Employment of the Thermometer at the Bedside.*)

FRANCIS DELAFIELD

SOME FORMS OF DYSPEPSIA

Editor's Note

Francis Delafield (1841–1915) was born in New York, where his father was a successful teacher and practitioner; he thus belonged to that first generation of American physicians who helped transform medicine into a laboratory science as well as a bedside art. He spent much of his time doing what we would call pathology. In addition to numerous papers on a variety of subjects, Delafield was the author of a widely used text, *A Hand-book of Post-mortem Examinations and of Morbid Anatomy*, and co-author of *A Hand-book of Pathological Anatomy and Histology*, with T. M. Prudden, that went through a sixteenth edition as late as 1936.[1]

Dyspepsia, literally bad digestion, is a term still found in a variety of forms in modern medical dictionaries. In clinical practice today one does not often encounter it, although until fairly recent times it was a common diagnosis. In the nineteenth century some even called it the typical American disease. In the severer form of gastric or duodenal ulcer, of course, it is still common, and, if we are to believe Madison Avenue, hyperacidity is still the great American disorder.

Austin Flint, in his 1866 *Treatise on the Principles and Practice of Medicine*,[2] devoted more than eleven pages to dyspepsia, calling it also by several terms still used by laymen today: a fit of indigestion, sick headache, or bilious attack. In contrast to Delafield, Flint pointed out the relationship of dyspepsia to the mental condition of the patient. Proper diet, avoidance of excesses and irregularities of meals, psychological support, and some drugs were his recommended remedies.

By the time of William Osler's famous textbook of medicine in the 1890's the disease was referred to as chronic gastritis and gastralgia (painful stomach). The latter Osler subsumed under the heading "Neurosis of the Stomach."[3]

Series of Am. Clin. Lectures 2 (1876): 67–80.

[1] Francis Delafield, *A Hand-book of Post-mortem Examinations and of Morbid Anatomy* (New York: Wood, 1872); Francis Delafield and T. Mitchell Prudden, *A Hand-book of Pathological Anatomy and Histology* (New York: Wood, 1885).

[2] Austin Flint, *A Treatise on the Principles and Practice of Medicine* (Philadelphia: Lea, 1866), pp. 364–74.

[3] William Osler, *The Principles and Practice of Medicine* (2nd ed.; New York: Appleton, 1895), pp. 374–90.

We see during every year at the college clinique, a considerable number of patients suffering from dyspepsia. In other words, they are patients suffering from a number of unpleasant symptoms, and these symptoms are due to the fact that their food is not properly digested.

In treating these patients, we can sometimes determine which of the viscera concerned in the digestive process is in fault. You know that the digestion and absorption of our food is effected by the physiological action of the stomach, the small and large intestine, and the liver. You will find, in practice, that you can distinguish cases of dyspepsia dependent upon diseased function of the stomach, others due to the condition of the small intestine, others to that of the large intestine, others to that of the liver. Of the pancreas, our knowledge does not enable us to speak.

It is not by any means always, however, that you can make the diagnosis of stomach dyspepsia, intestinal dyspepsia, liver dyspepsia, as the case may be; you will find some patients in whom none of the viscera act normally, and other patients in whom the symptoms do not enable you to locate the disease.

After excluding all these cases, however, you will still find many persons in whom only one of the digestive organs is at fault.

Now let us see what are the characteristic symptoms of the different anatomical varieties of dyspepsia and, first, what are the symptoms of dyspepsia dependent on an abnormal state of the stomach.

The symptoms are nausea and vomiting, pain, loss of appetite, eructations of gas and of sour fluid.

The nausea and vomiting follow the ingestion of food and seem to be directly due to the presence of the food. There may be only slight nausea after each meal or every meal may be followed by vomiting. Both the nausea and vomiting may follow every meal or they may select some part of the day—morning, noon, or evening—and only occur after the meal taken at that time. In some patients, such a condition of nausea and vomiting will continue for years. The vomited matters consist only of food or of food mixed with a sour fluid; of this, the patient may vomit several quarts during each attack.

The pain also follows eating: it varies from a mere feeling of oppression to the most intense agony. The pain, like the vomiting, seems to be due to the presence of food in the stomach and is usually relieved if the stomach is emptied. The pain is regularly followed by a desire to vomit, and after this is done the pain ceases. A fragment of bread not larger than a chestnut, remaining in the stomach, is sometimes sufficient to keep up the pain and retching for hours until it is expelled. The appetite is usually small, capricious, and unnatural. The patients often dread to take food on account of the pain and vomiting which they know will follow. In the older cases, there are frequent eructations of gas from the stomach. These may be so frequent and noisy as to be a serious annoyance. If the stomach be dilated, as is sometimes the case, this can be distinguished by percussion and palpation.

If the disease is of long standing and severe, the patients lose flesh and strength and present a very deplorable appearance.

The lesions consist in a chronic inflammation of the mucous coat of the stomach, with a loss of power in the muscular coat. The inner surface of the organ is constantly coated with an increased quantity of tenacious mucus. The connective tissue between the gastric tubules is increased in amount, and the tubules themselves become atrophied. The stomach is sometimes found very small, in other cases much dilated.

The milder cases of the disease can often be cured by regulating the diet and life of the patient, without much resort to medical treatment. The severer cases are only temporarily benefited by such means.

The patient whom we shall discuss to-day is an example of the more severe form of stomach dyspepsia. She is an Irish servant girl, forty years old. About two years ago she began to have pain and vomiting after her meals. After nine weeks these symptoms ceased, and she enjoyed tolerable health until eight months ago. At that time, she again began to vomit about fifteen minutes after eating. At the same time, there was a dull boring pain in the epigastric region and extending into the back. She has never vomited blood. The pain and vomiting continued; she became much emaciated and was so feeble as to remain in bed much of the time. Her appetite continued to be good; her bowels were somewhat constipated. I saw her for the first time five months after the commencement of her illness. She was then very feeble and emaciated. She had been put under a variety of medical treatment and had been kept on a milk diet for some time, but without relief. The pain and vomiting would cease for a few hours or a few days and then return.

In the epigastric region was a globular tumor, tympanitic on percussion, which I supposed to be the dilated stomach. At that time, three months ago, I stopped all drugs and washed out her stomach with the stomach pump every day. This treatment was continued, with occasional intermissions, for two months. The pain and vomiting became less frequent and then ceased entirely. She has steadily recovered her strength and flesh and is now able to work. For the past month the pumping has been discontinued, and her health has continued good.

As a companion to this case, let me read you the history of a gentleman who has been under my care for a considerable length of time. He is a man forty-five years old, by occupation a broker. About sixteen years ago he began to have attacks of pain and discomfort in the epigastric region, lasting several days, and ending in an attack of vomiting. These attacks occurred about once in four weeks. At that time his habits were irregular. His food was often eaten hastily, he worked hard during the day, used stimulants pretty freely, and frequently ate late dinners and suppers. In this condition he continued until about six years ago. At that time the attacks of pain and vomiting gradually became more frequent, were more readily excited by indiscretions in diet, and left the patient feeble and prostrated for several days. Any preparation of alcohol was almost certain to bring on one of these attacks. From time to time he consulted different physicians and followed out several plans of treatment. On several occasions he became so much better as to think himself cured, but, sooner or later, the old symptoms always returned. The attacks of pain and vomiting gradually became more and more frequent, until they occurred almost every day. The pain was always the most distressing symptom, and the patient would often voluntarily excite vomiting in order to relieve the distress.

Finally, he was placed on a milk diet. This diet he carried out strictly for six months. For the first four months the attacks of pain and vomiting ceased, but after that time again recurred.

In the summer of 1874 he came under my care. I commenced to wash out his stomach with the pump, at first, every other day, and then every day. He soon learned to use the instrument himself and has continued to use it up to the present time. He eats all the ordinary articles of diet, has gained much in flesh and strength, and with ordinary prudence in diet could easily give up the pump altogether. But, as he finds he can always prevent the bad effects of improper food, he is apt to take good dinners and suppers as he pleases and pump himself out afterwards.

These two cases will give you an idea of what I mean by dyspepsia confined to the stomach.

You will observe that in both cases we have the same set of symptoms—attacks of pain and vomiting, coming on, first at long, and then at short intervals. The attacks always excited by the ingestion of food, and the pain ceasing when the stomach is emptied; the disease lasting for years, and growing steadily worse. Medical treatment alleviates the symptoms for longer or shorter intervals, but never permanently.

For these cases I believe the most rational and effectual treatment to be the systematic use of the stomach pump.

The cause of the attacks seems always to be the presence of undigested food in the stomach. The longer the disease lasts, the less tolerant does the stomach become of any such substance, until, at last, every day there is an attack of pain and vomiting.

Why the stomach should become so irritable and intolerant of the presence of food, I do not know. Autopsies of such cases show only the lesions of chronic gastritis.

The vomiting in these cases seems to be the effort made by nature to effect a cure. By the use of the stomach pump we do the same thing, but much more easily and effectually. . . .

Now let us consider those cases in which the symptoms are due to functional derangement of the small intestine, the stomach being unaffected.

In these patients the symptom which is apt to be the most troublesome is pain. This pain may be referred to any part of the abdominal cavity. It is usually described as a constant dull pain, not like that of colic. It has no special relation to the ingestion of food or to its quality. It occurs when the stomach is full or empty; whether the food is spare and simple, or abundant and rich. The use of liquor will usually stop it for a short time. There may be some particular time of the day at which the pain comes on with tolerable regularity; very often this will be late in the afternoon.

There may be nausea but not vomiting. The nausea does not follow eating, but is apt to occur in the morning.

The appetite often remains good. Food is taken with relish and causes no distress.

The bowels may continue to act with perfect regularity. Flatulence is a common, but not a constant symptom.

The patients are up and about and able to attend to their business, but they feel languid and good for nothing. Sometimes they become much alarmed about themselves and imagine that they are suffering from cancer or some other serious disease.

Not infrequently persons have several attacks of this condition, at intervals of several months. The earlier attacks only last a few days, the later attacks are more severe and may last weeks and months.

Some of the cases are very easily relieved by treatment, others prove very obstinate.

The drugs usually indicated are cubebs, ipecac, and asafoetida. Cubebs may be given in the form of powder or of tincture. Ten grains of the powder or twenty minims of the tincture is the usual dose to be given three or four times a day. Ipecac is given at first in small doses—one-eighth of a grain—and then increased gradually up to one to four grains three times a day. Asafoetida may be given in four-grain sugar-coated pills or in the shape of the compound Galbanum pill.

Riding on horseback is often of very great service; walking, on the other hand, does not seem to be of as much benefit. Traveling for several months from place to place may effect a cure when all other remedies fail.

I am unable to show you any case illustrating this variety of dyspepsia. It is rare among clinique and hospital patients, although in private practice it is sufficiently common.

Dyspeptic symptoms dependent upon disordered function of the liver are very common. The great majority of cases of dyspepsia coming to this clinique are cases of liver dyspepsia, either alone or combined with disorders of the other digestive organs.

In this variety of indigestion the symptoms are variable and often very intractable to treatment.

Physiologists teach us that the liver performs several important functions. These functions are very well summed up by Murchison as follows:

1st.—The formation of glycogen, which contributes to the maintenance of animal heat and to the nutrition of the blood and tissues and the development of white blood corpuscles.

2d.—The destructive metamorphosis of albuminoid matter and the formation of urea and other nitrogenous products, which are subsequently eliminated by the kidneys; these chemical changes also contributing to the development of animal heat.

3d.—The secretion of bile, the greater part of which is re-absorbed, assisting in the assimilation of fat and peptones, and probably in those chemical changes which go on in the liver and portal circulation; while part is excrementitious and in passing along the bowels, stimulates peristalsis and arrests decomposition.

It is not easy in any given case to say which of these functions of the liver is disordered and gives rise to the existing symptoms. I have found it convenient, however, clinically to divide these patients into two classes, according to their general condition. In the first class I include those of florid complexion and with well-developed adipose and muscular tissues. In the second class I include those of pallid complexion, spare figure, and feeble muscles.

It has seemed to me that in the first class the symptoms are due to the derangement of those functions of the liver which should effect the destructive metamorphosis of albuminoid substances, so that the patients receive a full supply of the nutritious portions of the food, but do not get rid of the excrementitious.

In the second class of cases, on the other hand, there is no failure of these destructive and excretory functions, but those functions which should effect the assimilation of fat and peptones are disordered so that the patient is imperfectly nourished.

In the one case, the tissues are over-manured, but badly drained; in the other, they are well enough drained, but not manured at all.

I will show you first an example of the second class.

This man is thirty years old, a policeman by occupation. He tells us that his health has been good until within the last year. During this time he has gradually lost flesh, strength, and color. His appetite is sometimes good, sometimes not; occasionally there is slight nausea in the morning. He has a dull, uncomfortable feeling in the head much of the time. There is a dull pain in the right hypochondriac region. His bowels are constipated. During the year he has consumed a large quantity of medicine at different times. His urine is normal, except for an increased amount of oxalate of lime.

His face is thin, pale, and anxious. He is very much alarmed about himself. This man's condition I believe to be due to the fact that his liver does not properly perform its functions of excreting bile. This is felt in two ways. There is insufficient assimilation of fat and peptones, and the large intestine does not feel the natural stimulus of the excrementitious bile.

Some of the patients belonging to this class are much troubled with flatulence.

Headache is a very common symptom and often very distressing. Curious nervous feelings in different parts of the body are often complained of. The patients say that the top of their heads feel like ice, or that they have cold chills down the back or limbs, or pricking sensations in the skin, or a feeling of constriction about the body. Very often they are much troubled by sleeplessness. They are very apt to be much disturbed about their own condition and even to become very hypochondriacal.

There may be irregular action of the heart and pain in the precordial region. There is also often dull pain in the right hypochondriac region, which may extend into the back and shoulder.

The bowels are usually constipated. The patients lose flesh and strength. The urine is normal, or contains an increased amount of oxalate of lime, or sometimes stellate crystals of phosphate of lime.

This condition is often very intractable to treatment and always requires continuous and systematic care.

The diet is to be carefully regulated, but should be full and nutritious. Wines, ales, and spirits are often of service. Cream and even cod-liver oil are sometimes indicated.

To relieve the constipation, strychnia, aloes, sulphate of magnesia, rhubarb, and podophyllin answer a good purpose. Bromide of potash, asafoetida, and guarana are of service in allaying the nervous symptoms and restlessness. To improve the appetite and act as a tonic nothing is better than the mineral acids. Exercise in the open air is to be insisted upon and, in young persons, bathing the entire body every day with cold water.

The general principle which you bear in mind in treating these cases is that their symptoms depend on the failure of the liver to perform its share in the process of digestion, and as a result of this, the entire body is insufficiently nourished.

You must also remember that the various pains and uncomfortable feelings from which these patients suffer give rise to many errors of diagnosis. Congestion of the brain, paraplegia, uterine disease, heart disease, pulmonary phthisis, are all ascribed, not so very infrequently, to patients suffering from liver dyspepsia alone.

In the first class of cases of abnormal liver function, the appearance of the patients differs widely from that of the patients of whom we have just been speaking. These patients are stout and well-developed, often of rosy, florid appearance. They are usually persons who live well, drink, and use tobacco freely. They may even be in the habit of taking a good deal of exercise.

In spite of their healthy appearance, however, we find the same depression of spirits and tendency to hypochondriasis. They are less liable to headache, but more so to attacks of vertigo. These attacks of vertigo may be so severe that they fall to the ground and lose consciousness.

The appetite is usually good. The bowels are sometimes constipated, sometimes regular. There is often an occasional diarrhea from very slight causes. The urine is very apt to contain an excess of uric acid or of the urates.

In many cases, the first symptoms of which complaint is made are the vertigo and the uncomfortable feeling about the head, sometimes also an inability to apply the mind to business, and a partial loss of memory.

These patients sometimes discover that a brisk purgative makes them feel much better for several days, and they become regular customers of the venders of the different kinds of purgative pills. . . .

I have endeavored thus to sketch out roughly for you some of the cases of dyspepsia in which only one of the digestive viscera is involved. I think that in your future practice you will be able to recognize some of these cases when you see them, and I think it will add much to your satisfaction in the treatment of all cases of dyspepsia, if you make the attempt to analyze the mass of symptoms and assign them to the different viscera to which they belong.

PART V

SURGERY

INTRODUCTION

In this section it is surgeons who are commenting on their specialty. Many nonsurgical writers of the nineteenth century, however, were perhaps in a better position to evaluate surgery's position and accomplishments. The Englishman Robley Dunglison, whom Jefferson brought to the new University of Virginia to teach medicine, told medical students in the 1840's about "the present improved condition of surgery." There was much to admire, he believed. "The major operations have been simplified by the invention of appropriate instruments, and the bold daring of the modern surgeon has led him to perform operations which were totally unknown even in the middle of the last century."[1] As an example, Dunglison cited the ligature of large arteries in cases of aneurysm. Heretofore these patients would have been allowed to go on to a fatal end without surgical interference.[2]

For the most part, surgeons and their art were exempted from the doubts and criticisms applied to their nonoperating colleagues. After the introduction of effective and relatively safe anesthesia in mid-century, and especially after the advent of antisepsis, surgeons were able to bring about more readily apparent results. The higher esteem in which the public held surgeons was not lost upon the medical men, and many, such as Elisha Bartlett in the *Inquiry on the Degree of Certainty in Medicine*[3] dealt with it directly (see Section IV).

Alfred Stillé, a Philadelphia physician and author of a widely used text on therapeutics,[4] agreed with Bartlett that the general immunity of surgery from detractors was owing to its mechanical processes, "which appeal so directly and forcibly to the senses of the unskilled."[5] Stillé further complained that: "The

---

[1] *The Medical Student, or Aids to the Study of Medicine*, (rev. ed.; Philadelphia: Lea & Blanchard, 1844), p. 208.

[2] Dunglison did not mention the post-operative mortality, which prior to antisepsis was discouragingly high.

[3] Elisha Bartlett, *An Inquiry into the Degree of Certainty in Medicine* (Philadelphia: Lea and Blanchard, 1848).

[4] Alfred Stillé, *Therapeutics and Materia Medica*, 2 vols. (Philadelphia: Blanchard and Lea, 1864).

[5] Review of "Bartlett on degree of certainty," *Am. J. Med. Sci.* 16 (1848): 398–406; 404.

surgeon is commonly judged by his *operation*, i.e., his prescription; . . . . The public form a notion of the comparative value of surgery and medicine, by contrasting the *agents* of the one with the *results* of the other. A comparison of nutritious food and strong men would be just about as rational, and lead to an equally correct idea of their respective merits."[6]

Henry J. Bigelow, himself a surgeon and professor of surgery, warned his students that surgeons were prone to foster and to encourage undue appreciation by the public. The exaggerated interest and adulation, he claimed, were not altogether healthy:

> Why is the amphitheatre crowded to the roof, by adepts as well as students, on the occasion of some great operation, while the silent working of some well-directed drug excites comparatively little comment? Mark the hushed breath, the fearful intensity of silence, when the blade pierces the tissues, and the blood of the unhappy sufferer wells up to the surface. Animal sense is always fascinated by the presence of animal suffering.[7]

According to the *Seventh Census of the United States*, 1850, the state of New York had 5,060 physicians for a population of 3,097,394. What is of greater interest, however, is that in addition to the physicians, surgeons are noted separately in the list of occupations, 54 having been counted in the state.[8] Five years later, in a census of New York State, New York City claimed 1,252 physicians and 19 surgeons.[9] This division between physicians and surgeons is interesting because we usually think that in this country no such distinction was made. In the absence of more knowledge about the men listed as surgeons it is difficult to say much, except that the government acknowledged the existence of specialists who called themselves surgeons. From what we do know of men who were professors of surgery in medical schools, one can surmise that the surgeons also practiced nonsurgical medicine.

As late as 1876 Samuel D. Gross of Philadelphia, one of the country's best known surgeons put it quite succinctly:

> . . . there are, strange to say, as a separate and distinct class [of surgeons], no such persons among us. It is safe to affirm that there is not a medical man on this continent who devotes himself exclusively to the practice of surgery. On the other hand, there are few physicians, even in our larger cities, who do not treat the more common surgical disease and injuries, such as fractures, dislocations, and wounds, or who do not even occasionally perform the more common surgical operations. In short, American medical men are general practitioners, ready, for the most part,

---

[6] Ibid.

[7] *Introductory Lecture* (Boston: Mussey, 1850), p. 21.

[8] *Seventh Census of the United States*, 1850 (Washington: Armstrong, 1853), pp. lxxiv, lxxviii, 91.

[9] *Census of the State of New York for 1855* (Albany: Van Benthuysen, 1857), pp. xxiv, 189, 193.

if well educated, to meet any and every emergency, whether in medicine, surgery, or midwifery.[10]

More and more, as the nineteenth century progressed, surgery was done by those who called themselves surgeons. While most practitioners probably did what we call minor surgery, the major procedures were usually performed by specialists. This distinction held especially true for the bigger cities. In rural areas, which during much of the nineteenth century still represented more Americans than did the cities, there was undoubtedly less specialization among physicians.[11]

Bibliographical Note

The general history of surgery in America has not been well served by historians. Packard, Shafer, and Shryock do of course treat it in their books on the development of medicine as a whole. Samuel D. Gross's long paper of 1876 is a gold mine for references. An old, but still useful, history of surgery that includes the American story is John Shaw Billings, "The history and literature of surgery," in Frederic S. Dennis, ed., *System of Surgery*, 4 vols., Philadelphia: Lea, 1895, vol. 1, pp. 17-144. Also Stephen Smith, "The evolution of American surgery," in *American Practice of Surgery*, 8 vols., New York: Wood, 1906-11, vol. 1, pp. 3-67. There are a number of biographies of nineteenth-century surgeons of this country, as well as autobiographies that are of interest. See also the general review by Courtney R. Hall, "The rise of professional surgery in the United States, 1800-1865," *Bull. Hist. Med.* 26 (1952): 231-62.

Three recent books have appeared. Most to be recommended is A. Scott Earle, ed., *Surgery in America*, Philadelphia: Saunders, 1965; this includes classical papers and very useful editorial notes. Audrey D. Stevens, *America's Pioneers in Abdominal Surgery*, American Society of Abdominal Surgeons, 1968, is available as a paperback. Allen O. Whipple's *The Evolution of Surgery in the United States*, Springfield: Thomas, 1963, is too brief, but useful for the story of surgery of various organs.

George Rosen has described the rise of specialization in his *The Specialization of Medicine with Particular Reference to Ophthalmology*, New York: Froben, 1944.

---

[10]"A century of American medicine, 1776-1876, II. Surgery," *Am. J. Med. Sci.* 71 (1876): 431-84; 432.

[11]Historians, unfortunately, must base much of their knowledge of what happened on reports of the men who went to the trouble of publishing their experiences. The medical journals, then, reflect only a small segment of the practice of medicine at any given time. Careful research may reveal a much different picture than the one we usually accept as reasonably accurate. See, for instance, Erwin H. Ackerknecht, "A plea for a 'Behaviorist' approach in writing the history of medicine," *J. Hist. Med.* 22 (1967): 211-14; and Charles E. Rosenberg, who carried out Professor Ackerknecht's prescription in "The practice of medicine in New York a century ago," *Bull. Hist. Med.* 41 (1967): 223-53.

EPHRAIM McDOWELL

THREE CASES OF EXTIRPATION
OF DISEASED OVARIA

Editor's Note

Ephraim McDowell (1771–1830) has achieved immortality, though he wrote very little. Born in Virginia, McDowell grew to manhood in Kentucky. Little is known of his medical education, but he did attend some classes while in Edinburgh for the 1792–93 session. He was not, however, awarded a degree. He began to practice medicine in Danville, Kentucky in 1795.[1]

McDowell's accomplishments in ovarian surgery, while facing the frontier conditions of early nineteenth-century Kentucky, have long captured the American imagination. As much courage and skill with which McDowell must surely be credited, his first patient, Mrs. Jane Todd Crawford also deserves great praise.

On that Christmas day in 1809 McDowell not only successfully completed the removal of Mrs. Crawford's large ovarian tumor, but he did so while his patient endured the process without anesthesia. The drama of the time must have been intense, for outside his house a large group of men were waiting, rope in hand. Should McDowell have failed, he would have been a martyr to his art.

Bibliographical Note

The story has been particularly well told by James Thomas Flexner, in *Doctors on Horseback*, Dover, 1969.

McDowell's 1817 paper and a second one describing two more cases published in the same journal in 1819 have recently been reprinted by A. Scott Earle, ed., *Surgery in America*, Philadelphia: Saunders, 1965, pp. 60–70. See also Irvin Abell, "Professional attainments of Ephraim McDowell," *Bull. Hist. Med.* 24 (1950): 161–67, in which McDowell's paper is also reprinted.

In December 1809, I was called to see a Mrs. Crawford, who had for several months thought herself pregnant. She was affected with pains similar to labor pains, from which she could find no relief. So strong was the presumption of her

---

Eclectic Repertory 7 (1817): 242–44.

[1] Emmet F. Horine, "The stagesetting for Ephraim McDowell, 1771–1830," *Bull. Hist. Med.* 24 (1950): 149–60.

being in the last stage of pregnancy, that two physicians who were consulted on her case requested my aid in delivering her. The abdomen was considerably enlarged and had the appearance of pregnancy, though the inclination of the tumor was to one side, admitting of an easy removal to the other. Upon examination, per vaginam, I found nothing in the uterus; which induced the conclusion that it must be an enlarged ovarium. Having never seen so large a substance extracted, nor heard of an attempt or success attending any operation such as this required, I gave to the unhappy woman information of her dangerous situation. She appeared willing to undergo an experiment, which I promised to perform if she would come to Danville (the town where I live), a distance of sixty miles from her place of residence. This appeared almost impracticable by any, even the most favorable conveyance, though she performed the journey in a few days on horseback. With the assistance of my nephew and colleague, James McDowell, M.D., I commenced the operation, which was concluded as follows: Having placed her on a table of the ordinary height, on her back, and removed all her dressing which might in any way impede the operation, I made an incision about three inches from the musculus rectus abdominis, on the left side, continuing the same nine inches in length, parallel with the fibers of the above named muscle, extending into the cavity of the abdomen, the parietes of which were a good deal contused, which we ascribed to the resting of the tumor on the horn of the saddle during her journey. The tumor then appeared full in view, but was so large that we could not take it away entire. We put a strong ligature around the fallopian tube near to the uterus; we then cut open the tumor, which was the ovarium and fimbrious part of the fallopian tube very much enlarged. We took out fifteen pounds of a dirty, gelatinous looking substance. After which we cut through the fallopian tube, and extracted the sack, which weighed seven pounds and one-half. As soon as the external opening was made, the intestines rushed out upon the table; and so completely was the abdomen filled by the tumor, that they could not be replaced during the operation, which was terminated in about twenty-five minutes. We then turned her upon her left side, so as to permit the blood to escape; after which, we closed the external opening with the interrupted suture, leaving out, at the lower end of the incision, the ligature which surrounded the fallopian tube. Between every two stitches we put a strip of adhesive plaster, which, by keeping the parts in contact, hastened the healing of the incision. We then applied the usual dressings, put her to bed, and prescribed a strict observance of the antiphlogistic regimen. In five days I visited her, and much to my astonishment found her engaged in making up her bed. I gave her particular caution for the future, and in twenty-five days she returned home as she came, in good health, which she continues to enjoy.

Since the above case, I was called to a negro woman who had a hard and very painful tumor in the abdomen. I gave her mercury for three or four months with some abatement of pain, but she was still unable to perform her usual duties. As the tumor was fixed and immovable, I did not advise an operation; though from the earnest solicitation of her master and her own distressful condition I agreed to the experiment. I had her placed upon a table, laid her side open as in the above case; put my hand in, found the ovarium very much enlarged, painful to the touch, and firmly adhering to the vesica urinaria and fundus uteri. To extract I thought would be instantly fatal, but by way of experiment I plunged the scalpel into the diseased part. Such gelatinous substance as in the above case, with a profusion of blood, rushed to the external opening, and I conveyed it off by placing my hand under the tumor, and suffering the discharge to take place over it. Notwithstanding my great care, a quart or more of blood escaped into the abdomen. After the hemorrhage ceased, I took out as clearly as possible the blood, in which the bowels were completely enveloped. Though I considered the case as nearly hopeless, I advised the same dressings, and the same regimen as in the above case. She has entirely recovered from all pain, and pursues her ordinary occupations.

In May 1816, a negro woman was brought to me from a distance. I found the ovarium much enlarged, and as it could be easily moved from side to side, I advised the extraction of it. As it adhered to the left side, I changed my place of opening to the linea alba. I began the incision, in company with my partner and colleague Dr. William Coffer, an inch below the umbilicus and extended it to within an inch of the os pubis. I then put a ligature around the fallopian tube and endeavored to turn out the tumor, but could not. I then cut to the right of the umbilicus, and above it two inches, turned out a scirrhous ovarium (weighing six pounds) and cut it off close to the ligature put around the fallopian tube. I then closed the external opening, as in the former cases, and she complaining of cold and chilliness, I put her to bed prior to dressing her—then gave her a wine glass full of cherry bounce and thirty drops of laudanum, which soon restored her warmth, she was dressed as usual. She was well in two weeks, though the ligature could not be released for five weeks, at the end of which time the cord was taken away, and she now, without complaint, officiates in the laborious occupation of cook to a large family.

HENRY J. BIGELOW

INSENSIBILITY DURING SURGICAL OPERATIONS PRODUCED BY INHALATION

Editor's Note

Henry J. Bigelow (1818–90) was born in Boston, the son of Jacob Bigelow. Henry was educated primarily at Harvard where he received the M.D. degree in 1841. In later years he became one of the leading surgeons of New England and made several contributions to surgical technique and surgical anatomy.[1]

Henry Bigelow was a junior member of the surgical team that introduced ether in 1846. A new epoch in the history of surgery was thus begun. By most estimates the first public use of ether in the surgical amphitheater of the Massachusetts General Hospital on that October day in 1846 was the single most important contribution made to medicine by Americans of the nineteenth century.

The story of anesthesia and of the controversies over priority that followed its introduction has been told by a number of historians for over a hundred years. Suffice it to say here that the introduction of anesthesia was not only a boon to patients but broadened the scope of the surgeon's work as well. No longer was speed in operating a primary factor, nor did the surgeon now have to operate on a struggling patient. Not for more than thirty years, however, did surgery become safe as well as painless.

Bibliographical Note

Most of Bigelow's paper appears in A. Scott Earle's *Surgery in America*, Philadelphia: Saunders, 1965, pp. 152–58. No book on American medicine of the nineteenth century is complete without mentioning anesthesia, thus it seemed worth while to include parts of the Bigelow article.

Bigelow again wrote on the subject in 1876 in "A history of the discovery of modern anesthesia," in "A century of medicine," *Am. J. Med. Sci.* 71 (1876): 164–84, in which he tried to untangle the claims of Wells, Jackson, and Morton. See also J. T. Flexner, *Doctors on Horseback*; Thomas E. Keys, *The History of Surgical Anesthesia*, New York: Dover, 1963; and Henry R. Viets, "The earliest printed references in newspapers and journals to the first public demonstration of ether anesthesia in 1846," *J. Hist. Med.* 4 (1949): 149–69.

Boston Med. Surg. J. 35 (1846): 309–17. Read before the Boston Society of Medical Improvement, November 9, 1846.

[1] The Y-ligament of the capsule of the hip joint is often called Bigelow's ligament. He clearly demonstrated its importance in hip-joint surgery. The Bigelows are the only father and son to be represented in this book, although many other single members of famous medical families are included.

For additional biographical details of Bigelow see the sketches in Kelly and Burrage, *Dictionary of American Medical Biography* New York: Appleton, 1928; and *A Memoir of Henry J. Bigelow*, Boston: Little, Brown, 1900.

-------------------------•-------------------------

It has long been an important problem in medical science to devise some method of mitigating the pain of surgical operations. An efficient agent for this purpose has at length been discovered. A patient has been rendered completely insensible during an amputation of the thigh, regaining consciousness after a short interval. Other severe operations have been performed without the knowledge of the patients. So remarkable an occurrence will, it is believed, render the following details relating to the history and character of the process not uninteresting.

On the 16th of Oct., 1846, an operation was performed at the hospital, upon a patient who had inhaled a preparation administered by Dr. Morton, a dentist of this city, with the alleged intention of producing insensibility to pain. Dr. Morton was understood to have extracted teeth under similar circumstances without the knowledge of the patient. The present operation was performed by Dr. Warren and, though comparatively slight, involved an incision near the lower jaw of some inches in extent. During the operation the patient muttered, as in a semi-conscious state, and afterwards stated that the pain was considerable, though mitigated; in his own words—as though the skin had been scratched with a hoe. There was, probably, in this instance, some defect in the process of inhalation, for on the following day the vapor was administered to another patient with complete success. A fatty tumor of considerable size was removed by Dr. Hayward from the arm of a woman near the deltoid muscle. The operation lasted four or five minutes, during which time the patient betrayed occasional marks of uneasiness; but, upon subsequently regaining her consciousness, professed not only to have felt no pain but to have been insensible to surrounding objects, to have known nothing of the operation, being only uneasy about a child left at home. No doubt, I think, existed in the minds of those who saw this operation that the unconsciousness was real; nor could the imagination be accused of any share in the production of these remarkable phenomena.

I subsequently undertook a number of experiments, with the view of ascertaining the nature of this new agent, and shall briefly state them, and also give some notice of the previous knowledge which existed of the use of the substances I employed.

The first experiment was with sulphuric ether, the odor of which was readily recognized in the preparation employed by Dr. Morton. Ether inhaled in vapor is well known to produce symptoms similar to those produced by the nitrous oxide. In my own former experience the exhilaration has been quite as great, though perhaps less pleasurable than that of this gas, or of the Egyptian *haschish*.* It seemed probable that the ether might be so long inhaled as to produce excessive inebriation and insensibility; but in several experiments the exhilaration was so considerable that the subject became uncontrollable and refused to inspire through the apparatus. Experiments were next made with the oil of wine (ethereal oil). This is well known to be an ingredient in the preparation known as Hoffman's anodyne, which also contains alcohol, and this was accordingly employed. Its effects upon the three or four subjects who tried it were singularly opposite to those of the ether alone. The patient was tranquilized, and generally lost all inclination to speak or move. Sensation was partially paralyzed, though it was remarkable that consciousness was always clear, the patient desiring to be pricked or pinched with a view to ascertain how far sensibility was lost. A much larger proportion of oil of wine and also chloric ether, with and without alcohol, were tried with no better effect.

It may be interesting to know how far medical inhalation has been previously employed. Medicated inhalation has been often directed to the amelioration of various pulmonary affections, with indifferent success. Instruments called *Inhalers* were employed long ago by Mudge, Gairdner, and Darwin, and the apparatus fitted up by Dr. Beddoes and Mr. James Watt, for respiring various gases, has given birth to some octavo volumes. More recently Sir Charles Scudamore has advocated the inhalation of iodine and conium in phthisis, and the vapor of tar has been often inhaled in the same disease. The effects of stramonium, thus administered, have been noticed by Sigmond.

The inhalation of the ethers has been recommended in various maladies, among which may be mentioned phthisis and asthma. "On sait que la respiration de l'ether sulfurique calme souvent les accidents nerveux de certains croups," is from the *Dict. des Sc. Med.*; but I find that mention of the inhalation of this agent is usually coupled with a caution against its abuse, grounded apparently upon two or three cases, quoted and requoted. Of these the first is from Brande's *Journal of Science*, where it is thus reported: "By imprudent respiration of sulphuric ether, a gentleman was thrown into a very lethargic state which contained from one to three hours, with occasional intermissions and great depression of spirits—the pulse being for many days so low that considerable fears were entertained for his life." Christison quotes the following, from the *Midland Med. and Surg. Journal*, to prove that *nitric* ether in vapor is a dangerous poison when too freely and too long inhaled: "A druggist's maid servant was found one morning dead in bed, and death had evidently arisen from the air of her apartment having been accidentally loaded with vapor of nitric ether, from the breaking of a three gallon jar of the Spiritus AEth. Nitric. She was found lying on her side, with her arms folded across her chest, the countenance and

---

*Extract of Indian hemp.

posture composed, and the whole appearance like a person in a deep sleep. The stomach was red internally and the lungs were gorged." The editor of the journal where this case is related, says he is acquainted with a similar instance, where a young man was found completely insensible from breathing air loaded with *sulphuric ether*, remained apoplectic for some hours, and would undoubtedly have perished had he not been discovered and removed in time. Ether is now very commonly administered *internally* as a diffusible stimulant and antispasmodic, in a dose of one or two drachms. But here also we have the evidence of a few experiments that ether is capable of producing grave results under certain circumstances. Orfila killed a dog by confining a small quantity in the stomach by means of a ligature around the oesophagus. Jager found that ℥ ss. acted as a fatal poison to a crane. It was for a long time supposed to be injurious to the animal economy. The old *Edinburgh Dispensatory*, republished here in 1816, explicitly states that it is to be inhaled by holding in the mouth a piece of sugar containing a few drops, and also that regular practitioners give only a few drops for a dose; "though," it adds, "empirics have sometimes ventured upon much larger quantities, and with incredible benefit" (p. 566). Nevertheless, it was known to have been taken in correspondingly large doses with impunity. The chemist Bucquet, who died of scirrhus of the colon, with inflammation of the stomach and intestines took before his death a pint of ether daily, to alleviate his excruciating pains (he also took 100 gr. opium daily):—and Christison mentions an old gentleman who consumed for many years ℥ xvi. every eight or ten days. Such facts probably led Merat and De Lens, in their *Matiere Medicale*, to question its grave effects when swallowed. Mentioning the case of Bucquet, they say, even of its inhalation, that it produces only "un sentiment de fraicheur que suit bientôt une legère excitation."

This variety of evidence tends to show that the knowledge of its effects, especially those of its inhalation, was of uncertain character. Anthony Todd Thomson well sums up what I conceive to have been the state of knowledge at the time upon this subject, in his *London Dispensatory* of 1818. "As an antispasmodic, it relieves the paroxysm of spasmodic asthma, whether it be taken into the stomach or its vapor only be inhaled into the lungs. Much caution, however, is required in inhaling the vapor of ether, as the imprudent inspiration of it has produced lethargic and apoplectic symptoms." In his *Materia Medica and Therapeutics*, of 1832, however, omitting all mention of inhalation, he uses the following words: "Like other diffusible excitants, its effects are rapidly propagated over the system and soon dissipated. From its volatile nature its exciting influence is probably augmented; as it produces distension of the stomach and bowels and is thus applied to every portion of their sensitive surface. It is also probable that it is absorbed in its state of vapor and is therefore directly applied to the nervous centers. It is the diffusible nature of the stimulus of ether which renders it so well adapted for causing sudden excitement and producing immediate results. Its effects, however, so soon disappear that the dose requires to be frequently repeated."

Nothing is here said of inhalation, and we may fairly infer that the process had so fallen into disrepute, or was deemed to be attended with such danger, as to render a notice of it superfluous in a work treating, in 1832, of therapeutics.

It remains briefly to describe the process of inhalation by the new method and to state some of its effects. A small two-necked glass globe contains the prepared vapor, together with sponges to enlarge the evaporating surface. One aperture admits the air to the interior of the globe, whence, charged with vapor, it is drawn through the second into the lungs. The inspired air thus passes through the bottle, but the expiration is diverted by a valve in the mouthpiece, and escaping into the apartment is thus prevented from vitiating the medicated vapor. A few of the operations in dentistry, in which the preparation has as yet been chiefly applied, have come under my observation. The remarks of the patients will convey an idea of their sensations.

A boy of sixteen, of medium stature and strength, was seated in the chair. The first few inhalations occasioned a quick cough, which afterwards subsided; at the end of eight minutes the head fell back, and the arms dropped, but owing to some resistance in opening the mouth, the tooth could not be reached before he awoke. He again inhaled for two minutes, and slept three minutes, during which time the tooth, an inferior molar was extracted. At the moment of extraction the features assumed an expression of pain, and the hand was raised. Upon coming to himself he said he had had a "first rate dream—very quiet," he said, "and had dreamed of Napoleon—had not the slightest consciousness of pain—the time had seemed long;" and he left the chair, feeling no uneasiness of any kind, and evidently in a high state of admiration. The pupils were dilated during the state of unconsciousness, and the pulse rose from 130 to 142.

A girl of sixteen immediately occupied the chair. After coughing a little, she inhaled during three minutes and fell asleep, when a molar tooth was extracted, after which she continued to slumber tranquilly during three minutes more. At the moment when force was applied she flinched and frowned, raising her hand to her mouth, but said she had been dreaming a pleasant dream and knew nothing of the operation.

A stout boy of twelve, at the first inspiration coughed considerably, and required a good deal of encouragement to induce him to go on. At the end of three minutes from the first fair inhalation, the muscles were relaxed and the pupils dilated. During the attempt to force open the mouth he recovered his consciousness and again inhaled during two minutes, and in the ensuing one minute two teeth were extracted, the patient seeming somewhat conscious, but upon actually awaking he declared "it was the best fun he ever saw," avowed his intention to come there again, and insisted upon having another tooth extracted upon the spot. A splinter which had been left afforded an opportunity of complying with his wish, but the pain proved to be considerable. Pulse at first 110, during sleep 96, afterwards 144; pupils dilated.

The next patient was a healthy-looking, middle-aged woman, who inhaled the vapor for four minutes; in the course of the next two minutes a back tooth was extracted and the patient continued smiling in her sleep for three minutes more. Pulse 120, not affected at the moment of the operation, but smaller during sleep. Upon coming to herself, she exclaimed that "it was beautiful—she dreamed of being at home—it seemed as if she had been gone a month." These cases, which occurred successively in about an hour, at the room of Dr. Morton, are fair examples of the average results produced by the inhalation of the vapor and will convey an idea of the feelings and expressions of many of the patients subjected to the process. Dr. Morton states that in upwards of two hundred patients, similar effects have been produced. The inhalation, after the first irritation has subsided, is easy and produces a complete unconsciousness at the expiration of a period varying from two to five or six, sometimes eight minutes; its duration varying from two to five minutes, during which the patient is completely insensible to the ordinary tests of pain. The pupils in the cases I have observed have been generally dilated, but with allowance for excitement and other disturbing influences, the pulse is not affected, at least in frequency; the patient remains in a calm and tranquil slumber and wakes with a pleasurable feeling. The manifestation of consciousness or resistance I at first attributed to the reflex function, but I have since had cause to modify this view.

It is natural to inquire whether no accidents have attended the employment of a method so wide in its application and so striking in its results. I have been unable to learn that any serious consequences have ensued. One or two robust patients have failed to be affected. I may mention as an early and unsuccessful case, its administration in an operation performed by Dr. Hayward, where an elderly woman was made to inhale the vapor for at least half an hour without effect. Though I was unable at the time to detect any imperfection in the process, I am inclined to believe that such existed. One woman became much excited, and required to be confined to the chair. As this occurred to the same patient twice, and in no other case as far as I have been able to learn, it was evidently owing to a peculiar susceptibility. Very young subjects are affected with nausea and vomiting, and for this reason Dr. M. has refused to administer it to children. Finally, in a few cases, the patient has continued to sleep tranquilly for eight or ten minutes, and once, after a protracted inhalation, for the period of an hour. . . .

The process is obviously adapted to operations which are brief in their duration, whatever be their severity. Of these, the two most striking are, perhaps, amputations and the extraction of teeth. In protracted dissections, the pain of the first incision alone is of sufficient importance to induce its use; and it may hereafter prove safe to administer it for a length of time, and to produce a narcotism of an hour's duration. It is not unlikely to be applicable in cases requiring a suspension of muscular action; such as the reduction of dislocations or of strangulated hernia: and finally it may be employed in the alleviation of functional pain, of muscular spasm, as in cramp and colic, and as a sedative or narcotic.

The application of the process to the performance of surgical operations is, it will be conceded, new. If it can be shown to have been occasionally resorted to before, it was only an ignorance of its universal application and immense practical utility that prevented such isolated facts from being generalized.

It is natural to inquire with whom this invention originated. Without entering into details, I learn that the patent bears the name of Dr. Charles T. Jackson, a distinguished chemist, and of Dr. Morton, a skilful dentist, of this city, as inventors—and has been issued to the latter gentleman as proprietor.

It has been considered desirable by the interested parties that the character of the agent employed by them should not be at this time announced; but it may be stated that it has been made known to those gentlemen who have had occasion to avail themselves of it.

I will add, in conclusion, a few remarks upon the actual position of this invention as regards the public.

No one will deny that he who benefits the world should receive from it an equivalent. The only question is, of what nature shall the equivalent be? Shall it be voluntarily ceded by the world, or levied upon it? For various reasons, discoveries in high science have been usually rewarded indirectly by fame, honor, position and, occasionally, in other countries, by funds appropriated for the purpose. Discoveries in medical science, whose domain approaches so nearly that of philanthropy, have been generally ranked with them; and many will assent with reluctance to the propriety of restricting by letters patent the use of an agent capable of mitigating human suffering. There are various reasons, however, which apologize for the arrangement which I understand to have been made with regard to the application of the new agent.

1st. It is capable of abuse and can readily be applied to nefarious ends.

2nd. Its action is not yet thoroughly understood, and its use should be restricted to responsible persons.

3d. One of its greatest fields is the mechanical art of dentistry, many of whose processes are by convention, secret, or protected by patent rights. It is especially with reference to this art, that the patent has been secured. We understand, already, that the proprietor has ceded its use to the Mass. General Hospital, and that his intentions are extremely liberal with regard to the medical profession generally, and that so soon as necessary arrangements can be made for publicity of the process, great facilities will be offered to those who are disposed to avail themselves of what now promises to be one of the important discoveries of the age.

EDMUND ANDREWS

THE SURGEON

Editor's Note

Edmund Andrews (1824 – 1904) was born in Vermont, studied in Michigan, and early in his career moved to Chicago. In 1855 he joined the faculty of the Rush Medical College, but soon collaborated with Nathan Smith Davis and others in establishing Lind University Medical School, later to become Northwestern University. Here in 1859 the first three-year medical course was instituted, an important reform at the time. He served as professor of surgery at Northwestern for forty-six years and was a leader of the Chicago medical profession.

Andrews had good reason to stress to the young men in his class the qualifications of surgeons. The Civil War was to severely test the entire profession, but the surgeon's work on the battlefield and in the military hospitals was the most visible to all. Many experienced surgeons were horrified with what they saw when they went to the front. Stephen Smith of New York, a professor of surgery and editor of the *American Medical Times*, wrote several editorials decrying sloppy and unnecessary surgery. In a letter from Virginia in 1862 he was more blunt: "Surgically, I am digusted with N.Y. and other surgeons. Everyone came with the determination of performing all the operations he could, and as a consequence hundreds of operations have been needlessly performed, with the most shocking results."[1]

We live in an hour, such as comes to men but once a lifetime. Medical science and art, which have hitherto illumined the hours of peace, are summoned to the battlefield to front the grim realities of war; and not only our profession, but all others are mingled in a struggle which moulds the characters of millions and which will stamp the impress of the coming century.

Chicago Med. Examiner 2 (1861): 587–98. Introductory lecture delivered before the Medical Department of Lind University, October 14, 1861–published by request of the students.

[1] Letter, Stephen Smith to Lucie Smith, 18 May 1962. This is not to say that much good and heroic work was not also done. Smith's letter is quoted only to corroborate what Andrews said.

At such a time, I cannot talk to you of common petty interests apart from the influence of the great convulsion. It is War that speaks, not I. I must talk to you as men to be moulded by the influence of this tremendous hour for the destinies of another age than that which has just past.

War is a moral tonic. It comes to the social world as the whirlwind and the earthquake come to the natural. It finds many flimsy social fabrics in its path, erected for the time of peace. They are cheaply glorious with paint and gorgeous with stucco, but the sweep of the tempest bears them away like chaff in its passage, until that which is truly strong and giantlike alone remains.

In times of long peace, men lose their hold on strong first principles. They plan flimsy and insecure schemes of business; their social fabrics are artificially painted and stuccoed and bedizened with nonsensical observances. Education grows out into distorted and strange forms, and even the learned professions spin theories frailer than cobwebs and take to forming artificial rules of conduct and false notions of their relations to the rest of the community.

So then, I, for one, rejoice that this war has come. Not only *our* profession, but others, and the social and civil organizations themselves, have grown up too rank and luxuriant for safety. They need the tossing of the blast to harden their limbs and the shock of war to consolidate their strength.

I know that the evils of war are great. There is paleness on many brows. For the first time the nation is shaken by a real danger and sees, flapping over her stars, the wings of a tempest whose thunders mutter of final dissolution. But in hours like this, God renovates communities and purges away their errors, their luxury, and their corruption. It is with throes like these that heroes are born— amid convulsions such as these, nations grow giant-like and renew their vigor, their youth, and power.

Americans had come to fancy that all their institutions were to be established forever, without a struggle. They verily thought that the duty of defending their country was one which could never be practically exercised. Even our civil freedom, since the throes of her birth, has not been put to serious peril. Her infancy was cradled among the green valleys of the east; in childhood she sported securely on the shores of the great lakes; and on the prairies of the west, we have watched with pride the rounding cheek of her youth; but now her majority is attained, the hour of her bridal draws near; this day freedom weds with the sword, and pours out on the battlefield, the red wine of her marriage feast.

In times like these, there are not sluggards: the very air is full of electric life, and honest vigor of action becomes a luxury. Let us, therefore, who are not called to the battlefield, where some of us may lay our bones before another year, let us take a new view of our privileges, responsibilities, and duties with the truthful vision imparted by this auspicious hour.

If I am equal to the occasion and the theme, I wish to portray to you tonight, the character of the *True Surgeon* for the present and the coming time.

First, then:—What is demanded to constitute a good surgeon? I answer,—
the primary requisite for a good surgeon, is *to be a man*,—a man of courage, a
man of moral rectitude, a man of broad views and noble sentiments. Narrow-
minded, mean-souled, little-brained men ought never to plunge into the learned
professions. Their circumstances bewilder them; they become entangled in their
learning like a fly in a cobweb; their language is barbarized by technical phrases;
their mental vision is obscured by professional squints, and their hearts, cut off
from the great life-current of humanity, dry up to nonentities. Such men never
grasp the grand and inspiring truths at the core of their profession, but flounder
bewildered among its accidental surroundings. Hence, we have lawyers learned in
statutes and decisions and reckless of justice; clergymen deep in theology and
devoid of religion; and surgeons skilled in anatomy and profoundly stuffed with
technicalities, but perverted in judgment, rotten in morals, and destitute of
sympathy. In one word, they are *not men*; they are only the dried-up shells of
preachers, lawyers, and doctors with all the manhood blown out of them.

Among the particular traits which go to make up a manly character, one of
the first, and one which is eminently necessary to a good surgeon, is courage. In
battle, a portion of the surgeons go with the line and dress the wounded under
fire. In the Crimea, the British surgeons dressed the wounded in the trenches
were they fell; and the results, both in their wars and our own, show that bullets
have no natural repugnance to killing medical officers. Unless, therefore, a man
can tie up an artery with a cool head and steady hand, while the bullets are
singing past him, he will not do for a surgeon. Again, he must sometimes walk
his hospital day by day, when it is filled with contagious and pestilential disease,
breathing an air more deadly than that of the battlefield. If he cannot do this
without flinching, he will not do for a surgeon.

And, again, in civil practice there are cases which quick, skilful, and daring
action alone can save; an instant only is given for a human life, and the surgeon
who is aghast and hesitates at the emergency loses his patient. I tell you, gentlemen, these moments will test your courage more severely than bullets whistling
across the line of battle.

Another requisite of high professional quality is breadth of knowledge, not
only of the practical branches, but of those general and preliminary topics which
are necessary to constitute a well-educated man. The intensely practical character of the American mind has unfortunately misled many students as to the
real requisites of high success. Every year, medical teachers receive applications
from men who desire the honors of a diploma, but wish to be excused from
attention to, what they call, the nonpractical branches. They imagine that but
little more is necessary for a physician than theory and practice, materia medica,
and obstetrics; and for a surgeon, than anatomy, surgery, and a case of instruments. One man who claimed to be eminent already in surgery, objected to
pathology as not practical; it was not necessary to study the nature of the
disease, the practical thing was to cure it. God help his patients; I think they had
better send for a butcher, as being the more practical man of the two. . . .

There is no doubt, whatever, that if circumstances permitted, it would be better for every young man to take a four years' college course, before commencing his proper medical studies, though at present, such an extensive preliminary course is out of the reach of many, who may yet become superior surgeons and physicians. But, fortunately, knowledge is power, however obtained, and the man, who, by industry will acquire it, though it be by hours and moments, stolen from other occupations, may reap its full fruits. Now, gentlemen, the way to commence is very plain. It is perfectly easy to point out a course by which a young physician, even of deficient preliminary education, can become the recognized superior over most of his fellows of equal natural talent. He must, like Elihu Burrit, the learned blacksmith, make up by after study his lack of early advantages.

The first years of a practitioner's life are not usually fully occupied with business. Of the leisure hours on hand, let one-half be devoted, for six years, to general literature and science, and the other half to reading, writing, and hard thinking directly upon his profession. I guarantee to any young practitioner of fair capacity who will do this faithfully, a superiority over his fellows which will be publicly known and recognized during the rest of his lifetime. A good education necessarily implies a variety of knowledge. Each kind of study leaves only its own special mark on the mind, and, hence, acquisitions of several kinds are necessary to a full development. The languages are of constant use in prescriptions and in technical terms; but besides this, the exercise of translating gives a man ease of grasping thought and facility in expressing it. Mathematics confers precision of reasoning, and accuracy in mechanical contrivance, which a surgeon especially requires; while natural sciences give breadth and scope of thought. I earnestly urge a liberal knowledge of these various branches. But beware of becoming so entangled in the meshes of your studies that they become master of you and not you of them. A few men become so fascinated with these pursuits as to follow them to the exclusion of all professional improvement and to the loss of public confidence in business. You should pursue them not as an end but as a means, in order that by self-culture you may bring to your professional duties a finer and more powerful mind—that you may become more perfect men, more splendid surgeons.

Some physicians have become so enamored of literature, as to actually forsake their profession for it. Some have studied mathematics and forgotten physic, and others have followed metaphysics until they have lost sight of earth altogether. . . .

Among the qualities of a true surgeon, not the least important is his enthusiasm, for on this depends his enjoyment and, consequently, his diligence in his work. You occasionally hear men say that the *study* of medicine and surgery is very interesting, but the practice is tedious and dull. Now I can assure you, that to a well-trained mind this is an unmitigated lie. Practice is dull only to those who do not think, reason, and study about their cases; in short, who are routine practitioners, not acting from the deductions of a living reason, but raking forever among the ashes of a dusty memory. Make your practice a perpetual study and it will be a perpetual enjoyment. To him who attentively thinks of all his cases, the truths of nature unfold themselves in wider and wider fields. Every day you reach a higher stand-point, and a broader view, every week you master some practical difficulty, and every year you learn to conquer some bodily evil which before defied your efforts. Progress, like this, will make any man enthusiastic, and the enthusiastic man is happy.

But if a man considers his education complete when the seal is applied to his diploma—if, instead of continuing to develop, he merely subsides into a mechanical way of taxing his memory for rules of practice, he will certainly not find it agreeable. There is a class of such physicians who grow worse as they grow older. Their very experience is a danger to them!—they learn nothing by it and, in fact, are never as good practitioners as when they first graduated.

Gentlemen,—set it down as certain, that there is something wrong about an old physician who thinks that practice is not interesting. Among well-balanced minds there are, however, some which naturally give preference to medicine and others to surgery; so that, to a certain extent, this division of the profession into two parts, marks two classes of minds. This preference depends on differences of the two positions and the relative mental qualities brought in play. Thus medicine requires more breadth and philosophical depth of thought than surgery, but less precision and mechanical ingenuity; and, accordingly, minds seek the sphere which best indulges their favorite bent. There is a difference, too, in the social relations of the two classes. A good physician secures a warm, earnest attachment from his patrons. There is a circle of families who look on him as a permanent and confidential friend and whose attachment is not valued by him at its mere product in dollars and cents. A man of fine sensibility cannot but highly prize this steady and earnest regard which is the reward, peculiarly, of medical skill and, moved by its stimulus, he will naturally engross himself, more and more, in that kind of practice. The surgeon, on the other hand, has a less warm but a more glittering reputation presented to his ambition. His patrons are transient. They come, perhaps, hundreds of miles for a single operation and, being relieved, return to their homes and disappear from the circle of his acquaintance. Of course, they cannot stand in the relation of intimate daily friends. To balance this, they look upon an eminent surgeon much as they do upon a renowned soldier. They yield the tribute of high admiration to one who dares to put his hand to the machinery of life and can, with impunity, take out its living wheels. If a surgeon's renown is less warm than a physician's, it is wider and more splendid.

As might naturally be expected, surgeons and physicians, considered as classes, have each their peculiar faults and virtues. As surgical appliances are less complex and more easily understood than medical, so surgeons, on the average, are more clear and accurate in their ideas than physicians and less in danger of running away into obscure theories which neither are nor can be definitely proved. Even quacks are obliged to keep somewhere near the truth when they meddle with surgery. But, on the other hand, these very advantages draw many inferior men to the surgical ranks. As surgery is easier to comprehend, too many of its votaries are superficial and narrow—not possessed of sufficient philosophical power to grasp easily the truth of medicine. As its renown is glittering and brilliant, it attracts men, too often, who are more cold and selfish than physicians—men incapable of warm friendships, over eager for notoriety, and greedy of gain. So it has been in time past. I call upon you to take this stain away from the profession by bringing to it hearts full of generous emotions; hearts whose rich pulses of youth live on in riper age; hearts that love nobleness and despise meanness and that feel for the sufferings of the afflicted. . . .

JOHN ERIC ERICHSEN

IMPRESSIONS OF AMERICAN SURGERY

Editor's Note

Born in 1818, Erichsen received his medical training at University College, London, where he subsequently became professor of surgery. He was best known in this country for his large textbook of surgery, first published in 1853 as *The Science and Art of Surgery* (London: J. Walton). By the fifth edition of 1869 it grew to two stout volumes, a format retained through a tenth and final edition in 1895. *The Dictionary of National Biography* refers to Erichsen's view of surgery as a science to be studied rather than an art to be displayed.

American historians and American readers have long been interested in the comments made about our institutions, manners, customs, and countryside by European travelers.[1] Many of these visitors briefly commented upon American science and medicine, but few went into such detail as did John Eric Erichsen, one of Britain's leading surgical authors of the second half of the nineteenth century.

A word about conservative surgery is in order, because Erichsen lauds American surgeons for being very skillful in the management of resections. He refers here to removal of part of a bone, especially in a limb, leaving behind as much as is possible. Just as the physicians were maligned for their heroic dosing with calomel and antimony and for their bleeding, the surgeons were scoffed at for their heroic amputations. Under the influence of French surgeons, particularly, some Americans began to amputate less and less in the years just before the Civil War. As Stephen Smith noted in his *Handbook* for military surgeons in the Civil War:

> This branch of operative surgery has assumed the highest importance within the past few years, owing to the recognition of the fact that when the osseous substance is removed, and the periosteum is left in position, new bone is formed, and often in sufficient perfection to restore the symmetry as well as the function of the part.[2]

Lancet 2 (1874): 717–20. An address delivered at University College Hospital, London, November 9, 1874.

[1] One of the better known collections of this type is Oscar Handlin, ed., *This was America* (Cambridge: Harvard University Press, 1949; reprinted as a Harper Torchbook, 1964). The classic analyses of the United States are by de Tocqueville in 1835 and James Bryce in 1881, both available in two-volume paperback editions: Alexis de Tocqueville, *Democracy in America*, 2 vols. (New York: Schocken Books, 1961); James Bryce, *The American Commonwealth*, 2 vols., edited and abridged by Louis Hacker (New York: Capricorn Books, 1959).

[2] Handbook of Surgical Operations (New York: Bailliere, 1862), p. 170.

Samuel Gross also emphasized the fact that nowhere was conservative surgery more appreciated than in the United States. "Comparatively few knivesmen, properly so called, exist among us, and it is worthy to note that their career is usually as shortlived as it is inglorious."[3] Had not some surgeons heeded the call for conservatism, even more limbless veterans would have resulted.

It is also interesting to note that Erichsen urged his younger colleagues to visit America and to spend time visiting the schools and the hospitals here. As is well known, the reverse flow was at high tide in those years.[4]

I have been requested to give you an account of the impressions that I have formed of American surgery and surgical institutions during my recent visit to the United States; and although I did not go amongst our transatlantic brethren as "a chiel amang them takin' notes," and still less with any intention to "print 'em," but solely for recreation in my autumn holiday, yet I have no hesitation in complying with this request: partly because I believe that too little is known of American surgery in this country; and partly because the opportunity is thus afforded me, which might not otherwise occur, of publicly expressing my deep sense of the great honour that was conferred on me by the most flattering reception I met with from the medical profession collectively in every part of the Union that I visited. It would be unbecoming here to do more than allude to the many friendly and cordial acts of private hospitality that were extended to me by individual members of our profession, and which have left a deep and pleasing recollection in my mind. But I may, without restraint, express my acknowledgments to the profession in America for the warm and hospitable and hearty welcome that was given to me wherever I went, east or west, north or south, from New York to Chicago, from Boston through Philadelphia and Baltimore to Washington; and for the splendid hospitalities of which I was in most of these cities on several occasions the recipient, as the guest of institutions or of the general body of the profession. I can only explain the reception I thus met with—a reception unparalleled, I believe, in the social history of our profession—on the assumption that it was not to me individually that so much honour was intended to be done, but that a compliment was thus paid to the surgical profession of Great Britain, of which I was considered the representative, and which was thus honoured though one of its members by our American brethren. But I must leave these topics, agreeable as it may be for me to dwell upon them, and grateful as the recollections conjured up by allusions to them are, and

---

[3] "A Century of American medicine," *Am. J. Med. Sci.* 71 (1876): 431 –84; 484.

[4] See, for instance, Thomas N. Bonner, *American Doctors and German Universities; A Chapter in International Intellectual Relations, 1870–1914* (Lincoln: University of Nebraska Press, 1963).

proceed to tell you, in a few words, what my general impression is of the profession, the schools, and the hospitals of the United States.

And first, as to the profession, I may at once say that it appears to me to occupy in America, relatively to the rest of the community, a far higher social status than it does in this country. The reason for this seems tolerably obvious. In the absence of an exalted hierarchy in an established church and of great dignitaries of the law, these professions do not offer sufficient inducement for men of the highest intellectual caliber to enter them. Medicine, therefore, stands prominent as probably the best-educated, certainly the most scientific, and, consequently, in a country where education is so widely diffused and so much regarded, the most respected of the professions. And in the absence of all titled classes, it can socially more than hold its own in competition with the trading and financial elements which are such prominent constituents of the society of most of the American cities. Perhaps, also, the high position that medicine occupies is owing, in some respect, to the greater uniformity of practice that prevails amongst medical men in America than with us. For, just as in the law there is no division into barristers and solicitors, so in medicine there is none into physicians, surgeons, and general practitioners. Special aptitude, inclination, or opportunity will necessarily lead men to a greater eminence in particular departments of the profession. But the subdivision into classes and specialties, which is so prevalent here, is unknown in the United States. With the exception of hospitals for diseases of women, I know of no special hospital in any of the large American towns; and I think that no better proof can be adduced of the inutility of the multiplication of these pseudo-charities, which are too often established in order to foster private gain under the flimsy shelter of that much-worn "cloak" which "covers a multitude of sins," than this fact, that in a population larger than that of Great Britain, with a numerous, highly educated, and active profession, it has not yet been found necessary to institute such establishments.

Surgery in the United States certainly stands at a very high level of excel-lence. The hospital surgeons throughout the country have struck me as being alike practical, progressive, and learned in a very high degree. In practical skill and aptitude for mechanical appliances of all kinds they are certainly excelled by no class of practitioners in any country. They are thoroughly up to modern surgery in its most progressive forms, and I have never met with any class of men who are so well read and so perfectly acquainted with all that is done in their profession outside their own country. It would be a great injustice to American surgeons for it to be supposed that surgical skill is confined to the large cities or to the few. On the contrary, I know no country in which, so far as it is possible to judge from contemporary medical literature, there is so widely diffused a high standard of operative skill as in the country districts and more remote provinces of the United States. The bent of the mind of the American surgeon is, like ours, practical rather than scientific; in fact, there are the same mental characteristics displayed in him that we find here—the same self-reliance, the same practical aptitude, the same *curative* instinct which leads him to consider his patient rather as a human being to be rescued from the effects of disease or injury rather than as a scientific object to be studied for the advance of professional knowledge. How, indeed, can it be otherwise than that there should be such a resemblance? It is true that in travelling through America one is struck by the fact that there is a singular combination of the new and the old—of the strange and the familiar. That there are differences of a remarkable character between the New and the Old World there can be no doubt. I use the word "different" rather than "foreign," because I feel it impossible to apply the word "foreign" to anything American. There are differences in climate, differences in the physical configuration of the country. The verdure that clothes its hills and the vegetation that fertilises its plains are different from those that we meet with here; but man, in all his characteristics, is exactly the same. There appears to me, indeed, to be as great, if not a greater difference between the mental characteristics of an Englishman and some of the other inhabitants of Great Britain than there is between an ordinary Englishman and an American of the Atlantic cities. It may be truly said, though perhaps in a sense slightly different from that in which the poet used the words, that, "Coelum non animum mutant qui trans mare currunt." Those who have crossed the great ocean have changed their clime, but not their characters.

The similarity that exists between American and British surgery, and which has struck me very forcibly, arises not only from the great resemblance that exists between the American and the English character, but from two other causes which have largely contributed to this end. The art of surgery is in a great measure traditional. The method of doing things in surgery is transmitted directly from the master to the pupil. The American surgeon of a past generation acquired in this way the traditionary art of British surgery and has transmitted it directly to his descendants. Surgeons of both nations drew their inspiration from the same source and drank at the same fountain of knowledge. The names of Cooper and the Bells, of Liston and of Brodie, are as familiar to the ears of American surgeons as they are to those of this country. I was much struck when visiting the oldest hospital in the United States—the Pennsylvania General Hospital at Philadelphia—by seeing over the entrance to the operating theatre the portrait of a face I had often seen delineated in this country. At first I thought it must be that of one of the American surgical worthies of a past generation—of Physick or of Mott, of Warren or of Mutter; but on closer inspection I found that they were the well-known features of him who was in his generation *facile princeps* of British surgery—Sir Astley Cooper. Not only have British traditions thus penetrated deeply into the surgery of the United States, but the modern American surgeon derives his information from the same sources as does his British contemporary. *The Lancet* is reprinted and is as widely circulated in the States as in this country; and I find in my own case that my pupils in America are probably more numerous than those in Great Britain. One of the great advantages—and it is a very great one—that an English writer enjoys is that he addresses eighty millions of people and that his works are not only disseminated throughout his own country, but, if of any value or importance, are eagerly sought after by that still larger body of readers existing in the "Greater Britain" which now encircles the globe. And if it be true, as has been said, that the judgment of enlightened foreign contemporaries is an anticipation of that which posterity will give, he may possibly have a foreshadowing of the verdict that a future generation of his own countrymen will pass upon him, in the estimate in which he is now held amongst those who inhabit the regions beyond the Atlantic.

The mode of instruction in the medical schools of America is necessarily very much the same as here. But there are some differences. Thus the course of education required is generally shorter than with us, and no preliminary examination in the way of matriculation is required before a young man can enter upon his medical studies. This undoubtedly is a great evil, and as such is much deplored by many teachers to whom I have spoken on the subject; but I am told that, in the present state of things in America it would be impossible to sift the candidates for a profession, or to establish such an ordeal as a matriculation examination. About the systematic instruction I have nothing to say. There is no essential difference in this respect between England and America. It is everywhere much the same. Dissection is easy to be obtained, and the bodies used for that purpose are either furnished gratuitously to the students or supplied at a low cost. There is but a nominal fee required for hospital attendance. The whole system of medical education, indeed, is far cheaper than with us. The chief difference that I have observed is in the method of communicating clinical instruction. The medical schools in the principal cities of the States, especially in New York and Philadelphia, are so enormous that the classes would be too large to be conducted through the wards of a hospital. Classes numbering from 600 to 800 are not uncommon. At Professor Pancoast's introductory lecture at Jefferson College, Philadelphia, there were probably 600 students present; and at my last visit to the clinical theatre at Bellevue Hospital, New York, it was estimated that a thousand students were present. It therefore becomes necessary to bring the patient to the students, rather than, as with us, the pupils to the patient. This is done by raising him off the framework of his bed on a small platform running on wheels, and thus carrying him without any disturbance of position into the clinical theatre, where he is examined and the case discussed. I will give no opinion as to the value of this method of teaching in medical cases, but in many surgical cases it appears to me to be far more useful than that which is generally adopted in this country. The surgical disease or injury can be more readily displayed in this way to a large body of students than it can when they are crowding around a bed, standing in one another's way, and often hampering the proceedings of the surgeon. There is one peculiarity in the mode of instruction in American hospitals which deserves mention. It is this: that each surgeon of the hospital often only serves for a short period of the year—four to at most six months; each of his colleagues in rotation taking up the practice and the clinical teaching during the remainder of the term. The advantage of this system is that the teacher is not exhausted by continuous work, but returns with refreshed energy to his duties.

The hospitals in the United States are, as with us, supported by voluntary contributions or by endowments from wealthy benefactors. The Americans are munificent in their charity, and hence these institutions are numerous and well-organised. America has two sets of hospitals, the old and the new. Like England in some of its larger towns, it is still embarrassed by the hospitals erected in pre-sanitary days, under systems of construction which time, experience, and the advance of scientific knowledge have proved to be erroneous, in which septic diseases are readily generated and become largely destructive to the patients. These institutions are, however, undergoing a process of conversion which will speedily do away with many of the evils inseparably connected with such buildings. The Americans learned a hard lesson in the deadly struggle of the War of Secession—a lesson which is not likely soon, if ever, to be forgotten by so practical a people, unfettered by old prejudices and preconceived opinions. The lesson to which I allude was this: that wounded and injured soldiers could only safely be treated in the open, in hut or barrack hospitals. This lesson has been taught to Europe by the more recent experiences of the Franco-German war, with what results in the future remains yet to be seen. That the barrack or hut system is superior to any other for surgical cases there can be no question. The misfortune is that in large towns, where ground is expensive and difficult to be procured, this system is, owing to the space required, not easy of adoption. There are also certain obvious inconveniences connected with it in those cases in which clinical instruction is required to be carried on in the hospital. The problem, then, to be solved in the construction of modern hospitals in large cities appears to be, how to combine the best condition for the patient with economy of space and proper facilities for the student. This problem is in process of solution in America. Indeed, it has, I believe, already been satisfactorily solved. . . .

There is a peculiar system adopted in many of the modern American hospitals—having private rooms for the reception of patients who can afford to pay. The charge for these rooms varies from two to five dollars per day. The patient is under the case of one of the medical officers, who receives his fees as he would in an ordinary private attendance. The system is well suited, in cases of sudden emergency, to a country in which there is so large a floating population as in the States, but it is also adopted in cases of chronic disease as a matter of convenience by many who come from a distance for operation or treatment.

Surgical practice in America does not differ in any very essential respects from that adopted here. There are necessarily some modifications and many ingenious appliances; but essentially there is no greater difference between American and English surgery generally than is to be found between the practice adopted in any two London hospitals.

The treatment of wounds is sufficiently simple and presents nothing peculiar. I observe that American surgeons are careful about the drainage of wounds and employ drainage tubes or similar appliances freely.

"Antiseptics" do not appear to be much, if at all, employed; at least, in a methodical form. Carbolic acid in the form of lotion or wash is commonly used. Indeed, antiseptics are not so much needed in the American hospitals as in ours. The object of antiseptics is to prevent the contamination of a wound by septic impurities from without. These sources of contamination do not exist in such hospitals as those that I have been describing to the same extent that they do in less perfectly constructed and less hygienically conducted establishments, and hence antiseptics are proportionately less needed. In America it is attempted to accomplish by improved construction of hospitals and by close attention to hygienic requirements, those great results which we are here driven to attain by "antiseptic" methods of treatment. In consequence of the ignorance in all matters that relate to the hygiene of hospitals that prevails amongst the architects and managers of these institutions, an undue burden of anxiety, responsibility, and care is thrown upon the surgeon, who is now unceasingly engaged in combating septic disease; and in order to keep down that rate of mortality which is the direct consequence of septic hospital influences he is driven to the employment of elaborate and complicated methods of antiseptic treatment. Cleanliness in its broadest sense is the best and most efficient antiseptic. If the constructors and conductors of hospitals were acquainted with or would adopt those hygienic rules on which hospitals should be built and managed, if hospitals were not overcrowded, if the system of ventilation was perfect, if there was a continuous water-supply, a proper isolation of wards and distribution of patients, the causes of septic diseases would not be generated. Those foul and filth-begotten diseases, pyaemia and hospital gangrene, would disappear, and antiseptics, in the absence of septic influences, would become unnecessary. Contamination of hospital air would be prevented; we should not, as now under defective hygienic arrangements, first allow the pollution to take place and then be driven to the use of antiseptics in order to prevent infection of wounds by the already septic-laden atmosphere. Under the present system we begin at the wrong end. Instead of preventing the possibility of atmospheric contamination by perfect hospital hygiene, we allow the septic poison to be engendered, and then, before it can be implanted on the wound, seek to destroy it by the employment of chemical agents.

With regard to anesthetics I have little to say. Ether is invariably used at Boston, and is preferred to chloroform by many hospital surgeons in other American cities. I saw it given in some operation cases at the Massachusetts General Hospital, which has the great honour and privilege of being the institution in which anesthesia was first employed in any surgical operation; it was administered here on a sponge, without any apparatus or complicated contrivance. . . .

I have thus given you a very brief sketch of some of the impressions that I formed of our profession during my recent visit to America, and in so doing I have purposely, as far as possible, omitted mentioning the names of American surgeons, because I felt that there are so many so highly distinguished that it would be invidious and perhaps unjust to make a selection of a few amongst the juniors, and amongst the seniors it would be needless to name to you such men as that Nestor of American surgery, Gross, or of Pancoast, of Philadelphia; of Van Buren, Wood, Parker, or Sayre, of New York; Bigelow or Hodges, of Boston; Smith or Johnston, of Baltimore. I can only say that the surgical profession in America contains a phalanx of men alike distinguished for their skill and their knowledge, at least equalling what any European country can produce. And, in conclusion, I would advise those amongst you who wish to see and study the practice of surgery elsewhere than in the school in which you have been brought up in this country, who are not content throughout their lives *jurare in verba magistri*, to run in the one professional groove in which they have been launched, but who unfortunately have not acquired that fluency of the speech of Germany or of France that would render a residence in those countries profitable for the purposes of study, to take a trip across the Atlantic—a voyage in itself interesting, amusing, and health-giving—and to spend a few months in visiting the great hospitals and schools in the cities of the United States of America.

SAMUEL D. GROSS

THE FACTORS OF DISEASE AND DEATH AFTER INJURIES, PARTURITION, AND SURGICAL OPERATIONS

Editor's Note

Samuel D. Gross (1805–84) was one of America's leading surgeons of the nineteenth century. Part of his fame, no doubt, was owing to his ever-active pen. Born and educated in Pennsylvania, Gross taught in four medical schools, but was most closely identified with medicine in Philadelphia. As early as 1839 he published an important work on pathology, *Elements of Pathological Anatomy*,[1] that went through several editions and revisions. His large, two volume surgical text, *A System of Surgery: Pathological, Diagnostic, Therapeutic, and Operative*,[2] first appeared in 1859. It was a standard for years; the sixth edition appeared in 1882.

The following paper by Gross illustrates the difficulties which a theory and practice, such as antisepsis, faced in the years after its enunciation by Joseph Lister. Gross deals with a number of problems that interested the surgeons of his day: hospitals and hospital infection, theories of the etiology of infectious diseases, hygiene, and nursing. His paper is a good example of the kind of discussion that the germ theory received in the days when Pasteur had already demonstrated its scientific nature and Joseph Lister its practical application, but when the so-called golden age of bacteriology was still a few years in the future.

Gross, one must remember, was one of the leading medical men in the country at this time. Erichsen in 1874 called him the Nestor of American surgeons. The difficulties encountered by the germ theory, then, were no less when a man of Gross's stature said, regarding blood poisoning, that science was dumb. It would be unfair to say that it was Gross who was dumb, but certainly he was not among the earliest to accept what was becoming more obvious almost month by month. He was nearing the end of an illustrious career, and he had little need for a new method of treating wounds. As he tells us in the following paper, his results, measured in terms of his time, were very good indeed.

Bibliographical Note

Of Gross's many historical writings two are of most interest here: "A century of American medicine, 1776–1876, II. Surgery," *Am. J. Med. Sci.* 71 (1876) 431–84; and his *Autobiography*, 2 vols., Philadelphia: Barrie, 1887.

Reports and Papers, A.P.H.A. 2 (1874–75): 400–14. A discourse before the American Public Health Association at its meeting in Philadelphia, November 10, 1874.

[1] Samuel D. Gross, *Elements of Pathological Anatomy*, 2 vols. (Boston: Marsh, Capen, Lyon, Webb, and Drew, 1839).

[2] Samuel D. Gross, *A System of Surgery: Pathological, Diagnostic, Therapeutic, Operative*, 2 vols. (Philadelphia: Blanchard and Lea, 1859).

Science is the patrimony of mankind; she stretches forth her right hand and her left in her efforts to develop knowledge, and to utilize it for the benefit of the human race. Until within a comparatively recent period, philosophers and scientists were contented to occupy themselves with the study of the grosser elements of matter, as they appeared to the unassisted eye; but in our generation new objects have engaged their attention, and instruments, of the most delicate construction, have been devised for the investigation and examination of the most minute entities, the very existence of which was not even suspected by the most enlightened of our forefathers. How far the facts revealed by these re-searches have contributed to the extension of our knowledge of sanitary science is familiar to every intelligent person. Without their aid we should still literally be groping in the dark respecting many points of essential importance to the health and the lives of the people. The dangers which constantly beset us in our daily walks in city, town, and country are better understood; the noxious weeds which everywhere so cunningly intertwine their leaves with those of the rose and the lily are more easily discerned; and if, in consequence of the knowledge thus derived, we do not live longer, certain it is that we live more securely and more happily.

The great enemies to health and life, after injuries, parturition, and surgical operations, are septicemia, pyemia, erysipelas, and hospital gangrene, diseases all more or less intimately connected with, if not directly dependent upon, blood-poisoning, itself the result of the influence of vitiated air acting upon the part and system, the pernicious effects being so much the greater in proportion to the crowded condition of a hospital and the tainted state of the atmosphere gen-erated under these circumstances. Even healthy persons, subjected only for a short time to the foul emanations of the crowded wards of such an institution, must inevitably incur great risk to health and life; and, if this be the case, it is easy to perceive what must be the fate of those who, previously to their admis-sion, suffered from severe shock and loss of blood, the great predisposing causes to pyemia, septicemia, erysipelas, and gangrene. The systems of such persons may be compared to tinder which the slightest spark may kindle into a devour-ing flame which no human agency can arrest or control. Persons exhausted by protracted suffering, whether from inadequate supply of food, dissipation, in-temperance, unwholesome occupation, loss of sleep, hard study, mental anxiety, or any cause whatever, are, if brought under the influence of a contaminated atmosphere, liable to be affected in a similar manner; that is, the system is in a state predisposed to disease and only requires to be brought into contact with some poisonous material as, for example, that of scarlet fever, typhoid fever, small-pox, or some other zymotic malady to contract the specific distemper. When the air is unusually tainted, the stoutest and healthiest individuals may, even in a wonderfully short time, contract fatal disease, the system being liter-ally overwhelmed by the specific poison, as we see occasionally exhibited in seminaries, colleges, workshops, factories, and similar establishments. Man and the domestic animals are equally liable to suffer in this manner from these and other causes. The rinderpest, or cattle-plague; the epizooty, which prevailed so extensively two years ago among the horses of this and other cities; the hog-cholera, so well described by Dr. Sutton of Indiana; and the epidemics that occur, from time to time, among dogs, cats, rabbits, and poultry afford ample illustration of the truth of my statement. These distempers, which, like cholera, scarlatina, typhoid fever, and small-pox in the human subject, are all of a zymotic nature and are dependent for their development and propagation upon the existence of a peculiar poison supposed, by common consent, to be contained in the air.

The identity of erysipelas and puerperal fever—an opinion long ago entertained by certain pathologists—is now generally recognized as an established fact. I am myself thoroughly convinced of its truth, and I am equally satisfied of the identity of both these affections and of septicemia, pyemia, and hospital gangrene. The poison of any one of these diseases is capable of producing all the others. Puerperal fever is, in the parturient female, what erysipelas, pyemia, or hospital gangrene is in the male after serious wounds and injuries. The secretions of the overworked and irritated uterus and vagina find their way either by absorption through their mucous surfaces, or directly through the mouths of the dilated uterine veins into the system, poisoning thus both the blood and solids and producing a state of things speedily followed by death. The most irrefragable proof exists that puerperal fever is a contagious disease, communicable by direct contact or indirectly through the agency of the clothes worn by the medical attendants, nurses, and friends of the patient. Many a practitioner has carried the poison of this disease about on his hands, his gloves, or his clothes. A medical gentleman, at one time largely engaged in obstetric practice in this city, lost in the course of a few months upwards of thirty woman from having carried the virus from one house to another, while the patients of other practitioners, even of those living in the same neighborhood, entirely escaped. His paths were literally strewn with dead women, and such was the effect which these melancholy disasters exerted upon his reputation as a professional man that he lost all his practice, and drove him in disgust from the city. Many similar cases could be adduced if time permitted. It was in view of these occurrences, so appalling in their consequences, throwing not only whole families but sometimes even whole communities into mourning, that a Boston gentleman, Oliver Wendell Holmes, gave to a most admirable paper, which he published upon this disease in 1850, the significant title of "Puerperal Fever, Considered as a Private Pestilence." In every lying-in hospital puerperal fever occasionally prevails as an epidemic, carrying off large numbers of women. . . .

How long hospital gangrene has existed as a distinct disease we have no means of determining. That it has, in modern times at least, been the scourge both of civil and military hospitals is well known. During the last century it prevailed more or less extensively in some of the civil hospitals of France, assuming occasionally an epidemic character, and likewise on board of some of the English transports that visited our coasts during the Revolutionary War. In one of these vessels, stationed at New York, upwards of two hundred cases occurred, and of these many proved fatal, death in a considerable number having been due to gangrene of the stump after amputation. The disease also committed great ravages at the Cape of Good Hope, in the West Indies, and in Spain during the Peninsular campaigns. The French army suffered severely from it in the Crimea, and during our late war many of our military hospitals, especially those at Annapolis, Washington City, Baltimore, New York, Louisville, and Frederick, Maryland, were more or less extensively infested with it. In the Philadelphia Hospital sporadic cases of the disease occurred every winter during the seven years of my connection with that institution, chiefly among old, broken-down patients, the subjects of chronic sores, and of a scorbutic state of the system. . . .

As preventives of the diseases incident to persons laboring under wounds and injuries, confined in hospitals, of necessity more or less crowded, various kinds of dressings have lately come into use, a few of which, from the attention they have attracted, may be appropriately noticed here; promising that while some of them are exceedingly complex others are so simple as hardly to merit the name. The hermetically sealed dressing, as I shall call it, or, as it is generally designated, the *antiseptic* mode of treatment of wounds has been brought prominently forward by Professor Lister of Edinburgh. He has rendered himself famous by the advocacy of the method of treatment of wounds and compound fractures and dislocations; many surgeons, especially in Europe, have bowed at his shrine, and many controversies have taken place respecting it during the last six or eight years. Notwithstanding, however, all that has been said and written upon the subject, the utility of the antiseptic treatment is still as much as ever a matter of dispute. As for myself, I have long been of the opinion that its good effects are due, mainly, if not wholly, to the care which is taken in cleansing the wound of blood and foreign matter, in approximating its edges, deep as well as superficial, in excluding the air, and in keeping the parts and system at rest in a pure atmosphere, and the patient upon proper diet until union has occurred. That carbolic acid, carbolate of soda, and kindred preparations are excellent disinfectants and deodorizers is unquestionable; but that they possess the virtues ascribed to them by Mr. Lister and his followers is in the highest degree improbable. According to the Scotch surgeon, these agents act as germicides, destroying, as the term implies, the animalcules supposed to be floating about in the atmosphere, and to insinuate themselves at every opportunity into the interior of wounds and the cavities of abscesses after the evacuation of their contents. Now, I shall not stop here to reopen the question of the germ theory, or whether there are such entities as germs or not; it will suffice for my purpose to state that some surgeons, of at least equal intelligence with Mr. Lister and his disciples, discard dressings altogether, leaving the wound freely exposed to the air and relying solely upon rest, cleanliness, and other hygienic measures for a speedy and successful cure. This plan of treatment, which is extensively pursued at the great hospital at Vienna, in the words of Professor Billroth, has furnished admirable results in the hands of a number of English and Continental practitioners, and recommends itself by its great simplicity. Professor Rose of Zurich has employed it in upwards of one hundred cases with the most gratifying effects. . . . Much of the success of the treatment of wounds depends, first, upon the manner in which they are made; secondly, upon the care with which they are cleansed; and, thirdly, upon the manner in which they are approximated. All these circumstances have a direct and positive influence upon its future wellbeing and final result. It may be assumed, as a general law that, all other things being equal, the rapidity with which a wound heals will be in direct proportion to the absence of contusion, foreign matter, and rude handling. A wound made with the surgeon's knife will be more likely to do well if the tissues have been cut smoothly than if they be divided roughly, as when the knife is dull or rusty. A dirty knife may even inoculate a raw surface, and so also a dirty finger, with the poison of a specific disease. A dirty or unwashed ligature, or a ligature roughly applied, may prove a source of irritation, sadly interfering with the healing process. Modern surgeons the world over pay much attention to the cleansing of wounds. The slightest particle of extraneous matter, even the finest hair, will inevitably interfere with the adhesive process. Blood acts in a similar manner. If allowed to remain in the wound it is soon decomposed, and thus not only opposes union, but some of the putrescent particles being carried with the system and so poison the entire body, it may become a prominent factor in the production of metastatic abscess. For this reason a wound, whether the result of accident or made with the surgeon's knife, is always cleansed with the greatest possible care. . . . Great injury is often inflicted upon a wound in the attempts to approximate its edges. A blunt, dirty needle, coarse, unwaxed thread, and rude manipulation, are ill calculated to favor reunion. A bandage applied unevenly or too tightly cannot fail to act prejudicially. Then, again, rest is of paramount importance, and not only rest but elevation and easy position of the parts. If all these things are attended to, and the patient has, in addition, the advantage of good air, good nursing, and good medical attendance, it is difficult to conceive how, in ordinary cases, a wound should fail to do well, or the system incur any risk from the ingress of putrescent matter. Immense numbers of persons die from defective ventilation and cleanliness, and I am quite sure that far more mortality is occasioned, in cases of injuries and of parturient women, by bad nursing than there is by bad doctoring, bad as the latter unquestionably often is. . . . When foul animal or vegetable germs enter the system through a large wound, as, for example, the stump of an amputated limb, or when the foul secretions that are under such circumstances formed in a wound are carried into the system, they become at once factors of pyaemia, erysipelas, and gangrene, and, consequently, causes of death, particularly so if there be an impure state of the air from overcrowding, defective ventilation, or want of cleanliness; for, once admitted into the system, few, if any, ever recover. The baneful fluid acts either as a direct poison, weakening the powers of life, and more or less rapidly destroying it; or it causes death by decomposing the blood, and inducing the formation of blood-clots, technically called thrombi, which, obstructing the circulation, occasion death by arresting the functions of organs essential to life, or by becoming so many centres for the development of destructive abscesses, often so numerous as to have received the significant appellation of multiple.

The interesting question here arises, what is the essential nature of the poison generated in decomposing animal fluids, such, more especially, as are formed in wounds and in the open surface of compound fractures and dislocations? Is it a peculiar poison, similar in principle to that of vaccinia or small-pox, for example; or is it a poison the product of fermentation, of catalysis, or of living germs or organisms, as bacteria and vibriones, floating about in the air and liable to be generated, often in immense numbers, in the blood and the various secretions of the body in cases of so-called blood-poisoning, however induced? Unfortunately here science is dumb; we literally know nothing of these things, but we do know that these animal poisons, whatever they may be, possess an astonishing power of multiplying themselves, and thus augmenting their virulence or destructive agency. That this is true is unquestionable, and it may therefore be assumed that the germs or animalcules are derived immediately and directly from progenitor or parent cells. Experience has shown that the poison of contagious and infectious diseases retains its specific properties for a long time, if not indefinitely, thus bearing a striking resemblance to the virus of vaccinia, small-pox, and of some other secretions common to both sexes. . . .

If hospitals are liable to become pest-houses, it is equally certain that private dwellings in the country, adorned with every luxury that taste and money can command, also occasionally serve as plague spots. It not infrequently happens in such residences that the same wind which wafts to its occupants the fragrance of the rose and the honeysuckle, carries with it in the same breath the virus of the most deadly disease, due, in most instances, to defective sewerage, often little, if at all, suspected by the ill-fated inmates.[1]

The old houses in the dirty, narrow streets and alleys of our cities are so many plague spots, which it would be a real godsend to burn to the ground. The great fire of London which, in the seventeenth century, within four days and nights destroyed nearly the whole of its miserable and degraded districts, previously ravaged by the plague, was the greatest boon ever conferred upon that now mighty and majestic city. It completely eradicated that frightful disease, which has been so graphically portrayed by De Foe, and which in six months in 1665 swept away nearly twenty thousand inhabitants, or one-eighth of its population.

---

[1] In 1833, Lexington, Kentucky, until then one of the most salubrious towns in the Union, as it has always been one of the most beautiful and charming, had its population decimated by Asiatic cholera from this cause; and a number of other towns in the west and southwest suffered equally severely.

No person can walk through Alaska Street in this city, or the Five Points in New York, without a sigh that civilized society should permit the existence of such degradation, such hot-beds of disease and vice; or without a silent prayer that God, in his infinite mercy, would visit the wretched hovels with consuming fire, the greatest scavenger and house-cleaner known to man. When we consider the many valuable lives that are lost by disease engendered by the foul air of such polluted and pestilential districts, it is evident that there is no economy in retaining such tenements, hardly fit as habitations for our inferior animals, but every reason, sanitary and moral, why they should be torn down, and others erected in their stead at the public expense. When this cannot be done, they should be frequently cleansed and disinfected. Now, what is true of such wretched dwellings is hardly less true of the old and dirty stores, factories, workshops, school-houses, hotels, and coffee-houses of every town and city in the world. To carry out these measures, useful alike in a sanitary and moral point of view—for no people can be good or moral who do not habitually breathe pure air and enjoy the advantages of bodily cleanliness—there should be salaried inspectors who, under the supervision of a Board of Health, should at stated periods visit the more humble districts and look after their sanitary condition, a part of their duty being to instruct the residents how to live, cook their food, ventilate their houses, dress their children, and, above all, how to keep themselves clean and tidy. These ideas are not Utopian, but founded upon common sense and the broad principles of humanity. There are some persons who are naturally clean and tidy under any circumstances, persons who have an inborn aversion to filth of every description, and who, however poor they may be, are always respectable, people in whose presence a gentleman instinctively takes off his hat; as there are other persons who are naturally unclean and untidy, who have no love for water and soap, whatever may be their worldly condition. With them dirt is soil always in the right place. How much these and a thousand other sanitary matters are neglected the world over is as familiarly known as they are disgraceful and reprehensible; or, to put it in more just language, as they are criminal in the sight of God and of thinking man. We send missionaries into heathen countries and spend thousands upon thousands of dollars annually in our efforts to civilize and Christianize our Indians; but we let the poor of our towns and cities wallow in their mire, contaminating the very air we breathe and breeding disease and pestilence, which, in turn, cut off, often by an untimely death, many of our best citizens. We license coffee-houses to increase our revenues, and thus make drunkards and criminals whom we afterwards punish with fine, imprisonment, and the hangman's rope. We boast of our civilization and our Christianity and consider ourselves wise in our generation. Well may we exclaim, where are our philanthropists, our legislators, our philosophers, our Christians? Where shall we find men, ready and determined, to stir up the public mind to devise measures for refining and elevating the wretched creatures who, shut up in the narrow and filthy alleys and by-ways of our cities, are aliens from God and outcasts from society, often with hardly any of the natural attributes of human beings? I wish to God that some mighty Howard, armed with Gabriel's trumpet, would arise to teach us our duty; nay, not only teach, but compel us to perform it. Surely such apathy, such criminal indifference must attracted the notice of a beneficient Deity and be visited with his sorest displeasure.

From the foregoing remarks the following conclusions may, I think, justly be deduced:

1. That the maladies known, respectively, as erysipelas, pyemia, septicemia, hospital gangrene, and puerperal fever all owe their existence to the same or similar disease-germs.

2. That these disease-germs, whatever their essential nature may be, possess an astonishing proliferating faculty or power of multiplication and extension, especially apparent in overcrowded and ill-ventilated hospitals, asylums, prisons, ships, and similar establishments.

3. That these germs adhere with great tenacity to everything with which they are brought into contact, especially woolen articles; that, having once fastened themselves, they are destroyed with great difficulty; and, lastly, that they may readily be conveyed by the clothes, and even by the hands, from house to house and patient to patient, by the medical attendants, nurses, and friends of the sick.

4. That in dressing wounds the greatest possible care should be taken to employ clean hands, instruments, and sponges, to avoid rude manipulation, to remove all extraneous matter, to effect close approximation, to guard against the retention of secretions, and to change the dressings the moment they become soiled.

5. That hospitals, however well constructed, especially during the prevalence of epidemics, are, as a rule, pest-houses or breeders of disease-germs and, therefore, under such circumstances, unfit as receptacles for sick, wounded, and lying-in persons.

6. That when a zymotic disease breaks out in a hospital immediate steps should be taken to place the inmates in tents in the open air and to cleanse the wards with disinfectants, as chlorinated soda and permanganate of potassa, and, above all, by whitewashing and painting.

7. That the attendants upon the sick and wounded and upon lying-in women should make free use of disinfectants, keep their nails and hands perfectly clean, and never wear the same clothes in visiting their private patients that they wear in the performance of their hospital duties.

ROBERT F. WEIR

ON THE ANTISEPTIC TREATMENT OF WOUNDS, AND ITS RESULTS

Editor's Note

After Lister's appearance before the International Medical Congress in Philadelphia in September 1876 and his tour of eastern cities, more and more surgeons became converts to the new system. Robert F. Weir was one of these. He was born in New York in 1838, received his M.D. degree from the College of Physicians and Surgeons in 1859 and soon became a leader among the surgeons of the city. He was a prodigious contributor of articles to medical journals and held several teaching positions in the medical colleges of New York City. Part of his long discussion of the antiseptic system, its rationale, and his results, are included in the following selection.

As we have seen, Erichsen in 1874 reported that antisepsis was not used much by American surgeons because their hospitals and their operating habits were generally cleaner than those in Europe. In 1876 Samuel Gross voiced similar sentiments when he said, "Little, if any faith, is placed by any enlightened or experienced surgeon on this side of the Atlantic in the so-called carbolic acid treatment of Professor Lister, apart from the care which is taken in applying the dressing."[1] Admittedly, acceptance of antisepsis in the United States was rather slow, but Gross's statement must be read with caution.[2]

It is only lately that in America attention has been given practically to the teachings of Lister in respect to the treatment of wounds. In fact, aside from an article by Schuppert in the *New Orleans Medical and Surgical Journal*, little or nothing has appeared in our medical journals relative to the results of the so-called antiseptic method. Within the past year, however, a change has occurred, due probably both to the interest excited by the personal expositions of Lister at our late Medical Congress at Philadelphia, and also to the satisfactory results that have ensued from this treatment in the practice of many German surgeons with large hospital experience. The reason why American surgeons—who justly have the reputation of being eager to seize upon any improvement in their

---

New York Med. J. 26 (1877): 561–80; 27 (1878): 31–51. Read before the New York County Medical Society at their meeting on November 26, 1877.

[1] "A century of American medicine," *Am. J. Med. Sci.* 71 (1876): 431–84; 483.

[2] See my "American surgery and the germ theory of disease," *Bull. Hist. Med.* 40 (1966): 135–45.

art—have been tardy in testing the success of this mode of treatment may, perhaps, be stated at follows: 1. That the treatment, as enunciated by Mr. Lister, has been repeatedly changed in its details; 2. That it was too complicated, and demanded the supervision of the surgeon himself, or, in a hospital, of a carefully-trained staff of assistants; 3. That many who had tried it had been unsuccessful in the cases where the essay had been made. But the most weighty objection which was asserted or entertained, was the positiveness of the enunciation of the germ-theory in explanation of the process of decomposition in the secretions of a wound. Only the latter reason requires any attention at present, and, as a clearer conception of the intent of the many *minutiae* of the dressing may come from a synopsis of this theory, it will be succinctly given, notwithstanding the purpose of this evening's paper is to present the subject as far as possible from a clinical point of view.

It is, in a few words, this: 1. That in the dust of the atmosphere, and in matter with which it is in contact, there are the germs of minute organisms, which under favorable circumstances induce putrefaction in fluids and solids capable of that change, in the same manner as the yeast-plant occasions the alcoholic fermentation in a saccharine solution; 2. That putrefaction is not occasioned by the chemical action of oxygen or other gas, but by the fermentative agency of these organisms; 3. That the vitality or potency of the germs can be destroyed by heat or by various chemical substances, which are called, in surgery, "antiseptics."[1] The very definition of the "antiseptic system," as given in the words of Lister himself, is "the dealing with surgical cases in such a way as to prevent the introduction of putrefactive influences into wounds."[2] Nothing need here be added to these statements, in their verification or otherwise (though analogy and accumulating facts seem to lend support to them), except that from the standpoint adopted two important statements need to be referred to. I mean those of Thompson,[3] Weitzelbaum,[4] and others, that they had found living bacteria in the carbolic solutions as used by Lister, and of Linhart,[5] Fischer,[6] Ranke,[7] Schüller,[8] and Volkmann,[9] who, in several hundred observations, have found bacteria in the discharges of wounds that had been most carefully and satisfactorily treated by the antiseptic method. It was noticed, however, that the presence or absence of these bacteria (and such were only

---

[1] T. Smith, *Lancet*, March 25, 1876.

[2] "Transactions of the International Medical Congress," Philadelphia, 1876.

[3] Medical Times and Gazette, November 6, 1875.

[4] *Wiener Med. Presse*, 1876, Nos. 10 and 11.

[5] Schmidt's "Jahrbücher," vol. 174, 4.

[6] *Deut. Zeitschr. f. Chirur.*, vol. vi., p. 319.

[7] Idem, vol. vi., p. 63.

[8] Idem, vol. vii., 1876, pp. 5, 6.

[9] Schmidt's "Jahrbücher," vol. 174, 2, 1877.

considered as present when chain-bacteria were found) did not influence the progress of the wounds; and Fischer gives the opinion, in which many of his countrymen join, that the object of the dressing is not so much to keep the germs away as to keep the secretions in such a condition as to be as unfavorable as possible to the development of bacteria and thus prevent decomposition taking place.

It is only justice to append the remarks of Mr. Lister at the Congress in respect to these observations, or rather, correctly speaking, of Ranke's. They are, textually: "The statement that cell forms have been found beneath antiseptic dressings must be received with caution. I have," continues he, "recently met a gentleman who was with Ranke in Halle when he found, as he supposed, these organisms beneath antiseptic coverings; and when the gentleman pointed out to me the bacteria which he called putrefactive, I at once recognized them as of the non-putrefactive variety, and the gentleman was forced to admit that they differed from those found in decomposing masses."[10]

Passing from these facts (?) of the laboratory, let us consider those to be used and acquired at the bedside. In practicing this method, in order to form a proper judgment of its merits, it is essential that Mr. Lister's plan should be thoroughly known and be carried out even to its minutest particular. The chorus on this point is unanimous among surgeons who have successfully used it. Hagedorn, of Magdeburg, says that in every failure the surgeon himself is to blame and not the method; and Lindpaintner,[11] representing the experience of Munich with nearly a thousand cases treated antiseptically, states that it must be considered a precept that the minutest directions must be followed, and that he who does not get the result (desired) must certainly have made some mistake. This opinion is reiterated by all who have achieved success by the method, and the number of such is already large and increasing.[12] A second condition, which really should have come first, is that they who use the method should at least provisionally accept the theory on which the dressing is based; they should, so to speak, act as if they saw germs on everything. This, however, is not so imperative as the one just spoken of.

"For," remarks Lister, "those who are unwilling to accept the theory in its entirety, and choose to assume that the septic material is not of the nature of living organisms, but a so-called chemical ferment destitute of vitality, yet endowed with the power of self-multiplication. . . . such a notion, unwarranted though I believe it to be by any scientific evidence, will, in a practical point of view, be equivalent to the germ-theory, since it will inculcate precisely the same methods of antiseptic management. It is important that this should be clearly understood." . . .

---

[10]"Transactions of the International Congress," 1875, p. 540.

[11]*Deut. Zeitschr. f. Chirur.*, vol. vii., p. 18.

[12]*See* Schmidt's *Jahrbücher*, vol. 172, 4, and Hirsch's *Jahresbericht*, 1877, for an interesting summary of the antiseptic treatment.

STEPHEN SMITH

THE COMPARATIVE RESULTS OF OPERATIONS IN BELLEVUE HOSPITAL

Editor's Note

Stephen Smith's life (1823–1922) spanned the great epochs of anesthesia and antisepsis. Anesthesia had barely been introduced when he began to study medicine in 1847, and he himself was one of the early American champions of antisepsis. The author of numerous surgical papers and three surgical textbooks, Smith was an active member of Bellevue's staff for fifty years. During the Civil War years he edited a weekly medical journal through which he championed several reform causes. (See section on Hygiene.) In his later life he was active in lunacy reform in New York, serving as the State's Commissioner in Lunacy from 1882 until 1888 and on the State Board of Charities until he resigned, at the age of ninety-five, in 1918.

Smith was very interested in medical history and wrote several papers and two historical sections for surgical texts. The following paper is an example of what we would call contemporary history. It is informative because Smith describes the conditions he and his colleagues faced until Lister's system came into regular use.

Smith seems to understand the underlying rationale of Lister's method, the germ theory, but is careful to leave open the "final conclusion of scientific students as to the cause of putrefaction in wounds." He leaves no doubt that the earlier surgeons dressed their wounds expecting suppuration, but by 1885 they expected primary healing. It is interesting, too, that Smith specifically pointed out that "no bystander [is] invited to put his finger in the wound, but scarcely an attendant at Bellevue would allow such an intrusion." This, we must remember, is only four years after President Garfield was shot in Washington's Baltimore and Potomac Station, and his wound subsequently examined frequently by probe and finger. Some of the medical reports of the President's progress indicated that "Listerism was used throughout." Yet we know this could not have been the case. Had Garfield been admitted to Bellevue a short four years later, he might have had less secondary infection if what Smith tells us in this paper was indeed the universal practice in 1885.

As we drift with current events, we but imperfectly estimate the real advance which any art or science with which we are daily familiar has made within a limited period. It is only when we considerately pause and deliberately compare, in detail, past methods and results with those now practiced and obtained that

Med. Record 28 (1885): 427–31.

we fully appreciate the vast changes which have so insidiously and imperceptibly taken place.

Perhaps there is no better place in which to test the progress of practical and operative surgery than the wards of Bellevue Hospital. This ancient institution has within its walls and its immediate environments all the conditions that in modern times are regarded as unhealthful and unsanitary. It was built between the years 1811–16, on the made lands of a cove of East River, without drainage, or adequate sewerage, and without regard to ventilation. During nearly three-fourths of a century the sluggish tides have ebbed and flowed through the sodden soil of its foundation, depositing far more filth than they have removed. Since its occupation it has been used for a prison, an almshouse, and a hospital. Its wards have, from time to time, been crowded with patients suffering from all forms of contagious and infectious diseases. It has been the common receptacle of typhus and typhoid fevers, small-pox, puerperal fever, cholera, and yellow fever. Although many changes have been made in its interior, yet the great and most serious defects of location and construction have remained unaltered and may be regarded as permanent.

Bellevue may be regarded as having been a surgical hospital only since 1850, a period of about thirty-five years, during most of which period I have been personally very familiar with the practice in the several surgical divisions. The amount of surgery in the wards of Bellevue has been a gradual increase. With the removal of the New York Hospital, and during the long interval of its non-existence, the surgical practice of Bellevue became large and important and has remained so to the present time. The surgeons of Bellevue have always ranked among the best in the city, and, as much of their practice in the hospital has been public and clinical, it must be assumed that they have endeavored to the best of their ability to illustrate to their classes the highest type and best results of the science and art of surgery of their day. And yet the practice of surgery in Bellevue Hospital has, within the period mentioned, undergone so complete a revolution that one of the older surgeons would scarcely realize that he was in the same hospital where he had practiced a decade ago. He would see, with horror, operations fearlessly performed that he had formerly regarded as without the pale of legitimate surgery. He would witness procedures in the after-treatment of operations which would seem to him to be fantastic and even ludicrous. His astonishment would be extreme on finding that the first week passed without fever and that no change in the dressings had been made. But, perhaps, the most remarkable feature of modern practice would be the rapid convalescence and final complete recovery without the complication or exhaustion of ordinary operations, which formerly gave so much trouble and anxiety. To make more evident the change in practice, we may contrast in detail the several steps of operations in general, and of individual cases, the methods of treatment, and the results.

The older surgeons of Bellevue Hospital had practiced in the period anterior to the use of anesthetics. The most important general principle governing the operator was *celerity*—in order to limit as much as possible the amount of pain. Long after anesthetics came into general use surgeons dwelt with much emphasis upon the necessity of cultivating the habit of operating rapidly. The preparations for an operation were all made with reference to this one feature. So much did this thought absorb the operator that he often became excited and annoyed by the delay. One surgeon, noted for the rapidity of his operations, was often seen, during the last moments of preparation for an amputation, to seize involuntarily the saw and move it rapidly, as if sawing a bone. Now, while every surgeon aims to diminish the period of anesthesia, mere haste at an operation is only mentioned to be condemned. No part of the elaborate preparations are designed to render the operation simply more rapid. One thought and purpose occupy the mind of the surgeon, and that is recovery without suppuration. To this end all his preparations are made, and the entire procedure is subordinated. Formerly the surgeon prepared his instruments only by keeping them free from rust and giving them a fine edge. When he operated the instruments were taken from the case and, without any cleansing, were so placed that he could most readily select the one required. During the operation he laid them down, or dropped them, and without cleaning applied them again to the wound. Now instruments are not only protected from rust and all soiling and kept sharp, but long before the operation they are placed in a carbolic solution, in order that any possible septic matter on them on their handles may be destroyed.

During the operation one assistant devotes himself entirely to the duty of handling the instruments to the operator, and of receiving them from him and at once submerging them in the disinfectant liquid. To avoid the possibility of laying an instrument down on an unclean surface and then putting it in the wound soiled, towels wrung out of the antiseptic fluid are spread around the wound.

In preparing a part for an operation, as amputation, the surgeon used to do nothing farther than, perhaps, to have superfluous hair shaved off, and that, too, often without soap and water. Patients brought directly from the street or shop, with limbs begrimed with dirt and filth, were subjected to operations without bathing. Even when there was ample time for preparation, little or no thought was given to the immediate condition of the part about to be incised. The accumulated secretions of the skin and the dead epidermis, charged with poisonous animal matters, became part of the wound and its immediate surroundings. Through this layer of filth the surgeon passed his knife into the living tissues beneath, conveying to the deepest parts of the wound matters of untold septic virulence. In this simple failure to secure ordinary cleanliness of the surface more wounds were poisoned and induced to suppurate than from any other cause. In the closure of the wound the filthy margins were often brought in direct contact with the cut surfaces, and thus the propagation of the germs of fermentation or putrefaction were implanted in a fertile soil. Now, the greatest pains are taken to cleanse the part about to be operated upon. In addition to a general bath, the entire limb, including the hand or foot, is washed with soap and water, with a flesh-brush, and all the hairs are shaved cleanly from the part. This washing is followed by a douche of an antiseptic solution, and then all the parts adjacent to the wound are covered with towels wrung out of bichloride solution.

The personal preparation of the surgeon and his assistants for the operation was limited to self-protection against soiling their clothes or person. No special thought was ever given to the condition of the hands and nails. The assistants came directly from other ward duties, their hands soiled by contact with the thousand impure matters which they must handle, and with slight or no washing, engaged actively in the manipulations of the operation. Now the surgeon and his assistants take infinite pains with their hands. Soap and water and the flesh-brush are brought into active use, to be followed by a douche of bichloride solution. The nails, the most fertile source of filth in the body, are rendered scrupulously clean. Many will recall with a shudder the long claw-like nail of one surgeon, which penetrated, unwashed, every wound where he was present. Not only is no bystander invited to put his finger in the wound, but scarcely an attendant at Bellevue would allow such an intrusion.

The sponges of former times are universally believed to be the carriers of filth to the wounds, and yet little was done to purify them except to cleanse them in water. They may have been boiled at first to free them from sand, but they were not purified by any adequate means when first prepared nor after their use in suppurating wounds. Now, the process of purification of sponges is elaborate in the extreme and is so exact in details as to render them positively harmless in wounds.

The ordinary silk ligatures were formerly regarded as necessarily foreign bodies in wounds, and no care was taken of them to improve their condition. They were carried about in any convenient pocket, and at the operation the silk was cut to proper lengths, waxed, and then drawn through a buttonhole of an assistant, or laid on any convenient surface. Now the ligature thread undergoes a long process of cleansing and disinfection at the hands of a chemist and is then applied to a reel enclosed in a corked bottle filled with antiseptic fluid. From this bottle it is removed only as it is drawn out at the moment of using it. Considering the well-recognized fact that the ligature, as formerly used, was an intense irritant to wounds, it is not surprising that surgeons applied as few as possible. From time to time they resorted to other methods of closing arteries, as by torsion, or metallic wires, to avoid the use of silk. But all these devices bore no comparison to the simple and efficient antiseptic ligature of today. Reeled off from the bottle, clean, strong, and supple, the surgeon applies them without other limit than the complete suppression of hemorrhage.

Recognizing the silk ligature as an irritant, the surgeon always used to cut off but one end and left the other end depending from the wound, to be removed by traction when it had finally separated from the end of the vessel to which it had been applied. And well and faithfully did the ligature meet its indications, for, during the first week, the most critical period in the history of the wound, it did not fail to induce free and often profuse, suppuration. But now, not only does the surgeon freely apply the ligature, but he cuts off both ends and closes the wound as completely as if there was no foreign substance left between its surfaces. Nor is he disappointed. No suppuration follows the presence of the ligatures, and union takes place as promptly as if no ligatures had been used. The operation being completed in the shortest possible time, the operator concluded by exploring all parts of the wound with his unwashed fingers. If it was a hernia, he thrust his fingers as far into the abdominal cavity as possible, and explored it freely. This act completed, it was a very common occurrence, also, for the surgeon to invite any bystander to examine the wound with his fingers, and sometimes several persons would avail themselves of the opportunity to improve their tactual sensibilities. . . .

Surgical fever, with all its disastrous variations, is, in practice, rare in Bellevue Hospital. Pus, as an outcome of surgical operations, is a thing of the past. On one occasion last winter, a teacher in one of the medical colleges sent to the wards of Bellevue for a specimen of pus for exhibition to his class, but none was to be found in the four surgical divisions of the hospital, although there was at that time an unusually large number of wounds and operated cases under active treatment. The wound is now dressed with no expectation that fever will rise, or that suppuration will occur, or that the dressings will require renewal on account of the presence of pus. The patient sleeps and eats well from the first, and the surgeon removes the dressing, often only to find the wound united. This remark is true, not only of incised wounds, but equally of wounds of amputation, excision, ligation of arteries, etc.

If now we turn from this review of the several stages of operations in general to particular operations, we find many curious illustrations of the remarkable progress of practical surgery in this hospital. It must be understood that in every operation all of the general precautionary measures already described are scrupulously taken and carried out, and, therefore, only special differences in treatment will be mentioned.

Compound fractures were formerly regarded as proper cases for amputation, if the local injury exceeded a single fracture, with a simple penetration of the soft tissues. And even the simplest cases of compound fracture were reserved for treatment with many misgivings as to the result. The dictum of Hunter that "compound fractures commonly suppurate" was ever the guiding principle in the mind of the surgeon. If, therefore, the wound was extensive, or the bones comminuted, or a joint involved, amputation was the rule. If it were decided to endeavor to save the limb, the only measures adopted were sealing the external wound with some imperfect substance, and placing the limb in a comfortable position. The old fracture-box for the leg and the fenestrated gypsum bandage were the only measures employed. The fracture-box, with its bed of bran or sawdust, was regarded as a remarkable advance in the treatment of compound fractures of the tibia. Placed in the box, with the foot fixed to the foot-board, the wound was covered with bran and suppuration allowed to go on *ad libitum* and *ad infinitum*. The contrivance had no merit whatever. On the contrary, it greatly aggravated the suppuration by fixing the lower fragment, while it allowed the upper fragment to move freely upon it every time the patient moved. The gypsum splint and bandage had the merit of keeping, or aiming to keep, both fragments at perfect rest. This method of treating compound fractures was a real step in advance, but it did not prevent suppuration in some measure. Today compound fractures are welcomed to the wards of Bellevue as a class of cases which give the most satisfactory results.

Amputation is not thought of unless arteries and nerves are so far destroyed that death of the extremity must follow. Even when the wound involves a joint, the question of amputation is not more pressing. The treatment pursued is designed—1. to remove from the wound every particle of matter liable to injure the tissues and induce suppuration; 2. to place in fixed apposition all of the tissues composing the wound; 3. to cleanse and disinfect the wound and protect it from becoming soiled during recovery; 4. to protect the wound from any movement of the parts entering into it while the process of repair is going on. The procedure, so far as concerns the wound, consists in freely exposing the injured parts by incision, removing all effusions of blood, shreds of injured tissue, fragments of bone, and then wiring the bones together so that fractured parts exactly fit each other, next stitching together all cut or torn tissues with prepared catgut thread, as far as they can be brought together; then the final closure of the wound, except where a drainage-tube may be inserted into a cavity of the deep parts; and, finally, the external antiseptic dressings and a light bandage of plaster-of-Paris, and over all a wire-gauze splint for suspension. This treatment of compound fractures is so uniformly successful that the surgeon has none of that care and anxiety after the final dressings which formerly harassed him. If there should be symptoms indicating suppuration, the dressings are at once removed and the source of the trouble searched out and destroyed.

Amputation wounds rarely, if ever, recovered at Bellevue, except after long-continued suppuration. From the smaller amputations patients recovered in due time, but often greatly enfeebled by the drain of suppuration. The larger amputations were terribly fatal. A resident surgeon once made the statement that a recovery after amputation of the thigh had not occurred in Bellevue Hospital "since the time that the memory of man runneth not to the contrary." Though this remark was not strictly true, it had a painful significance to the surgeons of that period. Suppuration, with its sequelae, septicemic, pyemic, and hectic fevers was the scourge of the surgical wards. The open method of treatment of amputation wounds, advocated by Dr. James R. Wood, had only the merit of not confining the pus within the wounds, and of thus diminishing somewhat the liability of septicemia and pyemia. It did not prevent suppuration, the source of all the evil. The treatment consisted in closing the upper part of the wound, and placing the stump in such position that the pus flowed freely out into a vessel placed to receive it. The period of suppuration was undoubtedly diminished by this free exposure of the wound to the air, and the application of balsam of Peru, a favorite remedy with Dr. Wood. The open method was, therefore, a decided improvement upon the old method of closing wounds, but it came far short of the present method, which prevents suppuration altogether, or reduces it to a minimum. Except for the unfavorable conditions incident to the injury, amputations are now among the most successful operations at Bellevue. Death, by suppuration and its results, does not occur.

Excision of the larger joints was formerly a most doubtful and dangerous operation. The wounds were flooded with pus for months; and if the patient survived, it was only after the most desperate struggle. The specimens of exsected joints in the Wood Museum, honeycombed with channels through which pus flowed out from the deeper parts of the wound, will be lasting witnesses to the destructive pathological processes which the surgeons of a former period could not avert, and which brought to an untimely issue the best-planned operations. In dressing exsection wounds the older surgeons made ample preparation for suppuration. The wound was left open, and the limb was placed in such position as would allow the pus to escape most freely. For months the patient lay in the same position, wasting under the excessive drain, and often having as a dreaded complication extensive bed-sores. Now the surgeon completes the operation by firmly and accurately closing the wound at all points, except where the drainage-tube emerges. This tube is used only for the temporary purposes of relieving the wound of accumulating serous fluid and is soon removed. As a rule, excision wounds now do not suppurate; union takes place by rapid and healthy granulation.

During the past year or two we have had under observation many cases of excision of the knee joint, the hip joint, the elbow joint, and the ankle joint, which have been repaired without suppuration. In one instance of an old and destructive inflammation of the ankle joint, the articular ends of the tibia and fibula, the surfaces of the astragalus and os calces, and all of the surrounding tissues had to be thoroughly scraped to remove the dead bone and fungus granulations. When the cavity was prepared for dressing it was enormous. But as all diseased structures seemed to be removed, and the wound appeared everywhere clean, it was dressed for union without suppuration. The wound did heal without other suppuration than a slight amount of pus, which discharged from a small carious surface. The health of the patient began at once to improve, and in due time she was about the ward on crutches. We may now say of excisions, as of amputations, that they are regarded as simple and very safe operations.

The ligation of large arteries was formerly justly estimated as a very serious operation. The common silk ligature, prepared by unwashed hands, was left depending from the wound. To do its work properly it must in due time sever the strangulated artery by the ulcerative process and then be removed by traction. With the keenest and often most painful anxiety, the surgeon daily watched the wound to note the amount of suppuration and gently tested the firmness of the ligature. If after the separation of the ligature the suppuration diminished, and finally ceased, the surgeon was happy and boastful of his success. But far too often the suppuration did not diminish, and to the dismay of the surgeon a slight oozing or gush of blood indicated to his practiced eye a fatal issue by secondary hemorrhage.

How desperately yet vainly he struggled against fate by resorting to pressure, position, styptics, etc., the older surgeons can alone realize. The repeated hemorrhages, or uncontrollable outburst, at length placed the case in the category of unsuccessful operations. Now, how completely are all the conditions of the operation changed! It is no longer necessary to divide the artery by the ligature to accomplish our object and thus endanger life by hemorrhage; but, on the contrary, we seek, while we interrupt the circulation sufficiently to effect our purpose, to strengthen the artery by our operation. The indications now are the opposite of those which before obtained. The ligature now selected is nonirritating, and preferably absorbable, as catgut. When applied, it may or may not divide the internal coats of the artery. In either case the wound is completely closed and no suppuration occurs. . . .

Though this paper was to be limited to a review of the comparative results of the ordinary surgical practices of Bellevue, formerly and now, with a brief commentary upon the means and methods employed, I cannot pass unnoticed the success which attends the practice of gynecology in that hospital. The surgery of the pelvic organs of the female is based on the same principles as those which govern the general practice of surgery in Bellevue. And the results are equally remarkable.

Septicemia and pyemia are almost unknown in the pavilion devoted to this branch of surgery, and recovery after operations is rapid and complete, unless the case is complicated with conditions quite beyond control. The following statistics show the great success of operations in this branch of practice at Bellevue. Dr. Wylie states that since November, 1883, he has performed laparotomy thirty times, chiefly in the Marquand and Sturgis pavilions, with five deaths. Of the cases proving fatal, two were hysterectomies, one for cancer of the uterus and the other for a myoma weighing fifty pounds; two were cases of pelvic abscess, complicated with purulent collections in the fallopian tubes. All of the cases of ovarian cysts recovered.

In reviewing the surgical practice of Bellevue, it is not difficult to determine the essential feature of the present methods as compared with those of the past. Cleanliness is the one great object sought to be attained in all operations. Whatever may be the final conclusion of scientific students as to the cause of putrefaction in wounds, practically it is determined that the surgeon may, with the most absolute certainty, protect an ordinary open wound from suppuration. To effect this object he finds that he has simply to resort to those measures which are known to secure perfect cleanliness of the wound. The agents now relied upon and found efficient are: 1. Soap and water to external parts. 2. Carbolic solutions for the instruments. 3. Bichloride solutions to all surfaces and tissues. 4. Iodoform for external dressings. We may summarize the conditions regarded as essential to success as follows, viz.: *A clean operator; clean assistants; a clean patient; clean instruments; clean dressings.*

PART VI

PSYCHIATRY

INTRODUCTION

Of all the afflictions that beset man none is more threatening than mental illness. In the nineteenth century, as today, experts argued over its causes, its treatment, even over its definition and classification. The majority of patients were sent to county almshouses, where care was purely custodial, or to state hospitals that were usually over-crowded and understaffed.

The movement for reform in the care of the mentally ill was one of several humanitarian concerns at mid-century. The work of Dorthea Dix, for instance, is well known. But progress was very slow. She fought many battles in order to force reluctant state legislatures to spend more money for properly housing and treating their insane. Some states, notably Massachusetts and New York, built good state hospitals, but the cry throughout the century was that mental illness was rising at a rate faster than hospital beds to care for the patients became available. Dorman B. Eaton, the New York lawyer and social reformer, reflected the thought of his time when he wrote:

> Now, as never before in this country, it [mental illness] is arresting the thoughts of statesmen and moving the hearts of philanthropists. And none too soon. For while science and benevolence, by setting limits to disease and affliction, have extended the duration of human life; while ignorance and crime have diminished, and education has become more extended and profound, insanity, and insanity alone among our great afflictions, has become both more frequent and more fatal in this country.[1]

At the same time a group of reform-minded humanitarians, some of whom were leading neurologists, founded the National Association for the Protection of the Insane and the Prevention of Insanity. The history of this short-lived group is not of concern here; but its goals, what it stood for and against, clearly summarize the existing problems as seen by a group of perceptive observers. The Association wanted to educate the public to the needs of general asylum reform. Within the asylums it urged the abolition of mechanical restraints, which were

---

[1] Dorman B. Eaton, "Despotism in lunatic asylums," *North Am. Rev.* 132 (1881): 263–75; 263.

not as much in evidence around 1880 as ten years earlier. The Association pressed for stricter safeguards against illegal commitment and detention of insane patients, a problem of concern to many others as well. Within the asylums, the Association wanted to reduce the despotic rule of some of the superintendents of these institutions, while at the same time urging more scientific or clinical research. Linked with the latter was the plea for more instruction about mental diseases and the care of the disturbed within the curricula of medical schools. In a general way, then, these aims portray what was lacking in the area of the care and study of the mentally ill.[2]

Bibliographical Note

There were many debates in the nineteenth-century psychiatric literature revolving around such subjects as the physical or moral basis of insanity, state versus local control of asylums, moral treatment, and the legal responsibilities of the insane. These have been extensively discussed in the following references:

Albert Deutsch, *The Mentally Ill in America, A History of Their Care and Treatment from Colonial Times*, 2nd ed., New York: Columbia University Press, 1949—still the first place to look for a general description of the rise of psychiatry in America. As Deutsch and others have pointed out, the care of the mentally ill cannot be separated from the problems of public welfare. See especially, David M. Schneider and Albert Deutsch, *The History of Public Welfare in New York State*, 2 vols., Chicago: University of Chicago Press, 1941.

An older work on which Deutsch and others have often relied is Henry M. Hurd, ed., *The Institutional Care of the Insane in the United States and Canada*, 4 vols., Baltimore: The Johns Hopkins Press, 1916.

Two more recent books that explore psychiatric thought regarding etiology and treatment are Norman Dain, *Concepts of Insanity in the United States, 1789-1865*, New Brunswick: Rutgers University Press, 1964; and Ruth B. Caplan, *Psychiatry and the Community in Nineteenth Century America, The Recurring Concern with the Environment in the Prevention and Treatment of Mental Illness*, New York: Basic Books, 1969.

For a very thorough description and analysis of the status of psychiatry around 1880, especially for its medico-legal ramifications, see Charles E. Rosenberg's *The Trial of the Assassin Guiteau*, Chicago: University of Chicago Press, 1968.

A detailed history of one of the best state hospitals is Gerald Grob's *The State and the Mentally Ill, A History of the Worcester State Hospital in Massachusetts, 1830-1920*, Chapel Hill: University of North Carolina Press, 1966. See also J. Sanbourne Bockoven, *Moral Treatment in American Psychiatry*, New York: Springer, 1963.

---

[2] For a good discussion of the National Association for the Protection of the Insane and the Prevention of Insanity, see Albert Deutsch, "The History of Mental Hygiene," in *One Hundred Years of American Psychiatry* (New York: Columbia University Press, 1944), pp. 325-65. There are many other worthwhile chapters in this book.

PLINY EARLE

A GLANCE AT INSANITY, AND THE MANAGEMENT OF THE INSANE IN THE AMERICAN STATES

Editor's Note

Pliny Earle (1809–92) was one of those nineteenth-century physicians who truly could be called an alienist. He spent his professional life caring for and treating the insane. From 1864 until 1886 he was director of the Northhampton Lunatic Hospital in Massachusetts. Earle was concerned by the phenomenon that has been called the "cult of curability" by Albert Deutsch.

During the second quarter of the nineteenth century, the previous pessimism over the prognosis of mental illness changed to an attitude of extreme optimism. This was an era when expansiveness and progress were the ideals, and that, in part, may have accounted for the rise of the "cult of curability." The older system of "boarding out" the mentally ill, while adequate for custodial care, was now deemed inadequate because it lacked facilities for actual treatment. Curability of insanity was equated with institutionalization, so in the 1830's and beyond, more and more asylums were constructed.

Overcrowding and lack of sufficient facilities for treatment occurred almost immediately, and many insane patients continued to be sequestered in county poorhouses. As the state lunatic asylums reported their results, the public came to believe that treatment of acute cases was the only hope. But as Pliny Earle stresses in the essay below, this zeal gave the public "a false impression, from which sprang hopes and expectations that could never be fulfilled."[1] It was to this misleading optimism that Dr. Earle addressed himself. The service he performed was valuable in itself, the more so because as a superintendent of a large hospital he had a vested interest in portraying it in the best possible light.

Intimately linked to Earle's plea for more honest statistics was his fight against extravagant expenditure for hospital buildings. If the public were told the truth, then perhaps the high expenditures for fancy buildings might be curbed, Earle argued. Needless to say, these positions won him few friends among his colleagues. One biographer has written that after his Chicago paper of 1879 (reprinted below) the open and secret hostility soon ceased, for the truth of his remarks began to make things clear.[2]

Proc. Sixth Annual Conf. Charities and Correction, 1879 (Boston: Williams, 1879), pp. 42–59.

[1] Earle was not the first to question hospital statistics. Thirty years earlier Isaac Ray had posed the same questions. What can rightfully be called recovery? he asked. "The fact is, however," Ray claimed, "that in the present statistics of recovery, no conventional rule whatever, has been followed. Every individual has decided what should not be called recoveries, just as it seemed good in his own sight." "The statistics of insane hospitals," *Am. J. Insanity* 6 (1849): 23–52; 30.

[2] F. B. Sanborn, *Memories of Pliny Earle, M.D.* (Boston: Damrell & Upham, 1898), p. 269.

In coming before you, pursuant to the appointment for the honor of which I am indebted to the Conference of Charities of 1878, I make no pretension of attempting to present for your consideration anything new from that special field of labor in which I am employed, a comparatively small, although far from being an unimportant, part of the broad domain which legitimately comes within the purview of the association here assembled.

It is proposed to occupy your attention with a very brief consideration of the general subject of insanity in the United States, contemplated as historical, contemporaneous, and prospective; to lay before you the skeleton of an argument by which, through the experience of the past and a just comprehension of the present, the subject may be placed in such a light as to render more easy the selection of proper methods of meeting the grave responsibilities of the future.

Fifty years ago, in 1829, there were within the limits of the United States but eight institutions specially devoted to the care and the curative treatment of the insane. Only four of them were state institutions; and two of these had been in operation but a few months, since both of them were first opened in the preceding year. At about this time the people of the states began, more generally than theretofore, to take an interest in the subject of insanity, to recognize the fact of the measurable curability of the disease, to direct their attention to the condition of the insane, to perceive the inadequacy of provision for their suitable accommodation and treatment, and to discuss the importance of these questions in relation, not alone to humanity but also to the social compact and the governmental autonomy of the state.

The state hospital at Worcester, Mass., went into operation in 1833; and of all the institutions of the kind within the United States, the opening of which was within the half-century preceding the present year, it is the oldest. The time at which it began its work forms an important epoch in the history of the enterprise for the amelioration of the condition of the insane. Its superintendent, Dr. Woodward, was an enthusiast in the specialty; and although perhaps not more devoted than Dr. Wyman of the McLean Asylum, or Dr. Todd of the Hartford Retreat, he gave to the profession and to the world, by his detailed reports, vastly more than they of the results of his observation and practical experience. This information was widely disseminated and gave to the popular movement in favor of the insane an impulse such as it had never before received, and the importance of the consequences of which, extending as they do to the present day and as they will through all the future history of our nation, cannot now be estimated.

At a period not much later, Miss Dix began that long and laborious career of philanthropic devotion to the interests of the insane with which her name is indissolubly connected and to which the annals of all history furnish no parallel. To those two persons, Dr. Woodward and Miss Dix, more than to any other two, are the insane of our country indebted for the awakened interest of the people in their behalf and, consequently, for that rapidity of practical action manifested in the erection of asylums and hospitals for their benefit, which has in no other country been exceeded, even if it has been equaled.

In the course of the seven years from 1834 to 1840, both inclusive, no less than eight asylums and hospitals were opened for the reception of patients, thus doubling the number within the jurisdiction of the states, antecedent to the hospital at Worcester. Five of the new ones were founded by the states within which they are respectively situated. In the decennium from 1841 to 1850, inclusive, the number of institutions completed and put into operation was nine, of which six were founded by states; and in that from 1851 to 1860 it was no less than twenty, of which fifteen owe their origin to commonwealth provision. The remarkable increase during the decade last mentioned happily illustrates not alone the cumulative influence of agencies already mentioned, but of others which had been brought to bear upon the philanthropic enterprise. Not the least among the latter was the formation of the Association of Medical Superintendents of American Institutions for the Insane, an organization which, although sometimes accused of a persistent adherence to the methods of the past, uninfluenced by the results of experience, has nevertheless been a potent instrumentality for good.

The late Civil War was, naturally and necessarily, a serious check to the multiplication of curative and custodial institutions, and measurably so to all the activities engaged in the beneficent undertaking for the attainment of the ends of which those establishments are the most important practical agents. Yet, notwithstanding this, the area of the enterprise has continued to expand and the number of hospitals to augment until, at the present time we have within our national borders not far from eighty—a ten-fold increase during the lapse of half a century. . . .

But the imperfection and, consequently, the fallibility of human nature are such that the conduct of an enterprise, even though it be for charitable purposes, can no more be wholly free from mistakes that can the conduct of each individual life. And thus it happened that, in the early history of our specialty in this country, the zeal and the rivalry of those by whom it was prosecuted gave to the public mind a false impression, from which sprang hopes and expectations that could never be fulfilled.

As early as 1827, by a combination of fortuitous and favorable circumstances, Dr. Todd, of the Hartford Retreat, was able to report the recovery of twenty-one out of twenty-three recent cases of insanity received into that institution. This remarkable result was reduced to a formula; and the *percentage* (92.3) thus derived from *less than one-quarter of a hundred* of cases was published, and became more or less a criterion by which to measure the possibilities in *all* recent cases.

Dr. Woodward, at Worcester, adopted the fallacious method of calculating the proportion of recoveries upon the number of patients discharged, instead of upon that of the number admitted, and in this way had succeeded in reporting a percentage of 84.20 in 1836. Early in the following year, Dr. Bell took charge of the McLean Asylum, and Greek met Greek upon the arena of the professional specialty. The decennium last noted was soon entered upon, and the several superintendents above mentioned came successively into the lists. Before each of them stood the stimulating, the provocative precedent of erroneous percentages; and around each of them was the competitive ability of his colleagues in the specialty. It is no cause for marvel that under these circumstances a public opinion was formed, upon the curability of insanity, too favorable to be sustained by the experience of the future. This opinion was enunciated by a few superintendents at an earlier date; but considered as an established idea in the minds of the people, it was the fruitage of the decennium in question, more than of any other in the whole history of the past; and thenceforward it has very generally been claimed that of all cases of insanity of less duration than one year, from 75 to 90 per cent are susceptible of cure. For more than forty years in respect to a few, and more than thirty years in respect to many, this has been the shibboleth of the superintendents of the hospitals and of other writers upon the subject of mental alienation; and especially has it been depended upon as one of the crowning arguments in favor of the establishment of new hospitals and the enlargement of old ones, and of appeals to hesitating and reluctant legislatures for additional appropriations of money for the completion of unfinished ones, for which the purse of the commonwealth had already been taxed beyond the bounds of reason and of patient endurance.

But recent investigations have demonstrated the fallacy of the claim to a degree of curability so extensive. The experience of the hospitals during the last forty years has given to the statistician the results of a number of cases sufficiently large to form a basis of somewhat reliable general conclusions. In no single instance of the treatment of a thousand recent cases, has the recovery of even 66 per cent been reported. And in the most valuable and reliable statistics upon the subject, even the proportion reported was attained, in large measure, by the repeated recoveries of a few individuals from a multiplicity of attacks. The deceptive nature of the word *cases* was thus exposed. The superintendents reported the recovery of *cases*. The unprofessional readers of the reports, thoughtless of the technical use of the word, believed that *case* is equivalent to *person*, and, consequently, that the number of *cases* represented an equal number of *persons*. When the Bloomingdale Asylum reported, *without explanation*, six recoveries in one year, all of which were furnished by one woman, who was again brought to the asylum before that report was in print, and who finally died there, the public necessarily inferred that six different persons had recovered; and the same is true as applicable to the Worcester Hospital, when it reported, without explanation, seven recoveries in one year, of a woman whom it had reported as recovered no less than nine times in the course of the preceding two years—making sixteen recoveries in three years.

In order to impress the mind with an accurate estimate of the recoveries as annually reported at the hospitals, without analyzation or explanation, permit me to adduce a few further facts.

At the Northampton (Mass.) Hospital, five persons have recovered thirty-three times, an average of more than six recoveries to each.

At the Worcester (Mass.) Hospital, one woman (the one above mentioned) was discharged recovered twenty-two times.

At the Bloomingdale Asylum, New York, prior to 1845, a woman was admitted twenty-two times, and discharged recovered every time; and for another woman (the one who recovered six times in one year) forty-six recoveries were reported in the course of her life, and she died upon her fifty-ninth admission; and those forty-six recoveries are to this day published, unexplained, in the tables of the reports of that institution, as available material for all persons who wish to demonstrate, by the absolute infallibility of mathematical figures, which "cannot lie," the proportion of persons attacked with insanity who are again restored, by recovery, to health and to usefulness. When the Bloomingdale Asylum had been in operation fifty years, it had treated 6,325 patients, and the whole number of recoveries was 2,796. This one woman furnished 1.66 per cent, or one-sixtieth part, of all these recoveries.

At the Frankford Asylum, Pennsylvania, the aggregate of the recoveries of five persons was fifty-two, or more than ten recoveries to each person; and yet no less than three of those persons subsequently died in the asylum.

At the Worcester Hospital, in 1877, seven women had recovered ninety-two times, an average of more than thirteen recoveries to each; but, nevertheless, two of those women had died insane in that hospital; two of them were then present in the hospital, both of them insane, and one of them hopelessly so; and one was in another hospital, hopelessly insane. How admirably might those same ninety-two *recoveries* be used "to point a moral, or adorn a tale"! . . .

Of 1,061 cases of recent insanity treated at the Frankford (Penn.) Asylum, the proportion of recoveries was 65.69 per cent. But by an analysis of these cases it has been shown that the recoveries of *persons* were only 58.35 per cent; and that, of those that recovered, there were so many relapses that the *permanent* recoveries were but 48.39 per cent. Had it been possible to trace all the persons and obtain their history, it is not at all improbable—it is, indeed, only too probable—that the number of permanent recoveries would have been reduced to 40 per cent. These are the most reliable of all American statistics in regard to the results of treatment of so-called recent cases.

Of the true results of treatment of all the *persons* received into institutions, irrespective of the duration of the disease, the most valuable statistics are those for which we are indebted to Dr. Arthur Mitchell of Edinburgh, and the late Dr. John Thurnam, for many years superintendent of the Wiltshire Asylum at Devizes, England.

Dr. Mitchell informs us that, in the year 1858, 1,297 persons were admitted *for the first time* into the asylums in Scotland. Twelve years afterwards, in 1870, the intermediate history of 1,096 of them was ascertained. Of those 1,096, no less than 454 had died insane and 367 still lived insane; total, 821, or 74.91 per cent insane. And 78 had died *not* insane, and 197 still lived *not* insane; total *not* insane, 275, or 25.09 per cent. In general terms, three-fourths were insane, and one-fourth not insane.

Dr. Thurnam, having obtained the history until death of 244 *persons* admitted into the Retreat at York, deduced from the results the following general formula: "In round numbers, then, of ten persons attacked by insanity, five recover, and five die sooner or later during the attack. Of the five who recover, not more than two remain well during the rest of their lives; the other three sustain subsequent attacks, during which at least two of them die."

This formula, and the statistics from which it was derived, were published some thirty years ago; but in this country nearly all of the writers upon insanity have shunned them as if they were the fructified germs of pestilence.

Another mistake, or, more properly, a blunder—a species of error condemned by politicians as more censurable than crime—has been made in the enterprise for the treatment of the insane. From the initiation of that enterprise, the great ultimate object has been to provide, for all the insane requiring humane guardianship, adequate accommodations in either hospitals, asylums, or other places where such oversight and direction would assuredly be rendered. It was for a long time hoped to accomplish this object by well-equipped hospitals alone; and this hope was encouraged, and perhaps stimulated into expectation, by the constant iteration and reiteration of the assertion of the eminent curability of the disease. If ninety, or eighty, or even seventy-five, of each hundred of insane persons could be permanently cured—and such was the impression given—public benevolence would certainly properly provide for the comparatively small remainder, the more certainly so because it could be done at trifling expense. For these reasons the establishment of curative institutions, and curative institutions alone, was almost universally advocated, not merely by the medical superintendents but by other interested persons as well. In these establishments the curable could be cured and the incurable domiciled for life.

Then arose the not illogical argument, "The better the hospital, the greater will be the number of persons cured." But most unfortunately, not for the enterprise alone but for the treasuries of states and the purses of the payers of taxes, the word "better" in this proposition was in some places practically interpreted "more costly." Under this rendering, the ambition of architects, the pride of commissioners and superintendents, and the universal extravagance of the people during the years following the close of the late Civil War, strongly fortified and assisted this argument; and the practical consequences are now apparent in that class of hospitals—professedly *charitable* institutions—which have cost from twenty-five hundred to four, or perhaps five, thousand dollars for every patient to whom they can offer a comfortable domicile.

Such is a cursory view of the past. We come now to the absolute present. At this moment, pregnant with the problems of the future, what is the knowledge hitherto gained from experience?

We have learned, firstly, foremostly, and most importantly, that if reference be had to *persons* rather than to *cases*—and in the relations in respect to which the subject is here discussed such reference is the only one of importance—the proportion of recoveries from insanity is only about one-half as great as was formerly assumed as possible and was hoped to be attained.

We have learned that notwithstanding the general improvement of the institutions in the course of the last fifty years and the very lavish outlay of money upon some of those most recently established, ostensibly in the hope of increasing the proportion of recoveries, yet, with reference to all the cases admitted into those institutions, that proportion has not been increased, but has actually diminished.

We have hence learned one important reason—perhaps the most important of all—for the unintermitted and remarkable increase of insane persons among the people, in spite of the constant accumulation of hospitals—a fact which has been regarded by many as a marvel, if not a paradox.

We have likewise learned that this continual augmentation cannot be arrested by the ordinary human instrumentalities. It has become an established fact and must, apparently, be perpetual, unless the occult natural causes of the disease shall cease to operate or shall become essentially modified, or unless the human race attains a degree of wisdom and of self-abnegation not hitherto reached and abstains from or avoids those causes which are known and avoidable. . . .

S. WEIR MITCHELL

ADDRESS BEFORE THE FIFTIETH ANNUAL MEETING OF THE AMERICAN MEDICO-PSYCHOLOGICAL ASSOCIATION

Editor's Note

The eminent Philadelphia neurologist and writer Silas Weir Mitchell (1829–1914) was the son of the famed John Kearsley Mitchell. Weir Mitchell and his colleagues began their study of peripheral nerve injuries during the Civil War. In the postwar decades neurology began to grow as a specialty. Those who devoted themselves to this new field argued that there should be no difference between the study of peripheral nerve diseases and the study of the brain in all its manifestations.[1]

Mitchell's address to the fiftieth anniversary meeting of the American Medico-Psychological Association is one of the frankest and broadest criticisms that any society has invited upon itself. Only two years prior to his appearance the group had finally changed its outmoded name from the Association of Medical Superintendents of American Institutions for the Insane. (The Medico-Psychological Association became the American Psychiatric Association in 1921.)

Bibliographical Note

Ernest Earnest, *S. Weir Mitchell, Novelist and Physician*, Philadelphia: University of Pennsylvania Press, 1950.

Richard D. Walter, *S. Weir Mitchell, M.D.–Neurologist*, Springfield: Thomas, 1970.

I am here to-day under circumstances so unusual that I may be pardoned if I explain them in order to justify the frank language of this address.

When your representative, Dr. Chapin, asked me to be your speaker on this important anniversary, I declined. It is customary on birthdays to say only pleasant things, and this I knew I could not altogether do. I foresaw a struggle between courteous desire to follow a kindly custom and the duty to greatly use

Proc. Am. Medico-Psychological Assoc. 50 (1894): 101–21.

[1] Charles Rosenberg has discussed this issue in his *Trial of the Assassin Guiteau* (Chicago: University of Chicago Press, 1968).

a great occasion. When Dr. Chapin, after consulting some of you, came back to say it was still your desire that I should speak, I reflected that men who could thus ask the criticism, which they knew must come without mercy, were well worth talking to. I said, at last, that I would address you today, but that it would be boldly and with no regard to persons. That was a momentary insanity; I have been sorry ever since.

You are on the dividing year of your first century of life. You look back with just pride as alienists on the merciful changes made for the better in the management of the chronic insane. It is to be feared that you also have cause to recall the fact that as compared with the splendid advance in surgery, in the medicine of the eye, and the steady approach to precision all along our ardent line the alienist has won in proportion little. This is partly due to the nature of the maladies with which you have to deal; but there are many other causes at work to retard the wholesome progress. Just that which is impairing the usefulness of the lesser specialties in medicine has been more gravely enfeebling your value and retarding your development. I mean the tendency to isolation from the mass of the active profession. At first, as concerned the eye for instance, this separation seemed but too complete—the new terms, the methods, the instruments of the ophthalmologist were for a time absurdly unfamiliar. It is not so at present. The general practitioner has come again into touch with the oculist, and understands his terms and methods. In fact, every sudden advance of a brigade of our great line for a time appears to break our ranks; but soon we get up to it and go on as before.

With you it has been different. You were the first of the specialists and you have never come back into line. It is easy to see how this came about. You soon began to live apart, and you still do so. Your hospitals are not our hospitals; your ways are not our ways. You live out of range of critical shot; you are not preceded and followed in your ward work by clever rivals, or watched by able residents fresh with the learning of the school.

I am strongly of the opinion that the influence which for years led the general profession to the belief that no one could, or should, treat the insane except the special practitioner have done us and you and many of our patients lasting wrong.

Standing here in the home of Rush, I cannot forget that he was an alienist and a general practitioner; nor can I cease to lament the day when the treatment of the insane passed too completely out of the hands of the profession at large and into those of a group of physicians who constitute almost a sect apart from our more vitalized existence. What evil this has wrought, what harm it has done to us and to you I shall try to show. Why it has been so much more grave in its results here than in Europe is not clear to me, or would take too long to discuss.

I should, indeed, be easy enough in mind if I had only to criticize an uneducated public; ignorant legislators, and the boards which control our civic, state, and endowed institutions. But I shall have, frankly, to reproach as to certain

things many of those who still bear the absurd label of "medical superintendents." If any here think it pleasant to fire opinions into a crowd, not knowing
who are hit, whether his shot finds out the right man, or only annoys the
entirely efficient, I am not that man. Moreover abrupt statements are apt to be
needlessly annoying and to seem to lack good manners, and yet I have not time
to be other than brief to abruptness. . . .

The men before me see asylums from within. Some live on quietly. Some are
vaguely dissatisfied. Some are half-hopelessly striving to better things, which
only in part lie within their power to change. Outside, and of late years, your
asylums are relentlessly watched by one of the ablest groups of men known to
me, the neurologists and consultants of our cities. To thirty of these I addressed
the following letter:

> Dear Doctor: I have been asked to deliver, in May, the address on the
> occasion of the Fiftieth Anniversary of the Society of the Medical Superin-
> tendents of the Insane, now known under the name of the American
> Medico-Psychological Association. I have consented with the clear under-
> standing that I shall be free to represent the best professional opinion in
> the country to the gentlemen who are at the head of these institutions. I
> am told that I shall have full freedom. To enable me to carry out this plan
> I have addressed duplicates of this letter to a few of the leading American
> neurologists and to certain consultants not neurologists. May I ask you to
> answer the following questions:
>
> Do you think the present asylum management of the insane in America
> as good as it could be made?
>
> What faults do you find with it?
>
> If you had full freedom to change it what would you do?
>
> I do not want a written treatise on the subject, but within a reasonable
> time a reply of such brevity as will cover the ground for an expert.
>
> > Yours truly
> > S. WEIR MITCHELL

The men I called to my aid are physicians accustomed, in recent days, to
treat the insane. Some of them are familiar with asylums; most of them have
contributed largely and originally to neuropathology, symptomatology, and
therapeutics. No man can afford to set quite aside the criticism of their replies.
They are severe, but not unkindly; nor do they fail to point out how largely you
are trammelled by custom, lack of means, and above all, in some cases (and this
is saddest and most shameful of all), directly or indirectly by politics.

I have used also, certain communications from able asylum officers, which I
cannot print and, also, I have had in the past letters from intelligent people,
some of them doctors, who speak of their own experiences as patients in the
asylums and make reflections thereon.

But it is the arraignment of the neurologist which ought incessantly to
trouble you and the boards which you have to manage—for the management of
managers is an important business. It is this outspoken discontent which ought
to make you ask how far you, yourselves, are responsible. If we are right, neither

states nor boards nor you are ardently living up to the highest standard of intelligent duty.

And now as to boards of managers.

You know too well, I fear, how state boards are generally constituted. There the mischief begins. They meet at exceedingly variable intervals—some monthly and some every third month. When once they have decreed a superintendent physician for the asylum his reports must largely guide them. I approach a delicate matter when I say that in some states the selection, both of these boards and the appointment and continuance in office of a physician superintendent, is said to be more or less a question of politics. I am told that this inconceivably shameful thing is past doubt. But to accept such office as a mere bit of party spoil! Can a man do that and be fit for the work? Let us hope it is all mere scandalous gossip and turn from a too painful topic. Money changers in the temple! Ward politics at the bedside of the lunatic! How can one with patience even speak of it? . . .

I have said the ailments of hospitals begin, as a rule, in the governing boards; they do not end there.

In our general hospitals there is a diffused medical authority, but yours is a monarchy more or less limited. And now, my next query is as to whether you, who thus govern and make reports and live amongst your armies of the insane, are, in all respects, doing what you should and might do. We have done with whip and chains and ill-usage, and having won this noble battle have we not rested too easily content with having made the condition of the insane more comfortable?

The question we here ask at starting is if you, who are so powerful within these alien camps, are really doing all that might be done without serious increase of expenditure? Frankly speaking, we do not believe that you are so working these hospitals as to keep treatment or scientific product on the front line of medical advance.

Where, we ask, are your annual reports of scientific study, of the psychology and pathology of your patients? They should be published apart. We commonly get as your contributions to science, odd little statements, reports of a case or two, a few useless pages of isolated post-mortem records, and these are sandwiched among incomprehensible statistics and form balance-sheets; and this is too often your sole answer. Where, indeed, are your replies to the questions as to heredity, marriage, the mental disorders of races, the influence of malarial locations, of seasons, of great elevations, all the psychological riddles of a new land, a forming breed, never weary of quickening the pace, of inventing means of hurry—relentless workers? When I put such questions I am always met with the doleful reply. "We have no time; we want more money; we have not enough assistants." I am quite willing to admit that for the careful treatment of the possibly curable insane, none of you have enough help. I grant that, but it is not all. I could say the like of many a fertile man in this city. I can but partially admit this endless plea of overwork in extenuation of the charge of scientific unproductiveness; that serious symptom of a larger malady. Surely the immense and habitual hospital work among the sick which numberless city doctors do, their professional teaching, their clinics and societies, the endless cares, trusts, and social duties of a city life, do these make them fail of scientific productiveness? No, it is not time alone you people want. There is something defective besides number in your organizations. And as to this, what prevents your endowed suburban hospitals having any quantity of young resident physicians? It is only to choose with care and to feed them. There is much they can do, and be taught to do, which will relieve you and set you free for the higher work we ask of you.

But if your own institution is unhappily connected with a general hospital, do not let it send you residents for the first three months of their two-year term, as is done, I hear, in this city. Could there be a more senseless and thoughtless way of giving these young men a knowledge of insanity?

And then as to your paid assistants. You need as aids men who, first of all, have had long training in a general hospital, and here, the choice, I suspect, is left largely to you. Ask your boards to have competitions for your permanent assistants. Insist on hospital training, knowledge of psychology, of neuropathology, and then demand of your people original reports or product of some kind. I find myself that nothing is so useful as original research to urge on my aids. But then you must lead or they will not go the way you would have them go. I should insist, were I you, that your aids spend daily some hours outside of your walls and have a long summer holiday. There have been some among your best who have insisted that incessant contact with mental imperfection is not a wholesome thing.

Want of competent original work is to my mind the worst symptom of torpor the asylums now present. Contrast the work you have done in the last three decades with what the little group of our own neurologists has done. To compare your annual output with the great English or German work were hardly a pleasant thing to do. Even in your own line, most of the textbooks, many of the ablest papers are not asylum products. What is the matter? You have immense opportunities, and, seriously, we ask you experts, what have you taught us of these 91,000 insane whom you see or treat? You will point to certain books, some good work in this or that asylum, but, as we judge you, to no such amount of thoughtful output as your chances might lead us to expect.

There are other material failures by which we test as much of your work as we can see, and thence suspect the precision and general value of what we do not see. When we ask for your asylum notes of cases, or by some accident have occasion to look over your case books, we are too often surprised at the amazing lack of complete physical study of the insane, at the failure to see obvious lesions, at the want of thorough day by day study of the secretions in the newer cases, of blood-counts, temperatures, reflexes, the eye-ground, color-fields, all the minute examination with which we are so unrestingly busy. It is not thus in all your asylums, but you will see from the letters appended that I am not alone in this critical complaint. Not so many years ago in a certain asylum I could not get a stethoscope or an ophthalmoscope; and too often when we receive a patient and write and ask for his hospital record it is such as would surprise, for meagerness, the resident of a city hospital. I had, recently, occasion to see the printed schedule guide to symptom notes in an asylum; it was oddly defective, had been ten years in use, and would excite a smile from any of my clinical aids. If, as to all these defects, I am still told that they are due to lack of means, I make answer that our criticism applies as decisively to some of the amply endowed asylums as to those for the poor of the states. . . .

The cloistral lives you lead give rise, we think to certain mental peculiarities. I could tell you how to mend them; I shall by and by. You hold to and teach certain opinions which we have long learned to lose. One is the superstition (almost is it that) to the effect that an asylum is in itself curative. You hear the regret in every report that patients are not sent soon enough, as if you had ways of curing which we have not. Upon my word, I think asylum life is deadly to the insane. Poverty, risk, fear, send you of true need many patients; many more are sent by people quite able to have their friends treated outside. They are placed in asylums because of the wide-spread belief you have so long, and as we think, so unreasonably fostered, to the effect that there is some mysterious therapeutic influence to be found behind your walls and locked doors. We hold the reverse opinion, and think your hospitals are never to be used save as the last resource.

I have found some heads of asylums a trifle shy about discussing the question of the occasional use of mechanical restraint. There lingers a dislike to admit that it should never be used, as, we thank God, some of your best assistants earnestly believe. We think it a question settled past argument. Many years ago while using it I got a lesson never since forgotten. During the war, Drs. Morehouse, Keen, and I, had always about eighty to one hundred epileptics in charge, and some insane. We employed at times the camisole, or straps, in protracted convulsions. I tried them once on myself a half-hour for a purpose needless to mention. Before ten minutes had gone I began to have a half frantic sense of desire to fight for freedom. It was really very hard to conquer. Try it, and you will think long before you add to insanity this temptation to be violent.

We think, also, of your too constantly locked doors and barred windows, as being but reminder relics of that dismal system which we are pleased to think is gone forever. I presume that you have, through habit, lost the sense of jail and jailer which troubles me when I walk behind one of you and he unlocks door after door. Do you think it is not felt by some of your patients? . . .

Of the feeling of distrust concerning the therapeutics of asylums now fast gaining ground in the mind of the general public I have said nothing. This lack of medical confidence is of recent growth. Once we spoke of asylums with respect; it is not so now. We, neurologists, think you have fallen behind us, and this opinion is gaining ground outside of our own ranks, and is, in part at least, your own fault. You quietly submit to having hospitals called asylums; you are labelled as medical superintendents, and some of you allow your managers to think you can be farmers, stewards, caterers, treasurers, business managers, and physicians. You should urge in every report the stupid folly of this. Knowing what we do of the rate of the growth of medicine, does any man in his senses think that you can be even decently competent and have anything to do with outside business? You may be fair general practitioners in insanity, but productive neurologists of high class regarding disease of the mind organs as but a part of your work? No—I think not. That, you cannot be if you are also in business. It is a grave injustice to insist that you shall conduct a huge boarding house— what has been called a monastery of the mad—and keep yourselves honestly able to move with the growth of medicine and to study your cases or add anything of value to our store of knowledge. Some of you have, in a measure, shed this cumbersome coil of unprofessional business, but still declare yourselves over-weighted with letters to write, people to see, and so much to do that it is clear either that you do need help and more assistants, or that you are cursed by that slow atrophy of the energizing faculties which is the very malaria of asylum life. Asylum life! There is despair in the name as there is in the idea.

And the title "superintendent." Of what? You have let the word go as concerns this society. Insist to your managers that you are physicians and no more. There may be something to dread in a label.

The many grave questions which remain I can do no more than lightly mention. Some I may but touch and leave as texts for thought. I have notes of six cases dismissed as cured from great endowed hospitals without one written word of warning or direction as to the work, the play, the diet, holidays or future of these people. When you find a case getting well, and let it go home or elsewhere, is it as common as this would seem to make it that you no further concern yourselves with it? I never had much evidence that the reverse is often done, and yet with some of us mere outside practitioners the future of our convalescent, or cured, cases is a matter of the most thoughtful care and of the most anxious solicitude, of long written instructions how to live so as to avoid relapses.

As to work for the chronic and convalescent insane, I never yet saw in America the hospital where all was done that can be done in this direction. These alien people are relatively capable of bribery. Tobacco, later hours, better diet, larger freedom, a little wage, the use or non-use of certain privileged rooms, leave among women to wear this or that, putting some who shirk work with others who do work, the influence of example, all these helps may be more ingeniously varied than they are. But as long as you pay common nurses (whom, perhaps, you do well to describe as attendants), untaught and uninterested, to watch hordes of people, or to preside over men and women far better educated than those who watch them, you will do little with this essential means—work. I think there must be no effort to make this work pay. It is education we want.

Moreover, if you can make the work interesting and productive, it will be best. . . .

And now, a word more. I accepted this ungracious post from honest sense of duty. I have said no word of dispraise or critical annoyance that I did not eminently dislike to say. I may be wrong as to some men and to some hospitals. It would be strange if it were not so. But let me add this on parting. One preaches to a congregation. It is impossible to select individuals for blame or praise. Try not to be merely hurt or disgusted by the verdicts of my fellow neurologists and myself. If what we have said causes only bitterness and leaves you in thought, action, and purpose where it found you an hour ago, then I have assuredly failed as I do not want to fail and had better never have spoken. If it should happen, please God, that my words bear fruit of good I shall get more happiness out of this occasion than I ever thought could come out of a most distasteful task of a varied life. If I have hurt or personally annoyed any man here today I am, believe me, sincerely sorry. Perhaps many of you who do not feel vexed may yet rest sure that I am largely wrong in my censure and my theories; but fifty years hence, when we must all have been swept away, another will possibly stand in my place and tell your history, and to him and the bountiful wisdom of time I leave it to be declared whether I was right or wrong.

I have been very long and you as patient. I thank you.

PART **VII**
HOSPITALS

INTRODUCTION

Many towns at the beginning of the nineteenth century cared for their sick poor in small infirmaries attached to the local almshouse. Needless to say, the medical and nursing care dispensed in these institutions was usually inadequate. This, coupled with the often squalid conditions under which patients were kept, soon became one of the issues in a general humanitarian crusade of the mid-century years.

A safe generalization is that hospitals were founded for a variety of reasons beside their principal function of caring for sick and injured patients. They were the objects of charity, Christian and otherwise; they became, in the later nineteenth century, centers for specialized varieties of diseases and treatments; and finally, hospitals were important as centers for medical research and the training of medical students. As early as 1769, Samuel Bard of New York remarked that "the nature of diseases, and the practice of medicine cannot be taught but in a public hospital."

As more and more American physicians returned from study trips in England, and particularly in France, they brought back the conviction that medical research and education was properly placed in large hospitals. The examples of Laennec and Louis in Paris influenced the thinking of many of their American students.[1]

The average nineteenth-century physician, practicing before about 1885, probably did not have much direct contact with hospitals or their problems. The modern hospital as the primary center for dispensation of medical care is a much more recent phenomenon. In 1873 one survey revealed only 178 hospitals in the United States. Thirty-two were established between 1826 and 1850 and thirty-nine more between 1851 and 1860. The greatest rise in the number of hospitals occurred in the twentieth century and was related to increasing urbanization and

---

[1] See Erwin H. Ackerknecht's comprehensive book, *Medicine at the Paris Hospital, 1794-1848* (Baltimore: The Johns Hopkins Press, 1967); and the charming essay by William Osler, "The influence of Louis on American medicine," *Johns Hopkins Hosp. Bull.* 8 (1897): 161-67, reprinted in *An Alabama Student* (New York: Oxford University Press, 1908), pp. 189-210.

to those technical advances in surgery, radiology, and laboratory diagnosis, that make the hospitals the essential centers of medical practice.[2]

There is an interesting, and fairly obvious, relationship between surgeons, hospitals, and hygiene. A number of leading surgeons, such as Stephen Smith and Willard Parker in this country and John Simon in England, were sanitarians of note. The surgeons were also the logical ones to be interested in proper hygiene and design of hospitals, and some of the large surgical texts contained chapters on hospital construction.[3] W. Gill Wylie, in discussing the history of hospitals in 1876, specifically pointed to the fact that some of the professors of hygiene and surgery take up the construction of hospitals as a part of their course for students.

Under the rubric hospitalism, a term introduced in 1869 by James Y. Simpson in England, surgeons discussed erysipelas, septicemia, pyemia, and hospital gangrene.[4]

But more than widespread post-operative infection was at issue for those who strove for hospital reform. In the early 1860's a large city hospital such as Bellevue in New York was usually over-crowded and grossly unclean.

A sensational case in the spring of 1860 served to focus renewed attention on the conditions at Bellevue. A young Irish woman gave birth on a Sunday night. The following morning the infant was found dead next to the mother, who had been too weak to prevent rats from devouring the baby's nose, upper lip, toes, and half of the left foot.[5]

The introduction of anesthesia was of great importance in changing the primary locus of surgical operations from the kitchen table to the hospital operating room. Yet Simpson, and others too, could easily show that amputations performed in large city hospitals resulted in a much higher mortality than those done in the relative isolation of the country surgeon's practice. Although advance was made in surgical technique, much went for naught, because the crowd-

---

[2] Joseph M. Toner, "Statistics of hospitals in the United States, 1872–1873," *Trans. A.M.A.* 24 (1873): 314–33; E. H. L. Corwin, *The American Hospital* (New York: Commonwealth Fund, 1946), p. 6.

[3] E.g., J. R. Martin, "On Hospitals," in *A System of Surgery*, T. Holmes, ed., 4 vols. (London: Parker, 1860–64) 4: 983–1037.

[4] James Y. Simpson, *Hospitalism, Its Effects on the Results of Surgical Operations, etc.*, Edinburgh: Oliver and Boyd, 1869. For an American review that disagreed with some of Simpson's facts and figures see John Ashurst, Jr., "Hospitalism," *Am. J. Med. Sci.* 64 (1872): 162–72. For the most extended discussion of the subject see John Eric Erichsen, *On Hospitalism and the Causes of Death after Operations* (London: Longmans, Green, 1874). The problems of post-operative infections were linked to hospital design, location, ventilation, and the arrangement and classification of patients.

[5] *New York Tribune*, April 25, 1860. One should not be too smug about advances made since then. Recent investigations of Bellevue's condition reveal that it is still called a "dirty old hospital," *New York Times*, June 27, 1966. Bellevue's problems are those of many similar hospitals, and it is not fair to single out just Bellevue Hospital.

ing and poor hygienic conditions found in hospitals led to so much post-operative morbidity and mortality.

How much of the post-operative infection rate was related to the social class of patients is an intriguing question, difficult to answer. Undoubtedly in the large public hospitals, such as Bellevue in New York, where the paupers of the city were treated, the nutritional and general health conditions of the patients must be taken into consideration.

For much of the nineteenth century the hospital was a place to be treated only if you could not afford care at home, had no relatives to help provide nursing, or lived in such crowded tenement quarters that there was no room for a sick person. Laennec, in describing the circumstances surrounding his invention of the stethoscope, pointed out that he was looking for a better means of direct auscultation, more convenient to both physician and patient. But he also wrote that immediate auscultation (with the ear directly on the chest) was disgusting "in that class of persons found in hospitals."[6]

Stephen Smith, an acknowledged authority on hospitals, classified hospitals into three types: military, civil, and quarantine. The civil hospitals, he said in 1874, were "designed to furnish the sick poor comforts and care which they cannot obtain at home."[7]

Prior to 1860 most of the world's hospitals were constructed on the so-called block plan. Patients were crowded together in multistoried, poorly ventilated buildings in which mortality rates were high. The work of Florence Nightingale and others in England stimulated a number of hospital planners in this country. Her championing of the pavilion plan, by which patients were spread out in less congested, airy, and light quarters was followed with great success by the U.S. Army during the Civil War. After the war most of the new hospitals were built on the pavilion plan.

Bibliographical Note

Benjamin Franklin, *Some Account of the Pennsylvania Hospital, From its First Rise, to the Beginning of the Fifth Month, called May, 1754*, Philadelphia: Franklin & Hall, 1754; reprinted by The Johns Hopkins Press, 1954.

A fairly extensive history of hospitals, with emphasis on the American part of the story, is W. Gill Wylie, "Hospitals: History of their origin and development—their progress during the century of the American Republic," *Trans. New York Acad. Med.* 2 (1876): 251–85.

Leonard K. Eaton, *New England's Hospitals, 1790–1833*, Ann Arbor: University of Michigan Press, 1957, discusses the problems at the beginning of the century. The stout volume pertaining to the Johns Hopkins Hospital, *Hospital Plans, Five Essays Relating to the Construction, Organization and Management*

---

[6] C. N. B. Camac, *Classics of Medicine and Surgery* (New York: Dover, 1959), p. 162.

[7] "Hospitalism and the principles of hospital construction," *Reports and Papers, A.P.H.A.* 2 (1874–75): 396–99; 396.

of Hospitals, New York: Wood, 1875, is a good source for later nineteenth-century ideas about hospitals.

There are numerous books about individual hospitals, both general and psychiatric. For the latter, the large work edited by Henry M. Hurd *et al.* is still useful: *The Institutional Care of the Insane in the United States and Canada*, 4 vols., Baltimore: The Johns Hopkins Press, 1916.

Unfortunately, no over-all history of American hospitals has as yet been written. For the British story see Brian Abel-Smith, *The Hospitals 1800–1948, A Study in Social Administration in England and Wales*, London: Heinemann, 1964. See also Anthony King, "Hospital planning: revised thoughts on the origin of the pavilion principle in England," *Med. Hist.* 10 (1966): 360–73.

For a concise general history of hospitals see Edward D. Churchill, "The development of the hospital," in *The Hospital in Contemporary Life*, Nathaniel W. Faxon, ed., Cambridge: Harvard University Press, 1949, pp. 1–69.

JOHN JONES

APPENDIX TO *PLAIN CONCISE PRACTICAL REMARKS ON THE TREATMENT OF WOUNDS AND FRACTURES,* "CAMP & MILITARY HOSPITALS"

Editor's Note

John Jones (1729–1791), friend and physician to Benjamin Franklin and George Washington, was doubtless one of the foremost American physicians of his time. The little book from which the following selection was taken earned Jones the fond title of "Father of American Surgery." At any rate, his was the first surgical text published by an American. Certainly his British and French training left their mark in his thought and work.[1]

Jones added the remarks on hospitals in an appendix to his book, *Plain Concise Practical Remarks on the Treatment of Wounds and Fractures* (New York: Holt, 1775). The book was reprinted in Philadelphia the following year, and again, by James Mease, a student of Jones and his earliest biographer, in 1795. The two notes following the appendix come from Mease.

At the time of the Revolution, Jones was very pessimistic about the status of the country's hospitals. His discussion of hygienic and structural principles was, in tone and substance, a harbinger of the next century. Benjamin Rush, a generation later warned of similar problems when he wrote:

> Having finished the construction and organization of our hospital, we proceed next to speak of its application to the relief and cure of diseases. And here I am forced to acknowledge that hospitals have been much less effectual for that purpose than is commonly supposed; nay, further, they have in many instances created diseases and produced the mortality of such as seldom prove fatal in private practice. This has in a more eminent degree been the case in military hospitals. They were the passports to the grave of nearly one-half of all the soldiers who perished during the revolutionary war of the United States.[2]

As late as 1863 Florence Nightingale still felt it necessary to open her famous book with the somber warning, "It may seem a strange principle to enunciate as the very first requirement in a hospital that it should do the sick no harm."[3] Not until the twentieth century, with knowledge of asepsis, did hospitals really become relatively safe places in which to seek medical help.

New York: John Holt, 1775.

[1] For a discussion of his medical life and work see Edgar Erskine Hume, "Surgeon John Jones, U.S. Army, father of American surgery and author of America's first medical book," *Bull. Hist. Med.* 13 (1943): 10–32; and for his political views, Steven T. Charles, "John Jones, American surgeon and conservative patriot," *Bull. Hist. Med.* 39 (1965): 435–49.

[2] "On the construction and management of hospitals," *Sixteen Introductory Lectures* (Philadelphia: Bradford & Innskeep, 1811), pp. 182–209; 194–95.

[3] *Notes on Hospitals* (3rd ed.; London: Longmans, Green, 1863), p. iii.

Among the variety of public errors and abuses to be met with in human affairs there is not one, perhaps, which more loudly calls for a speedy and effectual reformation than the misapplied benevolence of hospitals for the sick and wounded.

We daily see persons of every rank and sex contributing to these charities with a spirit of liberality which does honor to humanity; while many of them, with the most becoming zeal, are devoting their time and sacrificing their private interest to the care of superintending the structure and management of the house; and yet an absurd, mistaken economy has hitherto not only rendered all this pious labor and expense, in a great measure, useless, but even fatal and destructive to the very end and aim of the intended purpose—that of healing the diseases of the sick poor.

To those who are unacquainted with the subject in question it will doubtless appear a very extraordinary assertion that there is not at present, in the capital of the kingdom, a single hospital constructed upon proper medical principles; yet it is a fact very generally acknowledged by the most eminent men in the profession of physic and surgery in England.

If we inquire into the causes of such glaring absurdities we shall easily trace them to those sources of darkness and ignorance from which most of our civil and religious abuses have originated; but how they should be continued, to disgrace the improvements of more enlightened times, can only be resolved by reflecting on the pride, obstinacy, and self interest which are too generally annexed to ancient errors.

If great and populous cities have been justly styled the graves of the human species, the large and crowded hospitals generally built in them may, with equal truth and propriety, be denominated the lazarettos or pest-houses of most of the unfortunate persons who, from ill directed motives of compassion, are carried into these charities. In the two great hospitals of St. Thomas and St. Bartholomew, in London, about six hundred patients die annually—which is about one in thirteen of those who are admitted as inpatients. [See note A.]

In Paris it is supposed that one-third of all who die there die in hospitals. The Hotel Dieu, a vast building, situated in the middle of that great city, receives about twenty-two thousand persons annually, one-fifth of which number die every year. It is impossible for a man of any humanity to walk through the long wards of this crowded hospital without a mixture of horror and commiseration at the sad spectacle of misery which presents itself. The beds are placed in triple rows, with four and six patients in each bed; and I have more than once, in the morning rounds, found the dead lying with the living; for, notwithstanding the great assiduity and tenderness of the nurses, some of whom are women of family, who take the veil and piously devote themselves to that office, yet it is almost impossible, from the vast number of patients, to bestow timely assistance upon every individual.

If we compare the number of patients who die in the county infirmaries of England with those of the London and Paris hospitals, the proportional difference will be greatly in favor of the former;* and, although the putrid air of great cities is more unfavorable to health in general than that of country towns, yet the greatest difference in mortality will be found, upon a close and fair examination, to arise from the structure and crowded wards of the hospitals in overgrown capitals.†

For, if to the comparison between the mortality in large city hospitals and those of country towns we further add the proportional difference between the last and that of private practice, it will be found to be in favor of the latter. From all which facts it evidently appears how essentially necessary pure fresh air is to the cure of diseases in general, and particularly those which arise from putrescent causes, either internal or external. [Note B.]

It is computed that a gallon of air is consumed every minute by a man in health, and much more must be necessary to one who is sick—as the morbid effluviae which are continually exhaling from all parts of the body and lungs must contaminate a larger portion of the surrounding atmosphere and render it less healthful to breathe in; for animals are observed to die much sooner in foul air than in vacuo.

But the preceding facts not having been sufficiently understood or attended to, a false economy has universally prevailed in the structure of hospitals for the sick; for those that have hitherto had a principal direction, both in the architecture and management of them, have confined their views entirely to objects of conveniency, cheapness or ornament; and, in one of the last hospitals built in London for lying-in women, there is more expense bestowed on an elegant chapel in it than would have furnished four wards.

In short, the physician and architect have, generally, two very opposite and incompatible views; the latter laying out his plan so as to contain the greatest number of persons in the least possible space; whereas the former always aims at having the utmost room which is consistent with use and conveniency. . . .

As to the disposition of hospitals, with regard to preserving the purity of air, the best rule is to admit so few patients into each ward that a person unacquainted with the danger of bad air might imagine there was room to take in triple the number. When the ceilings are low it will be a good expedient to remove some part of them, and to open the garret story to the roof—for Sir John Pringle says it is incredible in how few days the air will be corrupted in thronged and close wards; and what makes it harder to remedy the evil is the impossibility of convincing the nurses, or even the sick themselves, of the necessity of opening the doors and windows, at any time, for the admission of air.

---

*In the Northampton Infirmary one in nineteen dies annually, and in that of Manchester, placed in a more airy situation, one in twenty-two.

†It is to be hoped that the hospital lately built in this city will have fewer objections to its plan than any hospital hitherto constructed; the principal wards—which are to contain no more than eight beds—are thirty-six feet in length, twenty-four wide and eighteen high; they are all well ventilated, not only from the opposite disposition of the windows but proper openings in the side walls, and the doors open into a long passage or gallery, thoroughly ventilated from north to south.

The sick or wounded should, by no means, be put into common rooms without fire-places—as by that means the foul air is confined, and increased to a tenfold degree—nor will the usual ventilators answer the purpose of correcting or expelling the putrid effluvia.

Lastly, the utmost possible cleanliness is to be observed, both in the persons and bedding of the sick, whose discharges and dressings should be removed immediately out of the wards; and the floors, after being properly cleaned, may be sprinkled with vinegar—of which a large quantity should be allowed to every hospital.

With respect to those diseases which arise from improper diet, Sir John Pringle observes that no orders will restrain soldiers from eating and drinking what they like, while they have money to purchase it; and the only way to prevent excesses will be to oblige the men to eat in messes—by which means the best part of their pay will be bestowed on wholesome food, the choice of which may be left to their taste, as most men commit more errors in the quantity than quality of their food.

Pork has been sometimes forbidden in camps—being regarded as unwholesome. Sanctorius says it retards perspiration, and as it corrupts sooner than beef or mutton, it may be presumed to afford less proper nourishment where there is any tendency to putrefaction. However, it certainly constitutes more than one-half of the animal food consumed by the American peasantry and, when mixed with vegetables, is found to be a very nourishing and wholesome diet. . . .

NOTES BY DR. JAMES MEASE, IN HIS EDITION OF
DR. JONES' *WORKS,* PHILADELPHIA, 1795

[NOTE A]

Hospitals, and especially military ones, frequently defeat the very intention of their establishment, and, instead of proving the means of restoring the health of those confined within them, become the most certain sources of disease. Men shut up in the same room, all differing in customs, manners, and diseases, and deprived of the free circulation of that pabulum of life, *pure air*, have no chance of recovery from the diseases under which they labor, and acquire new ones from their situation. We are informed by the "Result of the Observations made in the Military Hospitals by Dr. Rush," that the principal diseases that prevailed were the *typhus, gravior* and *mitior,* and such was the prevalence of their contagion that men who came into the hospitals with other diseases soon lost the type of their complaints and became affected with the above mentioned fevers. Hence, hospitals have been styled by the same author the *Sinks of Human Life* in an army, and he also asserts that they robbed the United States of more citizens than the sword. In order, therefore, to render hospitals of that importance which they were intended to be of, the great object should be to prevent the progress of contagious diseases, by the greatest attention to cleanliness, free ventilation and frequent whitewashing. Of the efficacy of the latter means there are some remarkable facts in the works of Mr. Howard, and it was experienced in several instances in the military hospitals of the late war. The contagion of *typhus* fever, especially when it prevails with that degree of malignity observable in hospitals and prison ships, will adhere to the bed clothes and even walls and beams of the house, and can only be destroyed by the above means. That the contagion remained on the walls, and thus exerted its influence upon all those who were confined within them, was proved by people having been observed to die in great numbers while their beds were nigh the wall, while others, who lay in the middle of the room, recovered. (See *Trans. Med. Soc. of New Haven.*) So permanent was the nature of the contagion that it remained in one hospital for six months and affected healthy troops, who, at that distance of time, were quartered in it. As a means of counteracting the effects of contagion, or noxious air of any kind, Dr. Priestly recommends the muriatic acid gas obtained by the decomposition of that acid by means of vitriolic acid poured on common salt. Dr. William Fordyce also speaks highly of the efficacy of the muriatic acid, diluted with water, as an *internal* remedy in all diseases commonly called putrid.

M.

[NOTE B]

So essential an article is pure fresh air in the recovery of all those who labor under low contagious fevers, which so commonly prevail in military hospitals, that all medicine will prove ineffectual without it. Those, therefore, who attempt to cure these fevers, and neglect this important remedy, act as unwisely as the enervated and luxurious, who seek to obtain that strength from medicine which ought to be acquired by the more rational mode of temperance and exercise. So reanimating is fresh air to persons ill with low fevers, who breathe the noxious air of a hospital or confined room, that they will frequently recover by its influence alone. During the late war the *jail* or *hospital* fever prevailed to an alarming degree, and the houses appropriated for the reception of the sick were either so dirty or infectious as to render them very improper receptacles for sick people. By the judicious advice of Dr. Rush (who informed me of the fact) the patients were carried out every day and placed under apple trees, where they recovered with astonishing rapidity; for the miserable sufferers, notwithstanding the use of the most suitable medicines, could not be expected to recover while breathing an air which, from its impurity, would induce sickness in those who were in health, and that would act with double force upon those whose vital powers had been nearly exhausted by previous disease. But when removed from this situation, and by breathing the fresh air, rendered doubly refreshing by its mixture with the pure air and odors discharged from growing trees and fruits, they gained strength and recovered as fast as they would have been rendered worse by continuing in their former unhealthy situation.

M.

W. H. RIDEING

HOSPITAL LIFE IN NEW YORK

Editor's Note

W. H. Rideing (1853–1918), an American journalist and author, looked at some of the large hospitals of New York through the eyes of a nonphysician. Although his descriptions strike us today as somewhat overly sentimental, he probably reflected the views of the middle class readers of *Harper's* quite well. The picture we get of the ambulance surgeon, the hospital wards, and their staff and patients is more vivid than one usually finds in strictly medical writings.

Several points bear special notice. Rideing praised the nurses training school at Bellevue, established in 1873 with the aid of some of the surgical staff, especially James R. Wood and Stephen Smith. Despite the deplorable nursing that patients received prior to the presence of well-trained nurses, many medical men strongly opposed the innovation. Their main argument was that nursing was no occupation for genteel women, the other kind being too often pressed into service on public wards already, often to the detriment of patients. A second argument warned that a trained nurse would be prone to act as if she were a physician, a point Florence Nightingale specifically disclaimed.

Rideing, like Sir John Erichsen (see Section V) praised the Roosevelt Hospital. It was designed principally by the Bellevue surgeon Stephen Smith, who was one of New York's foremost authorities on hospital contruction and hospital infections. Rideing correctly pointed out Robert Weir's (whose name he misspelled) important work on antiseptic surgery. But he mistakenly credited Weir and the Roosevelt Hospital for being first in the country to adopt Listerism. Stephen Smith and William Van Buren used the system at Bellevue just as early, and there were individual surgeons elsewhere who introduced the methods of Lister when Weir did.[1]

Most of the hospitals of New York have two beginnings. The first is in the charitable forethought of the rich men who have endowed them. Inclosed by the privacy of his chamber or study, the millionaire has pondered over the disposi-

Harper's New Monthly Magazine 57 (1878): 171–89.

[1] I have discussed the problems associated with assigning the priority of introduction of antiseptic surgery in the United States in "American surgery and the germ theory of disease," *Bull. Hist. Med.* 40 (1966): 135–45.

tion to be made of his accumulated wealth and, feeling the hand of sickness upon him, has remembered the thousands of others whose pain could not know the alleviation that money can procure. The heavy damask curtains drawn in ample folds over the windows, the glowing fire, the mild light of the study lamp, the soft resoundless carpets, the ministrations of the most skillful physicians, and the attentions of trained servants—all these blessings might not take the sting away from death nor wholly disarm suffering, but they surely assuage both. Love can do more than money in smoothing the distressed pillow; the dying laborer in his attic, with his wife's hand in his, may cross the gloomy boundary with greater resignation than the millionaire, says the sentimentalist; but were the love that waits upon the laborer with tireless devotion supplemented with the means to do all that it craves, the fever might be allayed now and then, and life itself prolonged. In such meditations as these some of our hospitals have begun, and the total outcome of the endowments made through private munificence is a variety of establishments for the treatment of every imaginable ailment. A stranger is struck with the number and magnificence of the New York hospitals. Some are of the size and have the appearance of palaces. They are ornaments to the city and are among the largest buildings. The newer ones are built of warm red brick and, with their sunny windows, spacious pavilions, and galleries, are memorable objects to the city's visitors. There is no kind of physical suffering that may not find treatment in one or the other, as we have said. The penniless outcast who is overtaken by sickness, the haggard victim of hip-disease, the incurable consumptive, and the raving creatures stricken with fever are provided for with care and liberality; the patient with means may command all the luxuries a home could give, and those who are poor enjoy comforts impossible to them in their own narrow dwellings.

All hospitals began with Christ and belong to Christianity. The Greeks looked with contempt upon physical weakness, and other nations of antiquity thought it beneath them to make provision for the sick and infirm. But the Nazarene and His disciples taught men to compassionate suffering and, as the Church increased in wealth and influence, hospitals were founded—in the first place as houses for the shelter or refreshment of travellers, especially pilgrims, according to the Latin meaning of their name; and it was only with the multiplication of inns that they assumed their distinctive character as refuges for invalids.

The second of the two beginnings to the hospitals of New York that we spoke of above is in an episode with which all who walk the city streets must be familiar. There is a crash, a scream, a dull thud, and a crowd that momentarily chokes the traffic of the busy thoroughfare, the cause being an accident. The crowd presses around the horrible spot on the pavement baptized by the blood of a man who has fallen from a scaffolding aloft, out of a window, or through one of the trap-doors by which goods are hoisted into the lofts of the stores. "Give him air!" some cry, but the crowd hedges him in with morbid curiosity, only a few of weaker ones turning aside with pale faces. He lies there huddled up and deathly white, as though all the bones in his body were broken; his eyes are filmed and opaque, and his mouth is rimmed with blood. A telegram sent from the nearest police station brings an ambulance, which dashes up to the spot from the nearest hospital. The surgeon quickly binds the fractured limbs between splints; and while the crowd gapes with wonder and admiration at the dexterity and system, the sufferer is gently lifted into the vehicle and driven away. Such is the practical and beneficent beginning of the New York hospitals to the hapless thousands who are annually maimed in the turmoil of the city streets.

For the purposes of ambulance service the city is divided into three police telegraph districts, an independent wire connecting all the precincts with the hospitals that are provided with ambulances. These are the New York and Roosevelt hospitals on the west side, and the Bellevue Hospital on the east side. The New York has two ambulances, one stationed at the House of Relief in Chambers Street, and the other at the hospital in Fifteenth Street; the Roosevelt has one, stationed at the hospital in Fifty-ninth Street; and the Bellevue has several. When an accident is reported at a police station, it is immediately announced by telegraph to the hospital of the district, and an idea of what usually happens then may be gleaned from the following account of our personal experience.

We were loitering one morning last January in the apothecary's shop of the New York Hospital, which, besides the long rows of shelves filled with glass jars and bottles, contains a dial instrument, whose imperative tinkling suddenly put an end to our conversation. "The ambulance is wanted in Eighteenth Street," the surgeon in charge explained; and though his name was Slaughter—an obviously unfortunate one for an Esculapian—he proved himself to be one of the tenderest men that ever touched a wound. The apothecary's shop is in the basement, and from it a door opens upon a courtyard, at one side of which is a stable. A well-kept horse was quickly harnessed to the ambulance; and as the surgeon took his seat behind, having first put on a jaunty uniform cap with gold lettering, the driver sprang on to the box, where we had already placed ourselves, and with a sharp crack of the whip we rolled off the smooth asphalt of the courtyard into the street. Our speed was only pardonable in view of its object. As we swept around the corners and dashed over the crossings, both doctor and driver kept up a sharp cry of warning to the pedestrians, who darted out of our way with haste, or nervously retreated to the curb looking after us with faces expressive of indignant remonstrance, until they discovered by the gilt lettering on the panels what our vehicle was. The surliest car drivers and the most aggressive of truckmen gave us the right of way and pulled up or aside to afford us passage. People in a hurry stopped to look after us and strove on tiptoe to discover whether or not we had a passenger. We rattled over the uneven cobblestones of West Eighteenth Street, and at No. 225, where there is an iron gate before an alley-way with a small house at the end, an old man appeared and hailed us. We alighted, and followed him into the front room on the ground floor, the doctor carrying his instruments under his arm.

The case was not very serious. The occupant of the tenement, an old laborer, had slipped in entering and fractured his leg a short distance above the ankle. The room served as kitchen and parlor for him and his wife, who began to whimper as soon as she saw the doctor and refused to be comforted, with a determination worthy of a more reasonable cause. The furniture consisted of a few chairs, a table, some dishes, and a stove, upon which a kettle was steaming. "Where's the man?" inquired the doctor. The wife moaned, and we might have waited for an answer had not an expostulatory voice come from an inner apartment, "Hould yer noise, Mary." Obtaining a candle, we found the sufferer lying on a disordered bed with all his clothes on and a pipe in his mouth, the room having neither windows nor other light or ventilation than that which struggled from the kitchen through the door. He was a small, rosy old man from the north of Ireland and was not in the least discomposed by his accident. "If I'd had the laist dhrop of drink in me, I cud onderstand it; but faith I hadn't tasted," he exclaimed, as the doctor energetically threw his coat and cap on the floor, regardless of the gold lettering and gold buttons, and prepared for business. Two splints were selected, and a roll of cotton bandages taken from a sachel. "Hould on a bit, doctor; me pipe's out," the unfortunate called out, as the doctor rolled up his trousers. "Mary, me pipe's out; give us another draw, an' be quick about it. Maybe it'll be a long time till I get another one." The pipe was refilled with tobacco, puffed into a glow by an obliging friend and handed to him. "Yes, I must have another draw," he went on, as he put himself in position for the doctor, who gently raised the injured limb and applied the splints to it, packing them with oakum before binding them with the cotton ribbon. Once or twice and only once or twice, the old fellow winced. "Murther, doctor, don't touch me heel; that's where it hurts!" During the rest of the operation he quietly puffed his pipe, soothed his wife, and endeavored to flatter the doctor most outrageously. "Och, doctor, you're the greatest man in the world—mind me heel—be quiet, Mary—that's what ye are, doctor, the greatest man in the world."

"All comfortable, eh?" said the doctor, neatly cutting the last bandage.

"As nice as can be, Sor."

Finding that amputation was not immediately necessary, Mary smiled at last, and tidied her husband's dress before he was lifted by two burly policemen on to the stretcher, which had been brought from the ambulance into the outer room.

The stretcher, like all the appliances of the ambulance, is mercifully ingenious, and devised with the object of giving the sufferer the least possible pain in transportation. It consists simply of a strip of canvas about three feet wide and seven feet long, with a tube at each side, through which the wooden poles for carrying it are slipped. The poles are braced at each end of the canvas by iron cross-bars, which are easily detached; and the beauty of the whole arrangement is that it obviates the necessity of disturbing the patient again on his arrival at the hospital, the stretcher being put upon the bed and the poles being withdrawn.

A light mattress and several blankets were spread over the canvas, and the old man was tucked in as snugly as a baby in a crib. "Good-by, Mrs. Murphy," he cried to a neighbor who had come in as the policemen were bearing him to the ambulance.

"Good-by, Mr. Sullivan, and it's sorry I am to see ye l'avin' in this way," whereupon the wife burst into fresh tears.

The ambulance had been backed up to the curb, and the tail-board removed. We now discovered that it had two bottoms and the upper one, which was softly padded, had been drawn off on caster wheels so that it slanted from the end of the vehicle to the sidewalk. The padding was luxuriously yielding, and when the stretcher had been placed upon it, it was pushed into the ambulance and the tail-board closed upon it. The doctor took his seat behind and, as we drove off, a voice came from the blankets: "May I ta-ake another draw, doctor?" Assent being given, the blue wreaths of Mr. Sullivan's tobacco rolled upward from the blankets until we trotted under the archway of the hospital and pulled up before the door of the receiving ward, where two orderlies drew the stretcher out and deposited it on a bed in the manner previously described, while Dr. Slaughter reported the case to the house surgeon, who was thence responsible for it. . . .

To pass from it [the New York Hospital] to the Bellevue Hospital affords a contrast somewhat startling. The one combines in its structure and administration nearly everything that medical and sanitary science has revealed for the relief of the sick. Most of its patients are poor, but not so poor or alienated from brotherly affection that they are unable to pay the cost of their support; many of them are mechanics or small tradesmen; an impoverished actor or journalist may be found among them; and a few are prosperous and even wealthy. But the other is a hospital for the poorest of the poor, the dregs of society, the semi-criminal, starving, unwelcome class, who suffer and die unrecognized, and to whom charity at the best is cold and mechanical. This is a large and increasing constituency in New York City, where the word pauper is acquiring the dread significance and suggestion of hopeless misery that it has in Great Britain; and the wards are filled with wasted souls drifting through the agonies of disease toward unpitied and unremembered deaths, with no tenderer hand to clasp at the parting than that of the strange nurse, who has grown callous through long familiarity with such experiences. Many of the patients lie for months without receiving one friendly call except from the colporteur, the priest, or the ladies of the Flower Mission—lie and wait with the carelessness of result that makes the days blank and the future a matter of indifference. There is no luxury here; not much gentleness. The building was built for an almshouse or prison some fifty years ago, and its ponderous dull gray mass of granite is sullen looking and unadapted to its uses. The New York Hospital, with its sunny windows facing the south, and its pleasant surroundings, is less than a mile away; but to reach Bellevue we have to cross a district of tenement houses, plentifully dotted with shabby little stores and corner groggeries, where the garbage is piled up in the streets, the men are idle, the women slatternly, and the children as nearly nude as the weather permits. It is between Twenty-sixth and Twenty-seventh streets, and covers the whole block between them, First Avenue, and the East River. The river ebbing and flowing, shining and rippling in the sun, and bestirred by traffic, cheers the situation, and a few trees and a patch of grass—all that is left of the wide fields that once swept up to Murray Hill—soften the granite austerity of the eastern front. But Bellevue is still forbidding. A high brick wall isolates it from the thoroughfares. There is one medical college just within the boundaries, and another just outside. The windows of the dissecting-rooms shine until late hours in the night, for there is no scarcity of subjects in colleges which reap the harvest of a charity hospital. And at one end of the dispensary for the out-door poor, which is under the college within the ground, two downward steps lead into a low-roofed building, over the entrance of which hangs a dingy lamp inscribed with black letters, "The Morgue." The room within contains five marble slabs behind a glass partition, with sprays of water falling over them. The dead-house is close by, and several times a week the funereal little steamer bears the un-lettered coffins away to Potter's Field. It was a cold November morning when we last saw her leave the wharf, and the fog in which she was soon hidden symbolized the unrecorded lives, the cheerless deaths, and the unattended graves of her load. Suspicious looking men and untidy women haunt the neighborhood, attracted to it by the morbid curiosity of their diseased minds, and it may occur to them that if they do not die in prison, their death-beds will be here, or in the Charity Hospital on Blackwell's Island, which is visible from the grounds of Bellevue. . . .

The Training School for Nurses, which now possesses a substantial brick building as a residence in Twenty-sixth Street, opposite the hospital, was opened in May, 1873, to instruct intelligent women in hospital and private nursing. It began with a lady superintendent and a staff of six nurses, whose number has now increased to fifty-six, thirty-eight being actively employed at Bellevue and three at the Emergency Hospital. Many difficulties were experienced at the start, and though the committee in charge advertised and applied to physicians for aid, four women only were found capable of acting as head nurses, one of whom was soon discharged for inefficiency. Out of seventy-three applicants for admission to the school many were totally unfitted by mental incapacity, others by physi-cal weakness, and a large number withdrew because they would not spend two years in learning the profession. Accepting twenty-nine probationers, the com-mittee was compelled to dismiss three on account of ill health, five on account of inefficiency, and two on account of family claims upon them, leaving nine-teen who succeeded and proved the advantages of the school to themselves in affording them profitable employment, and to humanity generally in fitting intelligent women to become positive helps in the hospital and sick room. The requirements of the committee are exacting. Pupils must be from twenty-one to thirty-five years of age, unmarried, obedient, amiable, steadfast in purpose, in good health, having no kind of infirmity, neither deafness nor dimness of vision, and quick in observation. The candidates, having assured the committee of their excellence in these virtues, are admitted to the school on probation for one month, being boarded and lodged without expense, but not paid, and at the expiration of that period they engage themselves for a two years' course of instruction and service, with salary, provided they are satisfactory. The course includes lectures on the diseases of children, obstetrics, eruptive fevers, ventilation and bathing, hemorrhages and the circulation of the blood, arteries, respiration and temperature, superficial anatomy and uterine appliances—all of which are given by able physicians and surgeons. Lessons also are given in bandaging, in general ward work, in the management of a sick room, and in physiology. At the end of the first year an examination of the pupils is held, and at the end of the second year diplomas are issued to those entitled to them. The primary object of the founders was to improve the nursing in public hospitals, and no one can say that improvement was unnecessary or that it has not been effected. Previous to the opening of the school, Bellevue was a very much mismanaged institution; three patients sometimes slept on two beds, five patients on three beds, and it happened now and then that they slept on the floor. During two weeks of January, 1876, there was no soap in the hospital, and not enough clothing; many patients had neither pillows nor blankets, and forty-eight per cent of the amputations made proved fatal, owing, no doubt, to the poison in the walls. But the worst feature was the character of the nurses, who were profane, ignorant, careless, heartless, and in most cases utterly unfitted for their positions. We look back with extreme pity to the patients who were immured in the hospital and dragged through their illness to a long-deferred recovery or hurried to an avertable death at that period. The introduction of the young, intelligent, kindly nurses of the training school into the female wards, and a closer supervision of the orderlies in the male wards, have brought about a change for the better, however, and it is now possible to visit the hospital without having our instincts of humanity shocked. Instead of the untidy and often brutal creatures of old, such women as she to whom we spoke, gentle in manner and good to look upon, minister to the sufferers, who, paupers though they are, have claims that are eloquent from their helplessness. The ivy weaving its disks of green around the windows, the illuminated mottoes on the walls, the little odds and ends for diversion and recreation visible where the patients are most loathsome or least interesting, are testimony of the beneficence of the new era. . . .

The Roosevelt Hospital, at Fifty-ninth Street and Ninth Avenue, New York, is spoken of by the eminent English surgeon Erichsen as the most complete medical charity he has ever seen. It is near the Central Park and the Hudson

River, in a situation both quiet and salubrious. The material used is principally brick. It has a central administrative department with lateral pavilions, and a large detached barrack ward, which is erected in the garden and has no communication with the main structure, except by an open corridor. The administrative building contains the various offices; the apartments of the officers and their families; an apothecary's shop and a laboratory, in which all the drugs used are prepared; a very complete operating theatre; and small wards for patients requiring special accommodations. The barrack ward is devoted solely to the reception of acute surgical cases, and contains thirty-six beds, arranged two by two on each side of the interspaces between the windows. It has an open basement and a large ventilating space between the ceiling and the roof. Dr. Erichsen also stated, in his address on American surgery before the University College of London, that every appliance which modern science has discovered securing ventilation, cleanliness, and warmth has been introduced into it, and he recommends the adoption of the Roosevelt model in England. The garden contains, besides the barrack ward, an isolated hut for the reception of erysipelas cases; and in summer, when the flowers and shrubs are blooming, it is much frequented by the convalescent patients. Sixteen hundred and seventeen cases were treated in 1876, 1,451 of which were free; 602 were Americans and 558 were Irish. The death rate of all the cases treated is nine per cent or more than three per cent less than that of Bellevue.

The hospital is particularly interesting to the profession from the fact that it was the first in this country to adopt, through the exertions of Dr. Robert F. Wier, the antiseptic method of treating wounds invented by Joseph Lister, a celebrated Scottish surgeon. This method, which has been developed by years of patient research and has almost revolutionized surgery, is based on the experience that the inflammation which follows a wound, such as an amputation, is due to the decomposition of the discharges that are always formed on any cut surface. The substances formed by the decomposition give rise to erysipelas, hospital gangrene, etc., or they may be absorbed by the system with fatal result. Lister believes he has demonstrated that the cause of the putrefaction is due to the lodgment on the wound-secretions of minute living bodies floating in the air, and he discovered, after trying many other disinfectants, that carbolic acid would kill these germs. The principle, therefore, consists in surrounding a wound from its reception to its cure with an atmosphere charged with the vapor of the acid; and to accomplish this the surgeon operates amid a thin cloud of spray made by atomizing a weak solution, in which his hands, instruments, sponges, are also immersed. The blood vessels are tied by carbolized cords, the edges of the wound closed by carbolized stitches, and, finally, layers of gauze impregnated with carbolic acid and resin are bound over the wound and a considerable part of the adjoining skin, the resin causing the carbolic acid to be evolved slowly, so that the dressing need not be changed for several days. Dr. Wier considers the success of the method proven, and states that by its use the mortality resulting from serious operations has been noticeably reduced, and that under it the closure of the most serious wounds is truly wonderful.

The Roosevelt Hospital was the last gift of James H. Roosevelt to humanity. He made it the sole legatee of a princely fortune, with the exception of a few bequests to individuals; and as he left no near relatives, the heirlooms of his house are stored in the trustees' room, and his body rests under a plain monument in the garden, with the inscription over it: "Upright in his aims, simple in his habits, and sublime in his benefaction." The hospital is admirably managed by Dr. Horatio Paine, the gentlemanly superintendent; and there is no limit to the charity it dispenses, except in the extent of its funds.

We have not purposed being exhaustive, knowing that to be impossible within our space; and there are many hospitals in the city, such as the Presbyterian and the Mount Sinai, which for their extent and excellence of work deserve attention. The Fruit and Flower missions should also be remembered; but the most we have been able to do has been to describe some of the phases of hospital life by selecting representative institutions.

PART **VIII**
HYGIENE

INTRODUCTION

The nineteenth century witnessed the birth of sanitary science, or public health, as a professional specialty. As with most medical developments at that time, the movement for sanitary reform began in Europe, particularly in England. In recent years, more historians have been attracted to the history of public health in America. Their work has clearly demonstrated the importance of social history for the medical historian. Books such as Charles Rosenberg's *The Cholera Years* have taken the level of analysis an important step beyond the older, less imaginative histories of laws, health departments, or biographies. Medicine must always be seen in terms of the society in which it functions; nowhere is this more vivid than in the history of public health.

The early American sanitarians, most of whom lived in the large eastern cities where the sanitary problems were greatest, did much to improve their surroundings as well as the status of the medical profession. Their surveys and reports were widely read and reviewed, and in some cases led to civic action.[1]

One of the less well known, but important, American sanitarians was the New York physician John H. Griscom. His report on *The Sanitary Conditions of the Laboring Population of New York*, of 1845, was an attempt to "engage the attention of the magistracy" of his city to the problems of the public's health. He was obviously influenced and impressed by the work of Chadwick in England and Parent Du Chatelet in France, using the title of the former's report of 1842 for his own work. Beyond describing the stark conditions under which many of the citizens of New York had to live, Griscom also continued to work for an effective health department and for the establishment of a professional corps of health workers.[2]

---

[1] A number of these reports have become classics and have been reprinted in whole or in part (see references to McCready, Griscom, Shattuck). The 1837 paper by McCready and the 1850 Shattuck report are unfortunately again out of print. Perhaps the best of all the sanitary surveys was that carried out in New York in 1864 and published by the Citizens' Association in the next year. It has never been reissued, but the section by Stephen Smith that follows is based on that report.

[2] Part of Griscom's report has recently been reprinted in Charles N. Glaab, *The American City, A Documentary History* (Homewood, Ill.: Dorsey, 1963), pp. 117-28. See also Charles E. Rosenberg and Carroll S. Rosenberg, "Pietism and the origins of the American

Sanitary science, Griscom wrote in 1857, was a part of medical science yet distinguished by its special relation to society. Both medicine and sanitary science required a thorough knowledge of chemistry, pathology, and therapeutics:

> But for the sanitarian physician, superinduced, upon these, there is especially requisite a knowledge of forensic medicine, or the relations of the science of medicine to law; of meteorology, or the effects of climate and atmospheric influences on the body; of the physical character of dynamics of the atmosphere; of the philosophy and practice of ventilation; of various matters of a mechanical kind, bearing on sewerage, house building, street cleaning, and water supply; of statistics of life and mortality; of the literature of epidemics, and of all sanitary improvements. And, lastly, to be a good sanitarian, requires the possession of sound logical faculties.[3]

From this catalog one can readily see the main problems with which the sanitarians concerned themselves.

These problems of the public's health in nineteenth-century America existed in both rural and urban settings. The growth of the cities, however, by an influx of immigrants from the countryside and from abroad, led to more crises and greater sanitary evils. During times of epidemics, such as from cholera, typhus, or smallpox, it was the residents of the large city slums, or what we today somewhat more delicately refer to as the inner city, who were hardest hit.

The findings of the surveys by Shattuck, Griscom, or the Citizens' Association in the mid-century years revealed many tenements so crowded as to make poor health conditions inevitable. More than one hundred years later many similar conditions remain. That so many urban problems are still with us, illustrates the difficulty of their solution.

Technological developments have, of course, brought many health improvements, but, as with most progress, there goes paradox. The automobile, for instance, is a prime source of air pollution and cause of accidental death and injury, but it has also changed patterns of medical care and the disease picture. Horses, and their attendant flies, are no longer quartered in our cities. As a result the prevalence of diarrheal diseases, the greatest source of infant mortality during much of the previous century, has dwindled to insignificance.

Purification of water supplies has promoted better health, but as late as 1890 only 1.5 per cent of the urban population of the United States drank filtered water. By 1914 the figure rose to 40 per cent.[4]

---

public health movement: A note on John H. Griscom and Robert H. Hartley," *J. Hist. Med.* 23 (1968): 16–35.

[3] John H. Griscom, "Improvements of the public health, and the establishment of a sanitary police in the city of New York," *Trans. Med. Soc. State of New York* (1857): 107–23; 109.

[4] For these figures and a useful summary of social and economic changes and their effects on medicine and public health, see Bernhard Stern, *American Medical Practice in the Perspectives of a Century* (New York: Commonwealth Fund, 1946).

The health reforms and the many new health departments organized in the latter third of the nineteenth century were the fruits of long and hard labor. The work that these dedicated sanitarians performed did lead to lower mortality figures, longer life expectancy, and an improved general standard of living. As they ameleriorated health conditions, so too did they help to improve the image of medicine in the eyes of the public. Once again the profession's prestige began to climb, to reach somewhat unrealistic heights in the twentieth century.

Bibliographical Note

Benjamin W. McCready, *On the Influence of Trades, Professions, and Occupations in the United States, in the Production of Disease*, Genevieve Miller, ed., Baltimore: The Johns Hopkins Press, 1943; originally published in 1837.

Lemuel Shattuck was the moving spirit behind the *Report of the Sanitary Commission of Massachusetts, 1850*, reprinted in part by Harvard University Press, 1948.

Report of the Council of Hygiene and Public Health of the Citizens' Association of New York, Upon the Sanitary Condition of the City, New York: Appleton, 1865.

There are numerous books that deal with the history of public health in Europe. See especially George Rosen, *A History of Public Health*, New York: MD., 1958; the long introduction by M. W. Flinn to the reprint of Chadwick's *Report on the Sanitary Condition of the Labouring Population of Great Britain, 1842*, Edinburgh: Edinburgh University Press, 1965; and Royston Lambert's biography, *John Simon 1816–1904, and English Social Administration*, London: Macgibbon & Kee, 1963.

For a general survey of public health developments in this country see Rosen, *A History of Public Health*, op. cit.; Wilson G. Smillie, *Public Health, Its Promise for the Future*, New York: Macmillan, 1955; and Charles Rosenberg's *The Cholera Years*, Chicago: University of Chicago Press, 1962.

ROBERT TOMES

WHY WE GET SICK

Editor's Note

History abounds in recurring themes. One of the more fascinating is the supposed relationship of the hectic way of American life to various diseases. Robert Tomes (1817–82), a journalist, was an astute observer of the American scene a century ago. The following article appeared in a popular magazine in 1856, and much of it, except for some words and phrases that date it, could as readily appear today.

A short time after "Why We Get Sick" appeared, *Harper's Magazine* published an article entitled "How to Keep Well."[1] To settle the question, we need not call the doctor, the author (probably also Tomes) proclaimed. "When that learned gentleman drives up to the door, we step out and leave the case to him and the undertaker. Our office is to dispense the ounce of prevention, and thus save the necessity of swallowing the by no means agreeable or infallible pound of cure." Our way of life, our "living" in cities, our eating habits, all cause old age to come nearly a score of years earlier in America than elsewhere, the author informed his readers.

The popular health field was an active one in the mid-nineteenth century. Besides the many medical sects which published their own journals, there were also many health journals, such as the one edited by Sylvester Graham, who is now better remembered for his cracker.[2]

Articles on health, doctors, and medical discoveries, which still appear in the magazines of today, are, as in former times, probably the prime source of medical information for most of the public.

•

If, as some ill-natured fellow has said, sickness is a sin, we Americans are great sinners. That much of the ill-health of the world, and of our portion of it especially, may be directly traced to a positive disobedience of the laws of

---

Harper's Monthly Magazine 13 (1856): 642–47.

[1] *Harper's Magazine* 14 (1856): 56–61.

[2] See especially Richard H. Shryock's article "Sylvester Graham and the popular health movement, 1830–1870," reprinted in *Medicine in America* (Baltimore: The Johns Hopkins Press, 1966), pp. 111–25.

nature cannot be questioned; and that this disobedience is culpable, requires no casuist to prove. As, however, nature sufficiently vindicates its own justice by the heaviest penalties, there is no occasion for us to mock the criminal on his road to execution. Our object is to prevent, not to punish.

The Americans should be the healthiest people in the world; but, if we compare them with other nations, in the aggregate, they will be probably found to have no claim to this superiority. This, however, is not a fair comparison, as the condition of the masses with us more nearly approaches that of the prosperous classes than of the poor of foreign countries. Material advantages alone, apart from moral causes, have given the Americans a position far in advance of all other nations. Physical comfort is the rule with us, while it is but the exception elsewhere. If a potato patch, as in Ireland, were the only barrier between our people and starvation, there might be some excuse for our countrymen not being healthier; for a want of physical comfort is among the most powerful causes of disease. With abundance of food, and such liberal rewards of labor that humblest American can supply himself with those comforts of life which are only within the reach of the prosperous classes abroad, it is but fair to compare him with the latter. In this comparison he will be found very deficient on the score of health. Sickness is mostly a choice and not a necessity with us; and we now propose to show *why we get sick*, when we might as readily keep well.

The Americans work too much and play too little, and would that it were only with the usual effect of making Jonathan a dull boy. The result, however, is worse than this, for it tells very seriously against his health and vigor. If modern civilization has its blessings, it has its curses too, and of these the United States have a disproportionate share. There is a large class of diseases which were unknown to our forefathers, but which are fearfully wasting the health and happiness of the present generation. If our ancestors made the journey of life in slow coaches, they had the satisfaction of running less risks by the road. It is questionable whether, with greater speed and more frequent break-downs, our boasted progress is worth all we value it at. A host of diseases of the heart, the brain, nerves, and stomach, which exhaust the doctor's skill and fill his pockets, came in with modern civilization. To these diseases the Americans are far more subject than any other people, as might be naturally expected from the fact of their being more generally and powerfully brought under the influence of the intense activity of modern life.

With a brain in the delirium of excitement, with nerves like trains of gunpowder, ready to inflame at every spark, and with a heart in a tumult of passionate pulsation, driving its hot blood, which, like a current of lava, burns and destroys as it flows, American life is but the agony of a fever. There is no repose for us. We push on in frenzied excitement through the crowds, the noise, the hot glare and dust of the highways, without turning for a moment to refresh ourselves in the quiet and shade of the by-paths of life. We have but one object in our rapid journey, and that is to get the start of our fellow-travelers. Our political equality, offering to all a chance for the prizes of life, and thus encouraging everyone to try his speed in the race, is no doubt a spur to the characteristic hurry of Americans. Our institutions, however, are not responsible for the prize we choose to strive for. There is no reason that we know of why a republican should have no other aim in life but to get richer than his neighbor; but there are a thousand good reasons, if we value health and happiness, why we should pursue other and higher objects. When the pursuit of wealth is the great purpose of life in so rapidly a progressive state of material prosperity as exists in our commercial communities, it requires exclusive devotion and the highest strain of the faculties to succeed. A fair competence, however, is easily reached; and if we had learned to care for better things, we would not strive for more.

It is the excessive devotion to business, in order to compass that wealth that is so unduly prized, which is one of the chief causes of the ill health of Americans. Count the hours a man gives to work, if he be his own task-master—and he cannot have a more severe one—and how much time will be left—not to speak of enjoyment—for the mere requirements of health? Ten hours a day, with intervals of repose, is the allotment to the laborer in England, where to pause from work is to starve, while there is hardly an American in business who does not exceed this from choice. And his intervals of respose, what are they? Possibly half an hour for dinner, where, ten to one, he is clenching a bargain with his opposite neighbor in the short pause between bolted beef and bolted pudding.

Brisk, of the firm of Brisk and Smart, is a model merchant, eager for gain and constant in business. He hurries up in the morning and he hurries down impatient for his coffee and cakes, and gulping the one and bolting the other, he is soon whisked away in the omnibus to his dry goods in Pearl Street. Now he begins a day of intense activity, making a sale here and paying a note there, settling an account with one and beginning an account with another. Thus hurried along in the vortex of business, time passes without a thought of any thing but dry goods, bills payable and bills receivable, until he is reminded, by the approaching close of bank hours, that he has a deposit to make, when he is off in a heat, taking the only exercise in the day, by which he is as much benefited as an ox when driven to slaughter. The deposit made, the savory atmosphere of some neighboring eating-houses recalls to his memory the fact of the possession of a stomach and the possibility of its being hungry. He has not much time to spare for chops and brandy-water, as Smith, one of his best customers, always comes in in the afternoon and likes to be served by himself. Smith served, his bill must be made out and his goods packed; so the busy day is prolonged far into the night, when Brisk, finally, with a packet of letters in his hand, which must be answered and can be as well done at home, springs into an omnibus and is soon trotted up to the Fifth Avenue. As the children are in bed and Mrs. Brisk is dressing for a party, Brisk has a fine time of it, all to himself, his cigar, and his letters. This is a fair picture of the American man of business, and its original may be seen not only in the market and exchange, but in the forum and other busy departments of life.

Men who thus recklessly set at defiance all the laws of health must suffer the penalty of disease, and we are fast becoming, in consequence, a nation of invalids. Foreigners already affect to see in us a degenerate offspring of a nobler race, and with them a skeleton frame, a yellow-dyed bilious face, an uncomfortable dyspeptic expression, an uneasy spasmodic motion, and a general ghostlike, charnel-house aspect, serve to make up a type of the species Yankee. They put us all down as residents of the Dismal Swamp, and say that we have lost in that cheerless region our flesh and spirits, and have neither the heart nor the strength to laugh and make merry. They declare that our sides never shake but with the ague. . . .

A foreign medical observer, while traveling in this country, remarked, that the whole nation seemed to be suffering from a paroxysm of St. Vitus's dance. The peculiarity of this disease is the ceaseless and uncontrollable motion of the limbs of the patient, who appears to be possessed of a desire of being in half a dozen places at one and the same moment of time.

We care not, just now, to speak of the influence of this excessive nervous irritability—which, as it alternates with frequent fits of utter prostration, always craves for stimulants—upon American habits and character. We, however, firmly believe, were it not for our weakened and excitable nerves, there would be less occasion for the moralist to groan over the unconstitutionality of Maine laws, and to lament our occasional lapses in social and political ethics. Our business is with the physical results, and these become sufficiently alarming when we learn that dyspepsia, nervous disorders of all kinds and insanity, are so much more abounding in the United States than in any other country, as almost to become national characteristics. There are, doubtless, other concurrent causes of the ill health of our people, and of these we shall cursorily treat. It is, however, the causes within the control of the individual, and not those of climate and of public hygiene, for which the nature of the country and society are responsible, that we are considering at present.

Talleyrand said that England had a thousand religions but only one sauce, and that was melted butter. We may not be so rich in religion, but we are certainly no better off for sauces. The art of cooking, with us, is in its infancy, and a very unpromising infancy too. We are not only unskilled in sauces, but in every other branch of kitchen cunning. We want a Miss Coutts or a Lord Ashburton to teach us common things, and more particularly how to boil the pot. Our women are said to be very curious after knowledge and are known to be the most untiring listeners to the forced conceits of our itinerant New England would-be teachers. If these eloquent young gentlemen would descend occasionally from the clouds, where, sublimated by their own imaginings, they have lost all sympathy with daily flesh and blood, and hold communion with their audience in the body, their teachings might be possibly rewarded by the consciousness of doing some practical good. We suggest to our peripatetic philosophers a course of lectures for the coming season on cooks and cookery. There is more need just now of dietetics than aesthetics, and we promise a full house and a deluge of two shillings to the first New England philosopher who will hold forth on "Woman as Cook," "Soyer and Sauces," "Soups made Easy," "The Triune Dinner—Soup, Fish, and Meat," "The Age of Grease," "Buckwheat as a Civilizer," etc.

Lord Cockburn records the horror with which the word corn was first listened to by the Edinburgh philosophers, when Dugald Stewart, in his lectures on political economy, ventured, *ex cathedra*, upon so undignified a topic. But since that day corn has become in Great Britain a more imposing word, as it has always been a more important thing than Constitution and Commons, and we believe cookery worthy of as high an elevation. Liebig has not thought it below his dignity to teach us how to boil, roast, and fry. He tells us that bad cooking decomposes the food and produces certain compounds hard in name and harder of digestion. That philanthropic philosopher informs us, moreover, that frying, which, by-the-by, is a favorite American process, is the worst possible mode of cooking, as it requires so high a temperature as to decompose the food, and too large a quantity of fat. There are certain rules laid down by Liebig, founded upon the laws of chemistry, which we do not believe a single housekeeper in the United States knows in theory, or a single cook puts in practice. For example, is our meat ever boiled according to this canon of cookery? Put the meat into the water when it is boiling briskly, and keep it boiling some minutes, and then add cold water so as to reduce the temperature to $165°$ or $158°$, as this is the only way to make the meat juicy and digestible. Fancy Bridget, the cook, ordered to test the temperature of the water by putting a thermometer in it. We would probably find that valuable instrument served up like a boiled parsnip. . . .

The Americans are not epicures, but gluttons. They swallow, but don't eat; and, like the boaconstrictor, bolt every thing, whether it be a blanket or a rabbit. They take their food as if it were a part of their day's work. It startles a foreigner to see with what voracity even our delicate women dispose of the infinite succession of dishes on the public tables. We question whether this intemperance in eating harmonizes well with absolute temperance at dinner in drinking. Where the stomach is so much tasked, its powers require to be aided by the stimulus of wine. Wine, too, has the advantage of prolonging the feast and giving conviviality to what is otherwise but a gross indulgence of appetite.

We do not know why Americans are so averse to the convivial wine-drinking of the dinner table, while they are so given to swilling unsocially at the bar room. The bar room drink is more dangerous and more unhealthy, inasmuch as it is ordinarily stronger and taken into an empty stomach, upon the nerves of which it acts directly, while the beverage at the dinner table is weaker and, being mixed and digested with the food, hardly stimulates the nervous system at all. Our fashionable ladies, too, who are too delicate to take their glass of wine before the world, are accused of a growing fondness for the forbidden delights of the bar. The Newport, Saratoga, and Rockaway innkeepers have been obliged, it is said, to strengthen their establishments by an increased force of bar keepers, in order to keep up with the great female demand this season for sherry-cobblers. A stern moralist tells us that in coming down at break of day from his garret room at one of the watering places lately, he stumbled at almost every lady's door over an empty glass, the straw in which was very clear evidence how the wind had blown the night before. . . .

Life is too emotional in America either for strength of body or mind. Enough has been said of the enervating effects of the excessive devotion to business. Our diversions are ordinarily of a kind no less injurious in their influence. The American, with his irritable and diseased temper, knows but little enjoyment save in excitement. In fact, like an old epicure, he cannot taste his daily food unless it be well-peppered. Thus town is preferred to country life, and the dissipation of fashion to the simple pleasures of home. The robust amusements, which merely invigorate and do not excite, have become obsolete, and there is no country in the world nearer to us than Turkey or China where so many of the prosperous classes can be found who take such little manly physical exercise. There are thousands of our citizens who have both money and time to spare who never crossed the back of a horse, swam a stroke, pulled the trigger of a gun or the oar of a boat, and would be sorely puzzled to shoot a burglar or save a child from drowning. Yet strong exercise, such as most of these imply, is the best to invigorate the body and to secure our people against that effeminacy and ill-health into which they are fast lapsing.

Look at our young men of fortune. Were there ever such weaklings? An apathetic-brained, a pale pasty-faced, narrow-chested, spindle-shanked, dwarfed race—mere walking manikins to advertise the last cut of the fashionable tailor! With such weak heads and inconsiderable breadth of back it is hardly reasonable to expect that our young men of property should become the Atlases of the state, or, with such puny powers of locomotion, that they should make much progress in any of the walks of life. They are, however, the very class who have the leisure and means, and, if they were just to themselves, would have the power to give that manlier tone to society by which it might be strengthened and purified to noble influences. To urge those who are lying indolently night and day in the lap of pleasure "to scorn delights and live laborious days," for the sake of doing the world some service, may be a waste of labor. It may not be amiss, however, to remind such that their own health and happiness would be improved by some little exercise of those faculties with which nature has endowed them. To drink all day and to carouse all night are not the best means of cultivating even the physical functions, not to speak of the moral and intellectual powers. Such a career makes our young men animals, but ill-conditioned, scraggy lambkins at the best. Dissipation, of course, degrading and enfeebling everywhere, is more corrupting and destructive here than in any other country. It begins earlier and is less modified in its influence by refined tastes and habits of physical exercise. We have rakes at sixteen and worn-out debauchees at thirty. Our women are responsible to a great extent for this, in the encouragement they give to the juvenile weaklings of society, who have the time, and the means, and disposition for the dissipation of fashion, and not the heart for better things. Four-fifths of the beaux who do all the polking, waltzing, and flirtation of the gay world are boys who should be still under the ferule of the schoolmaster. The awaking of the emotions and passions, which seems the great purpose of fashionable life, is bad at any age, but infinitely worse in early youth, when to invigorate and not to excite is the only rule conformable with health.

A too early introduction to the excitements of social life is no less the ruin of the health of our young girls. To come out—which means the exposure of a youthful beauty at her earliest bloom in the public market-places of fashion—is the first thought of opening womanhood. How carefully, too, is the article manufactured and set off to suit the demand. All the education of the fashionable school is directed toward the early development of the emotions. Bodily exercise, the cultivation of the moral feelings, and the calm study of the lessons of household duty, if not utterly disregarded, are all made subordinate to the undue excitement of the intellectual faculties and senses. The excessive cultivation of music and dancing in early youth does more than any other cause toward exciting a morbid sensibility in young girls. Mothers, however, with an eye to the market, are more importunate in demanding these accomplishments than all the other elements put together of a good education. These anxious mothers will insist, with a pertinacity that no filial pouts or tears can overcome, on the hour's strumming of the piano, when they are perfectly indifferent whether their daughters spell that instrument with an -o or an -er. With such a preparation the young girl comes out all palpitating with sensibility and finds in the excitements of fashionable life those stimulants in abundance with which with an eager thirst she quickly debauches herself. Much of the ill health of our women has been attributed to early marriages, but physicians tell us that celibacy, with the emotional tendencies of our young girls, is more dangerous than matrimony. To believe that the only object in life is a husband, and to be educated in such a way as to be fit for nothing else than to catch one, may result in making useless wives, but its worse effect is in the production of a large class of unhealthy and miserable spinsters.

It is not easy to exhaust the subject of the causes of the ill health of our men, women, and children, nor to give in the compass of a single article all the reasons, some of which accordingly are held in reserve—"Why we get sick."

STEPHEN SMITH

NEW YORK THE UNCLEAN

Editor's Note

Stephen Smith the surgeon has already appeared in Section V. He was equally well known for his public health work, begun in New York in the late 1850's, when he was a member of the New York Sanitary Association. This group and the New York Academy of Medicine helped introduce health bills for the city into the state legislature in Albany (which had most of the control over city affairs). As editor of the *American Medical Times*, Smith frequently wrote about New York City's health needs.

When a group of prominent New Yorkers formed a Citizens' Association at the end of 1863, some of the leading physicians of the city were asked to form a committee on health. The doctors decided that in order to convince the public and the legislators of the need for a metropolitan health bill, a thorough sanitary survey should be carried out. Stephen Smith was the principal organizer of this survey, and when the thirty-one young physicians had finished their work, in the late fall of 1864, he and Elisha Harris put together the results in a large volume published the next year.[1] Harris wrote the long introduction for the book, but Smith went to Albany to report the findings. Armed with the extensive epidemiological data gathered in the survey, Smith appeared before the legislature on 13 February 1865. Andrew D. White, who two years later became president of Cornell University, presided over a joint committee of the Senate and Assembly that heard Smith's testimony.

It is not clear why the *New York Times* waited for more than a month to publish the testimony. When it did, however, the paper devoted the first two pages of the edition of 16 March 1865 to Smith's report. The *Times* favored a metropolitan health bill and the creation of a city health department. It seems likely that when the measure was in dire straits and the legislative session was entering its final month, the *Times* thought that all possible publicity was necessary.[2]

Smith's public health activities were by no means over when the legislature finally passed a health bill in 1866. In 1868 he became a Commissioner of Health for New York City, holding that position until 1875. Four years later

---

The City That Was (New York: Allaben, 1911), pp. 59–151. This chapter also appeared in the *New York Times*, March 16, 1865, pp. 1–2.

[1] *Report of the Council of Hygiene and Public Health of the Citizens' Association of New York, Upon the Sanitary Conditions of the City* (New York: Appleton, 1865).

[2] The version here reprinted was a slightly altered one that Smith included in his book, *The City That Was* (New York: Allaben, 1911).

President Rutherford B. Hayes appointed him to be one of seven civilian members of the newly created National Board of Health. Unfortunately, this forerunner of a cabinet department of health lasted only four years, when states' rights pressures forced its demise. Smith was also instrumental in the establishment of a state health department for New York in 1880. In 1894 he was one of the three American delegates to the International Sanitary Conference in Paris.[3]

Bibliographical Note

I have elsewhere described the fight for the Metropolitan Health Bill: "Sanitary reform in New York City: Stephen Smith and the passage of the Metropolitan Health Bill," *Bull. Hist. Med.* 40 (1966): 407–29. That paper contains numerous references to pertinent primary and secondary sources. Since its publication John Duffy has brought out his, *A History of Public Health in New York City 1625–1866*, New York: Russell Sage, 1968, tracing the history of health services in New York to the establishment of the modern department in 1866.

I have been requested to lay before you some of the results of a sanitary inspection of New York City, undertaken and prosecuted to a successful completion by a voluntary organization of citizens. There has long been a settled conviction in the minds of the medical men of New York that that city is laboring under sanitary evils of which it might be relieved. This opinion is not mere conjecture, but it is based upon the daily observations which they are accustomed to make in the pursuit of professional duties.

Familiar, by daily study, with the causes of diseases, and the laws which govern their spread, they have seen yearly accumulating about and within the homes of the laboring classes all the recognized causes of the most preventible diseases, without a solitary measure being taken by those in authority to apply an effectual remedy. They have seen the poor crowded into closer and closer quarters, until the system has actually become one of tenant house packing. They have witnessed the prevalence of terrible and fatal epidemics, having their origin in or intensified by these conditions, and many of their professional brethren have perished in the courageous performance of their duties of the poor and suffering.

Cognizant of these growing evils, and believing that they are susceptible of removal, they have repeatedly and publicly protested against the longer tolerance of such manifest causes of disease and death in our city. Large bodies of influential citizens have been equally impressed with the importance of radical

---

[3] All these activities will be described in greater detail in a biography of Smith that I am now preparing.

reform in the health organizations of New York and have strenuously labored, but in vain, to obtain proper legislative enactments.

To give practical effect to their efforts, it was determined in May last to undertake a systematic investigation of the sanitary condition of the city. For this purpose a central organization was formed, and when I mention the names of its leading members, I give you the best assurance that the work was undertaken in the interests of science and humanity. The president was Dr. Joseph M. Smith, one of the ablest writers on sanitary science in this country, and among its members were Drs. Valentine Mott, James Anderson, Willard Parker, Alonzo Clark, Gurdon Buck, James R. Wood, Charles Henschel, Alfred C. Post, Isaac E. Taylor, John W. Draper, R. Ogden Doremus, Henry Goulden, Henry D. Bulkley, and Elisha Harris.

In prosecuting this inquiry the Association was guided by the experience of similar organizations in Great Britain, where sanitary science is now cultivated with the greatest zeal and is yielding the richest fruits. As a preliminary step to the introduction of sanitary reforms, many of the populous towns of England made a more or less complete inspection of the homes of the people to determine their condition and to enable them to arrive at correct conclusions as to the required remedial measures. The English Government undertook a similar investigation through its "Commissioners for Inquiring into the State of Large Towns and Populous Districts," and the voluminous and exhaustive reports of that Commission laid the foundation of the admirable sanitary system of that country.

The first object of sanitary organization was apparently, therefore, to obtain detailed information as to the existing causes of disease and the mortality of the population, and as to the special incidence of that mortality upon each sex and each age, on separate places, on various occupations; in fact, to present a detailed account of what may be called, in commercial phrase, our transactions in human life.

Evidently the best method of arriving at such knowledge was by a systematic inspection. And that inspection must be a house-to-house visitation, in which the course of inquiry not only developed all the facts relating to the sanitary but equally to the social condition of the people. It must necessarily be required of the inspector that he visit every house, and every family in the house, and learn by personal examination, inquiry, and observation every circumstance, external and internal to the domicile, bearing upon the health of the individual.

To perform such service satisfactorily, skilled labor must be employed. No student of general science, much less a common artisan, was qualified to undertake this investigation into the causes of disease; however patent these causes might be, he had no power to appreciate their real significance. Minds trained by education, and long experience in observing and treating the diseases of the laboring classes could alone thoroughly and properly accomplish the work proposed.

Happily, experts were at hand and prepared to enter upon the task, viz.: the dispensary physicians. The daily duties of these practitioners have been for years to practice among the poor and study minutely their diseases; and thus they have gained an extensive and accurate knowledge of the sanitary and social condition of the mass of the people. Many of these practitioners have been engaged in dispensary service, and in a single district, for ten to twenty years. They have thus become so familiar with the poor of their district, though often numbering 40,000 to 50,000, that they know the peculiarities of each house, the class of disease prevalent each month of the year, and, to a large extent, the habits, character, etc., of the families which occupy them.

Everywhere the people welcomed the inspectors, invited them to examine their homes, and gave them the most ample details.

The plan of inspection adopted by the Council was as follows: The city was divided into thirty-one districts and an inspector selected for each, care being taken to assign to each inspector a district with which he was most familiar. The inspector was directed to commence his inspection by first traversing the whole district, to learn its general and topographical peculiarities. He was then to take up the squares in detail, examining them consecutively as they lie in belts.

Commencing at a given corner of his district, he was first to go around the square and note: 1. Nature of the ground. 2. Drainage and sewerage. 3. Number of houses in the square. 4. Vacant lots and their sanitary condition. 5. Courts and alleys. 6. Rear buildings. 7. Number of tenement houses. 11. Drinking shops, brothels, gambling saloons, etc. 12. Stores and markets. 13. Factories, schools, crowded buildings. 14. Slaughter houses (describe particularly). 15. Bone and offal nuisances. 16. Stables, etc. 17. Churches and school edifices.

Returning to the point of starting, he was to commence a detailed inspection of each building, noting: a. Condition and material of buildings. b. Number of stories and their height. c. Number of families intended to be accommodated, and space allotted to each. d. Water supply and house drainage. e. Location and character of water-closets. f. Disposal of garbage and house slops. g. Ventilation, external and internal. h. Cellars and basements, and their population. i. Conditions of halls and passages. j. Frontage on street, court, alley—N., E., S., or W. 18. Prevailing character of the population. 19 Prevailing sickness and mortality. 20. Sources of preventable disease and mortality. 21. Condition of streets and pavements. 22. Miscellaneous information.

He entered each room, examined its means of ventilation and its contents, noted the number of occupants by day and by night, and carefully estimated the cubical area to each person. Whenever any contagious or infectious disease was discovered, as fever, smallpox, measles, scarlatina, the inspector made a special report upon the dwelling. This report embodied specific answers to a series of questions, furnished in a blank form, requiring him: 1. To trace and record the medical history of the sick person. 2. To ascertain and record facts relating to the family and other persons exposed to the patients and to the causes of the malady. 3. To report the sanitary condition of the domicile, 4. To report the statistics and sanitary condition of the population of that domicile, 5. To report upon the sanitary condition of the locality or neighborhood and its population. 6. To preserve and make returns of these records. 7. To prepare on the spot the necessary outlines or data for the sketching of a map or descriptive chart of the domicile, block, or locality. . . .

Early in the month of May the work of thoroughly inspecting the insalubrious quarters, where fever and other pestilential diseases prevail, had been commenced, and the fact was soon ascertained that smallpox and typhus fever were existing and spreading in almost every crowded locality of the city. It was not until about the middle of July that the entire corps of inspectors was engaged. The work was then prosecuted with vigor and without interruption to the middle of November, when it was completed. The inspectors met regularly every Saturday evening to report to a committee on the part of the Council the progress of their work, and to receive advice and instruction in regard to all questions of a doubtful character.

On the completion of the inspection each inspector was required to prepare a final report embodying the general results of his labors. These reports have all been properly collated, under the direction of the Association, and are now passing through the press. They will soon appear in an octavo volume of about 400 pages, largely illustrated with maps and diagrams. It will be the first interior view of the sanitary and social condition of the population of New York and will abundantly demonstrate the fact that though a great and prosperous commercial center, she does not afford happy homes to hundreds of thousands. . . .

In reviewing the result of this inspection, I shall call your attention only to the more patent causes of disease found existing and to the preventable diseases discovered, and their relation to these causes. In this evidence you will find ample proof that radical reforms are required in the health organizations of New York.

I will first notice the causes of disease which exist external to our dwellings and which are the most readily susceptible of remedy. The first that attracts attention in New York is the condition of the streets. No one can doubt that if the streets in a thickly populated part of a town are made the common receptacle of the refuse of families, that in its rapid decomposition a vast amount of poisonous gases must escape, which will impregnate the entire district, penetrate the dwellings, and render the atmosphere in the neighborhood in a high degree injurious to the public health. In confirmation of this statement, I will quote the City Inspector, who, in a former communication to the Common Council, says:

> As an evidence of the effect of this state of things upon the health of the community, I would state that the mortality of the city, from the first of March, has been largely on the increase, until it has now reached a point of fearful magnitude. For the week ending April 27th, there were reported

to this department one hundred and forty more deaths than occurred
during the same week of the previous year. Were this increase of mortality
the result of an existing pestilence or epidemic among us, the public would
become justly alarmed as to the future; but although no actual pestilence,
as such, exists, it is by no means certain that we are not preparing the way
for some fatal scourge by the no longer to be endured filthy condition of
our city.

The universal testimony of the sanitary inspectors is that in all portions of the
city occupied by the poorer classes the streets are in the same filthy condition as
that described by the City Inspector, and that street filth is one of the most
fruitful causes of disease. . . .

The Inspector of the Eleventh Ward says:

As a rule, the streets are extremely dirty and offensive, and the gutters
obstructed with filth. The filth of the streets is composed of house-slops,
refuse vegetables, decayed fruit, store and shop sweepings, ashes, dead
animals, and even human excrements. These putrifying organic substances
are ground together by the constantly passing vehicles. When dried by the
summer's heat, they are driven by the wind in every direction in the form
of dust. When remaining moist or liquid in the form of "slush," they emit
deleterious and very offensive exhalations. The reeking stench of the
gutters, the street filth, and domestic garbage of this quarter of the city,
constantly imperil the health of its inhabitants. It is a well-recognized
cause of diarrheal diseases and fevers.

The Inspector of the Eighteenth Ward reports:

The streets in the eastern part of the district, east of First Avenue
especially, have, for the past six months, been in a most inexcusably filthy
condition. The pavement here is uneven, there are deep gutters at either
side of the streets, filled with foul slops, in which float or are sunk every
form of decaying animal and vegetable matter. Occasionally, at remote and
irregular intervals, carts come round, these stagnant pools are dredged, so
to speak, and their black and decayed solid contents raked out. If there be
anything on earth that is "rank and smells to heaven," these gutters do on
such occasions, especially in the summer months. The streets in this part
of the city are the principal depositories of garbage. In some instances
heaped up at the sides of the streets, in others thrown about promiscuously, the event in either case is the same, if it is allowed to remain day
after day, as it usually is. After having passed through every stage of decay,
after having corrupted the surrounding air with its pestilential smell, it
gradually becomes dessicated and converted into dust by the summer sun
and the constantly passing vehicles. And now every horse that passes stirs
it up, every vehicle leaves a cloud of it behind; it is lifted into the air with
every wind and carried in every direction. . . .

I will at this point simply allude to special nuisances. New York has within
the narrow limits of its present occupied area of about eight square miles, in
addition to its one million of people and all its commercial and manufacturing
establishments, a vast number of special nuisances which are, to a greater or less

degree, detrimental to its public health. There are nearly 200 slaughter houses, many of which are in the most densely populated districts. To these places droves of cattle, hogs, and sheep are constantly driven, rendering the streets filthy in the extreme, and from them flow blood and refuse of the most disgusting character.

In certain populous sections are fat-boiling, entrails-cleansing, and tripe-curing establishments which poison the air for squares around with their stifling emanations. To these must be added hundreds of uncleaned stables, immense manure heaps, etc., etc. But I shall not dwell further on these subjects and the evidence regarding them.

I pass from the consideration of the external to the internal domiciliary conditions. The poorer classes of New York are found living either in cellars or in tenement houses. It is estimated by the City Inspector that 18,000 persons live in cellars. This is also about the estimate of the police. The apartments of these people are not the light and airy basement rooms of the better class houses, but their homes are, in the worst sense, cellars. These dark, damp, and dreary abodes are seldom penetrated by a ray of sunlight or enlivened by a breath of fresh air. I will quote several descriptions from these reports. In the Fourth Ward many of these cellars are below tide water. Says the Inspector of that district:

> This submarine region is not only excessively damp, but is liable to sudden inroads from the sea. At high tide the water often wells up through the floors, submerging them to a considerable depth. In very many cases the vaults of privies are situated on the same or a higher level, and their contents frequently ooze through the walls into the occupied apartments beside them. Fully one-fourth of these subterranean domiciles are pervaded by a most offensive odor from this source, and rendered exceedingly unwholesome as human habitations. These are the places in which we most frequently meet with typhoid fever and dysentery during the summer months. I estimate the amount of sickness of all kinds affecting the residents of basements and cellars, compared with that occurring among an equal number of the inhabitants of floors above ground, as being about a ratio of 3 to 2.

The Inspector of the Fifteenth Ward reports: "In a dark and damp cellar, about 18 feet square and 7 feet high, lived a family of seven persons; within the past year two have died of typhus, two of smallpox, and one has been sent to the hospital with erysipelas. The tops of the windows of this abode are below the level of the surface, and in the court near are several privies and a rear tenant-house. Yet this occurred but a short distance from the very heart of the city."

The Inspector of the Ninth Ward writes: "At Nos. —, —, —, and — Hammond Street, and also at No. — Washington Street, are inhabited cellars, the ceilings of which are below the level of the street, inaccessible to the rays of the sun and always damp and dismal. Three of them are flooded at every heavy rain and require to be bailed out. They are let at a somewhat smaller rent than is asked for apartments on an upper floor and are rented by those to whom poverty leaves no choice. They are rarely vacant."

The Inspector of the Seventeenth Ward states that: "In 17 squares 55 houses contain 246 persons living in cellars entirely underground. As a matter of course such cellars are unhealthy dwelling apartments. Stanton Place has some of these miserable cellar-apartments, in which diseases have been generated. These cellars are entirely subterranean, dark, and damp." . . .

Such . . . is the external and internal sanitary condition of the homes of 500,000 people in the city of New York today, as revealed by this inspection. It requires no extraordinary amount of medical knowledge to determine the physical condition of this immense population, living under such circumstances. Even though no devastating epidemic is found ravaging the tenant house, yet the first sight of the wretched inmates convinces you that diseases far more destructive to health and happiness, because creating no alarm, are wasting the vital energies and slowly but surely consuming the very tissues of the body.

Here infantile life unfolds its bud, but perishes before its first anniversary. Here youth is ugly with loathsome diseases and the deformities which follow physical degeneracy. Here the decrepitude of old age is found at thirty. The poor themselves have a very expressive term for the slow process of decay which they suffer, viz.: "Tenant-house Rot." The great majority are, indeed, undergoing a slow decomposition—a true eremacausis, as the chemists term it. And with this physical degeneration we find mental and moral deterioration. The frequent expression of the poor, "We have no sickness, thank God," is uttered by those whose sunken eyes, pale cheeks, and colorless lips speak more eloquently than words, of the unseen agencies which are sapping the fountains of health. Vice, crime, drunkenness, lust, disease, and death here hold sway, in spite of the most powerful moral and religious influences.

Religious teachers and Bible readers are beginning to give this class over, as past all remedy until their physical condition is improved. Their intellects are so blunted and their perceptions so perverted by the noxious atmosphere which they breathe and the all-pervading filth in which they live, move, and have their being, that they are not susceptible to moral or religious influences. In London, some of the city missionaries have entirely abandoned the tenant-house class. There is, undoubtedly, a depraved physical condition which explains the moral deterioration of these people, and which can never be overcome until we surround them with the conditions of sound health. A child growing up in this pestilential atmosphere becomes vicious and brutal, not from any natural depravity, but because it is mentally incapable of the perceptions of truth. Most truly does the Inspector of the Fourth Ward say:

> There is a tenant-house cachexy well known to such medical men as have a practical acquaintance with these abodes; nor does it affect alone the physical condition of their inmates. It has its moral prototype in an

ochlesis of vice—a contagious depravity, to whose malign influence the youthful survivors of the terrible physical evils to which their infancy is exposed, are sure to succumb. We often find in persons of less than middle age, who have long occupied such confined and filthy premises, a morbid condition of the system unknown elsewhere. The eye becomes bleared, the senses blunted, the limbs shrunken and tremulous, the secretions exceedingly offensive. There is a state of premature decay.

In this condition of life the ties of nature seem to be unloosed. Maternal instinct and filial affection seem to participate in the general decay of soul and body. A kind Providence, whose hand is visible even here, mercifully provides that the almost inevitable decay and death which man's criminal neglect entails on the off-spring of the unfortunate who dwell in these dreary mansions, shall elicit comparatively feeble pangs of parental anguish. To the physical and moral degradation, the blight of these miserable abodes, where decay reigns supreme over habitation and inhabitant alike, may be plainly traced much of the immorality and crime which prevail among us. The established truth, that, as the corporeal frame deteriorates, man's spiritual nature is liable also to degenerate, receives its apt illustration here. . . .

Smallpox is the very type of preventable diseases. We have a safe and sure preventive in thorough vaccination. And yet this loathsome disease is at this moment an epidemic in New York. In two days' time, the inspectors found 644 cases, and in two weeks, upward of 1,200; and it was estimated that only about one-half were discovered. In many large tenant-houses, six, eight, and ten cases were found at the same time. They found it under every conceivable condition tending to promote its communicability. It was in the street cars, in the stages, in the hacks, on the ferry boats, in junk shops, in cigar stores, in candy shops, in the families of tailors and seamstresses who were making clothing for wholesale stores, in public and in private charities. I hold in my hand a list of cases of smallpox found existing under circumstances which show how widespread is this disease. Bedding of a fatal case of smallpox was sold to a rag-man; case in a room where candy and daily papers were sold; case on a ferry boat; woman was attending bar and acting as nurse to her husband who had smallpox; girl was making cigars while scabs were falling from her skin; seamstress was making shirts for a Broadway store, one of which was thrown over the cradle of a child sick of smallpox; tailors making soldiers' clothing, have their children, from whom the scabs were falling, wrapped in the garments; a woman selling vegetables had the scabs falling from her face, among the vegetables, etc., etc. Instances of this kind can be quoted at any length, but these examples are sufficient to show that smallpox spreads uncontrolled throughout our city. And they show, too, how this disease is disseminated abroad. . . .

Second only to smallpox as a preventable disease, but of a more fatal character, is typhus fever. Typhus is greatly aggravated by domestic filth and by overcrowding, with deficient ventilation. The inspectors found and located by street and number no less than 2,000 cases of this most contagious and fatal disease. Commencing in a large tenant house in Mulberry Street, it was traced from locality to locality in the poorer quarters, until it was found to have visited nearly every section of the city. It became localized in many tenant houses and streets, where it still remains, causing a large amount of sickness and mortality.

At Mulberry Street, in a notoriously filthy house, it has existed for more than four years. This house has a population of about 320, which is renewed every few months. During the period alluded to, there have been no less than 60 deaths by fever in this single house, and 240 cases. To-day this fever is raging uncontrolled in that house, creating more orphans than many well-fought battles. Every new family which enters these infected quarters is sure to fall a victim to this pestilential disease. . . .

Intestinal diseases, as cholera infantum, diarrhea, dysentery, typhoid fever, etc., which arise from, or are intensely aggravated by the emanations from putrescible material in streets, courts, and alleys, or from cess-pools, privies, drain pipes, sewers, etc., were prevalent in the tenant-house districts, creating, as usual, a vast amount of sickness, and a large infant mortality. Very generally these diseases were directly traceable to the decomposing filth, and in some instances were stopped by the removal of the nuisance.

The Inspector of the Eighth Ward reports: "Cholera infantum has probably consigned many more to the grave during the past summer than all other diseases in my inspection district. In every case examined I have found it associated with some well-marked course of insalubrity; vegetable and animal decomposition have been the most prominent causes. That fifty per cent die from preventable causes in my inspection district I do not doubt."

The Inspector of the Sixth Ward says: "The mortality among children is fearfully high, many families having lost all their children; others four out of five or six." . . .

It has been estimated by careful writers on vital statistics that 17 in 1,000 living persons annually die from inevitable causes. That is, in a community of 1,000 persons living under circumstances such that persons die only from old age, cancer, casualties, etc., 17 will die annually, and no more. And this number is the maximum that will die without the occurrence of some disease due to a removable cause. Taking this standard as the absolute necessary death rate, we can readily estimate the number of unnecessary or preventable deaths which occur in any community.

Says the Registrar-General of England (Twentieth Annual Report): "Any deaths in a people exceeding 17 in 1,000 annually are unnatural deaths. If the people were shot, drowned, burnt, poisoned by strychnine, their deaths would not be more unnatural than the deaths wrought clandestinely by diseases in excess of the quota of natural death—that is, in excess of seventeen in 1,000 living."

Taking this as the standard, let us see how the death rate of New York compares with it. It is claimed by the city officials that notwithstanding the vast accumulation of the universally recognized causes of disease, New York has a low death rate. It is not reasonable to suppose this statement true, nor is it true, as will presently appear. It is stated very truly in the City Inspector's Report for 1863, that "it is only by taking a connected view of a period of years that a correct judgment can be formed of the state of health of a city," and upon this basis let us determine what is the mortality of New York.

Take the eleven years preceding the last census, viz., 1860, excluding, however, 1854, the year of the cholera. I select this period because it includes the three last census returns, and it is only where we have the census returns with the mortality records that we have accurate data for our estimates. Now, the City Inspector's own records (reports of 1863, page 192) show that, during the period referred to, the death rate of New York City was never below 28 in the 1,000 and twice exceeded 40 in the 1,000, the average being as high as 33 in the 1,000. These deductions are made directly from the City Inspector's Reports, and, as they are claimed to be infallible, these conclusions cannot be controverted.

Now, when you remember that the highest death rate fixed by sanitary writers for inevitable deaths is 17 in 1,000, and that all deaths above that standard are considered preventable, it is apparent what a fearful sacrifice of life there is in New York. Estimated at the very minimum death rate of the last decennial period, viz.: 28 in 1,000, New York annually lost 11 from preventable deaths in 1,000 of her population, or upwards of 7,000 yearly, on an average, giving the enormous sum total for this period of 77,000 preventable deaths.

It may be urged that cities never can attain to this standard of healthfulness, but English writers maintain that the rate of 17 in the 1,000 is the true measure of the public health, and that even the most populous towns may yet be brought up to it. Nor can we doubt that there is much plausibility in the assertion, when we find the mortality in Philadelphia fall to 18 in 1,000, and that of London gradually descend from 30 in 1,000 to 22 in 1,000.

It is maintained, also, that New York has a lower death rate than London or Philadelphia. Let us see how far this assertion is sustained by the records of the health authorities of those cities. During the decennial period preceding but including 1860 and excluding 1854, as in the former comparison, the minimum mortality in London was 20 in 1,000, the maximum 24 in 1,000, the mean about 22 in 1,000. These figures are from the Registrar-General Reports.

The rate of mortality of Philadelphia for the same period was as follows: Minimum 18 in 1,000, maximum 23 in 1,000, mean about 20 in 1,000. These figures are from the report of Dr. Jewell, long the able health officer of that city. Placed in their proper relation, these mortality statistics read as follows: The number of deaths to the 1,000 living for the ten years, 1850–60 inclusive, but exclusive of 1854, is for

	Min.	Max.	Av.
London	20	24	22
Philadelphia	18	23	20
New York	28	41	33

If, then, New York had as low an average death rate as Philadelphia, she would have saved 13 in 1,000 of her population during that period, or in 1860, 10,577. These figures may seem excessive, but they are careful deductions from the annual returns of the several cities. And yet it is reiterated year after year by the City Inspector, that "New York City, at this day, can lay claim to the privilege of being numbered with the most healthy in the world."

With what consummate justice did Dr. Jewell administer this withering rebuke to our pretentious official. "It is unnecessary," he says, in his report of 1860, "to comment upon this extraordinary statement, when the above figures contradict so positively the assertion. It is to be regretted that the inspector had not availed himself of the above statistical information, which would have obliged him to have presented a widely different statement, although one indicating a more severe pressure of sanitary evils, upon the health of their population, than his report develops."

But excessive as is this death rate, it is not the full measure of the penalty which we pay to the demon of filth. A high death rate from the diseases which it engenders or intensifies, always implies a large amount of sickness. It is estimated by competent authority that there are 28 cases of sickness for every death. On this basis of estimate what an enormous amount of unnecessary sickness exists in our midst! Nor is this a mere supposition. I have an accurate census of many groups of families of that portion of our population who live immured in filth, and here we find the constant sickness rate excessive. It is no uncommon thing to find it 50, 60, and 70 per cent.

I wish now to call your attention to the fact that great as is our mortality and sickness rate, its excess is not equally distributed over the entire population, but falls exclusively upon the poor and helpless. One-half, at least, of the population of New York have a death rate no higher than the people of a healthy country town, while the death pressure upon the other half is frightfully severe. For example, the Seventeenth Ward, which is inhabited principally by the wealthy class and has but few tenant houses, has a death rate of but 17 in 1,000, or only the death rate from inevitable causes; but the Sixth and Fourth Wards, which are occupied by the laboring classes, have a death rate varying from 36 to 40 in 1,000.

Thus it appears that while the average death rate of the city is very high, it is principally sustained by those Wards where the tenant-house population is the most numerous. We find this excess of mortality just where we found the causes of diseases existing most numerously. And when we sift the matter further, we find that the excess of mortality is not even equally distributed over these populous poor Wards, but is concentrated upon individual tenant houses. For example, while the mortality of the Sixth Ward is nearly 40 in 1,000, the mortality of its large tenant houses is as high as 60 to 70 in 1,000. The following is a recent census of a large but not exceptional tenant house of that Ward: Number of families in the house, 74; persons 349; deaths, 18, or 53 in 1,000; constant sickness, 1 in 3; deaths of children, 1 in 6, or at the rate of 16 in 1,000.

The following table illustrates the distribution of the mortality of New York among the different classes of inhabitants at the last census:

Average mortality of entire city		28	in 1,000	
Mortality of better class	10	to 17	"	"
Mortality of tenant house	50	" 60	"	"

But I should not do justice to this branch of inquiry without noticing the alleged causes of the high mortality of New York. The first is the large foreign immigration. The reliance to be placed upon that scapegoat may be readily shown. Emigration occurs to this country under two conditions: 1. The emigrant is driven from home by famine, in which case the poorer class emigrate, or, 2. he is allured by advantages for labor or business, when the middle classes principally emigrate.

Now, it is under the latter circumstances that emigration generally takes place to the United States. This is seen in the vast sums of money which the emigrants now annually bring, and the amounts which they return to their friends as the result of their labor. This class is always very hardy and healthy, as is proved by the small mortality that occurs *in transitu* being but 4.31 per cent for ten years. Besides, we have the official statements of the Commissioners of Emigration that but 3 per cent remain in the city.

But the City Inspector himself shows the utter fallacy of this alleged cause of excessive mortality in his report for 1860, in which he makes the true explanation, and attributes to its proper cause whatever increased mortality arises from emigrants. He says:

> Most of the children who arrive in this city from foreign ports, although suffering from the effects of a protracted voyage, bad accommodations, and worse fare, do not bring with them any marked disease beyond those which, with proper care, nursing, and wholesome air could not be easily overcome. The causes of this excessive mortality must be searched for in this city, and are readily traceable to the wretched habitations in which parents and children are forced to take up their abode; in the contracted alleys, the tenement house with its hundreds of occupants, where each cooks, eats, and sleeps in a single room, without light or ventilation, surrounded with filth, an atmosphere foul, fetid, and deadly, with none to console with or advise them, or to apply to for relief when disease invades them.

Again, it is alleged that the floating population causes the excess of deaths. But it has been established by Dr. Playfair that the floating population is the most healthy. The same is true of wandering tribes, of a moving army, and equally of individuals. But when they fix their habitations or encamp, that moment the causes of disease begin to gather about them and, unless sanitary regulations are carefully observed, diseases, such as fever, diarrheal affections, etc., begin to prevail.

The poor population of New York is today but an immense army in camp, upon small territory, crowded into old filthy dwellings, and without the slightest police regulation for cleanliness. If this army should abandon its camp and begin a roving life in the country, all the diseases now prevalent would disappear. And, it must be added, that if these deserted and uncleaned tenements should immediately be filled by healthy people from the country, the new tenants would at once begin to suffer from all the pestilential diseases now indigenous to that part of the city.

I have now laid before you, as briefly as possible, the accumulated evidence that New York is today full to repletion with all the causes which originate and intensify the most loathsome and fatal diseases known to mankind.

This evidence proves that at least half a million of its population are literally submerged in filth and half-stifled in an atmosphere charged with all the elements of death. I have demonstrated that the legitimate fruits of her sanitary evils is an excessively high death rate and a correspondingly large sickness rate.

The all-important question which now concerns us as citizens, and you as practical legislators, is, can these evils be remedied? We answer, yes. In the first place the streets can be kept clean. Other cities accomplish this object and, therefore, New York can, and we have striking illustrative examples. In certain portions of the city the streets are as clean as this floor. They are swept daily, and scarcely a particle of dust is left in the streets or gutters the year round. But they are cleaned by private contract of the people residing upon them. What individual enterprise can do for whole squares, surely a corporation so lavish in money as New York ought to be able to do for the city at large.

The courts, alleys, cesspools, and privies can be cleansed and kept in good condition. There are tenant houses which are as clean in all their alleys, courts, and cellars as the best-kept private houses. These are dwellings for the poor in which the landlord takes especial interest. What is done for the surroundings of one of these houses, may be done for all. But the tenant houses of the worst class may be quickly placed in a good sanitary condition. . . .

Let the landlord be compelled to keep his house in good repair, supply it with an abundance of pure water, connect the privy with the sewer, open free ventilation, afford means for removal of garbage, and then keep a careful oversight of his tenants, enforcing cleanliness. If this were done, the tenant-house people would immediately improve, and the death rate, if we may judge from other cities, would fall one-fourth.

Again, the cellar population can be removed from their subterranean abodes and placed in better homes. Liverpool has solved this problem for us.

In 1847 that city had a cellar population of 20,000; an ordinance was passed forbidding the occupation of underground rooms as residences, with certain restrictions, and within three years the great mass of people in these subterranean haunts were removed to better tenements with a great reduction of the mortality of the city.

That city, formerly the most unhealthy in England, has continued the reforms thus inaugurated by compelling landlords to improve their tenant houses, and the result is that it has become one of the healthiest towns of Europe. London has recently taken similar action in regard to cellar tenements. What these cities have done, New York can and ought to do for her public health. . . .

The remedy for our evils must be apparent; and this remedy is suggested in such terse unqualified language by the City Inspector above quoted, that I call the attention of the committee especially to this remark, as a proper guide in your deliberations. In the City Inspector's report for 1861 we find the following:

> The stay of pestilence, to be effectual, must be prompt, and equally prompt must be the interposition of barriers against the introduction of disease, which may be kept back, but, once introduced, can with difficulty be checked or extirpated. For these reasons, there should be a power existing in other hands that may be ready to be used at the moment the exigency may arise. . . . The remedy, apparent to every one, must consist in the adoption of laws transferring the power of sanitary regulations to some other authority of a different order of instruction in sanitary science. . . . The first groundwork of reform, in the opinion of the undersigned, is to bestow upon some other body, differently constituted, all power over the sanitary affairs of the city; and, until this is done, all other proposals of reform will be deprived of their essentially beneficial features. To escape present complications is the first great point to be gained; and this point secured, simplicity, promptness, and efficiency may be substituted for inefficiency, complication, and delay.

Accepting this as the first step in reform, the practical question arises: How shall that body be constituted to which is to be confided the sanitary interests of New York?

If the experience of other large cities is of any value, or, indeed, if we rely simply on common sense, the following are indispensable prerogatives in any well-organized health board:

1. It should be independent of all political influence and above all partisan control.

2. It should combine executive ability with a profound knowledge of disease and the proper measures of prevention. To this end the board should be composed in part of men especially accustomed to the dispatch of business, and in part of medical men of great skill and experience.

3. It should have a corps of skilled medical officers as inspectors, which should be the eyes, the ears, in a word, the senses of the board, in every part of the city, searching out disease, investigating the causes which give rise to it, the conditions under which it exists, the means of its propagation, and the most effectual mode of its suppression.

4. It should have a close alliance with the police, which must be its arm of power in the prompt and efficient execution of its orders.

FREDERICK A. P. BARNARD

THE GERM THEORY OF DISEASE AND ITS RELATIONS TO HYGIENE

Editor's Note

It is perhaps unusual that a book of papers describing the development of medicine in America should include an essay by a layman on the germ theory, a scientific subject. Suffice it to say its author was an unusual man. Frederick Augustus Porter Barnard was born in Massachusetts in 1809, graduated from Yale in 1828, and then taught mathematics, natural history, and chemistry. In 1856 he became president of the University of Mississippi and eight years later was elected to the same office at Columbia University. He was a mathematician and an educator who possessed a good general scientific knowledge. These qualifications were ample preparation, then, for the President of Columbia University to lecture to the members of the American Public Health Association on the hottest scientific issue of the day. Perhaps it was even better that these words were spoken by one who had no vested interest in the theory's acceptance.

The sanitarians, along with the surgeons, had a very direct interest in the etiology of epidemic diseases and fevers of all sorts. For decades some hygienists had preached cleanups of cities, of dwellings, and of hospitals. They had done the right thing, but for the wrong reasons. Not until the advent of the germ theory and the discovery of numerous specific bacteria in the last two decades of the century did the filth theory of disease receive its proper rationale.

The arguments between contagionists and noncontagionists raged long and fierce. A substantial part of the 1859 National Sanitary and Quarantine Conference in New York was taken up by a discussion of the contagiousness of yellow fever; the noncontagionists prevailed on that occasion. At stake was much of public health practice. If a disease was contagious, then strict quarantine should be imposed. If, on the other hand, miasmatic or chemical influences in the environment were to blame, then proper cleanups were to be introduced. It is well known that many of the leading British sanitarians of the time were anti-contagionists. This group did not always accept cheerfully practices or theories that ran counter to their own.[1]

In his paper, Barnard touched on the scientific, the religious, and the philosophical implications of the germ theory, as well as its practical ones. One must remember that he was writing in the same year in which O. H. F. Obermeier of

---

Reports and Papers, A.P.H.A. 1 (1873): 70-87.

[1] See especially Lloyd G. Stevenson, "Science down the drain," *Bull. Hist. Med.* 29 (1955): 1-26, which is subtitled "On the hostility of certain sanitarians to animal experimentation, bacteriology, and immunology." Even at the end of the century George Bernard Shaw was still ridiculing the germ theory and vaccination.

Berlin discovered the spirillium of relapsing fever. Robert Koch's demonstration of the growth stages of anthrax was still three years in the future, and the so-called "golden age of bacteriology" was only a gleam in the eye of a few. Read in this context, Barnard's words are those of a perceptive and thoughtful man.

Bibliographical Note

William Bulloch, *The History of Bacteriology*, London: Oxford University Press, 1938; reprinted 1960.
John Simon, *Filth Diseases, and their Prevention*, 1st American ed., Boston: Campbell, 1876.
Phyllis Allen Richmond, "American attitudes toward the germ theory of disease (1860–1880)," *J. Hist. Med.* 9 (1954): 428–54.
Erwin Ackerknecht, "Anticontagionism between 1821 and 1867," *Bull. Hist. Med.* 22 (1948): 562–93.
Howard D. Kramer, "The germ theory and the early public health program in the United States," *Bull. Hist. Med.* 22 (1948): 233–47.

No more striking evidence can be adduced of the intellectual advancement characteristic of modern times, than the general recognition among men of the universal reign of law. It is true that this general recognition has not yet become quite universal. There are not wanting many, even in our enlightened age, to whom the advent of a comet still brings feelings of dismay and in whose belief the wind literally bloweth where it listeth every day. The belief in lucky and unlucky days has by no means disappeared, and among even the well educated there are yet some who would not willingly put to sea on the brightest Friday morning that ever shone. It is difficult to disabuse the mind of impressions which almost inevitably find a place there in the infancy of individuals and of peoples. Every event of which the causes are obscure is naturally attributed, by the ignorant or inexperienced, either to blind chance or to the purposed interference of some supernatural power; and such is the strength of the imagination that the feeling often survives long after reason has exploded the error.

There is no class of natural phenomena which the men of all times have been disposed to look upon as being more completely exempt from the dominion of law than those which concern sickness and health. The illness of an individual appears always to have been esteemed an event entirely fortuitous, which no human prescience could anticipate and no human precaution could avert; and the simultaneous sickening and death of multitudes has more frequently been regarded as an evidence of Divine displeasure, directly interfering with the usual order of nature, than as a grave and interesting phenomenon to be patiently investigated and rationally explained. The truth is, nevertheless, that the laws of health and of disease in living organisms are as fixed and invariable as, in abstract science, are those of mathematics. The difference lies in the greater difficulty of their discovery. This is well illustrated in the history of the subject which I have ventured, with a presumption which in this presence may seem like temerity, to select as the theme of my remarks this evening.

The germ theory of disease is not, as is commonly supposed, a theory which has originated in very recent years. More than two hundred years ago it was brought forward, at least as an hypothesis, by the celebrated Father Kircher, in his "Scrutinium Physico-Medicum contagiosae luis quae pestis dicitur," to account for the infectious propagation of the plague. However plausible this theory might at that time have seemed, it could then, nevertheless, claim no higher rank than that of a bare hypothesis; and it has only been in times comparatively recent that observation has brought to light a sufficient number of facts, apparently favoring it, to justify our advancing it in the arena of scientific discussion to the higher dignity of a theory.

GENERAL PRINCIPLES BEARING ON THE SUBJECT

Before proceeding to consider the evidences bearing on the truth of this theory, for or against, a few observations of a general nature may properly here find place. No living organism enjoys an existence of unlimited duration. Every such organism, under favorable circumstances, passes through three distinct stages, which are those of growth, vigorous maturity, and decline. The organism commences as a germ, and ends in dissolution and disintegration. Since the laws of life, as well as those of physics, are fixed and definite, there is reason to believe that all organisms of the same species, if placed in conditions equally favorable to their development, would be equally long-lived; yet, in point of fact, those which pass through the regular stages constituting their normal life are comparatively few. In the large majority, the vital functions are, earlier or later, more or less disturbed, if not arrested, by an endless variety of causes tending to produce disease and premature death. In the human race, life is often shortened by ignorant or willful disregard of the conditions necessary to the preservation of health. Accident, also, often exposes individuals to deleterious influences. Thus, in many cases, diseases arise from exposure to extremes of temperature, or from excesses in eating and drinking, persisted in until the organs of digestion become debilitated and fail to fulfill their proper functions. But besides these causes of disease, which may be classed under the head of "injurious conditions," there are other influences directly morbific, which, whenever they come into play, cut short the duration of life. Poisons belong to this class, but the effects of these are felt only in occasional and accidental instances. Other noxious influences, of which the pernicious consequences are more widely spread, are those which produce the diseases called zymotic. Such are malaria, contagion, and infection, instrumentalities to which are owing the wide-spread ravages of epidemics.

It may be remarked that there are many cases of disease in which the cause is not traceable directly to any of the sources above mentioned, but in which the disease has been transmitted by inheritance from a parent similarly affected. In such cases there is nevertheless every reason to believe that the disease in its first appearance was produced in a healthy organism by causes belonging to one or the other of the classes above named.

The diseases which it is the object of the present paper to consider, are only those which belong to the epidemic or contagious class.

THEORIES OF CONTAGION

No subject has occupied more the careful attention of physicians, or has been a subject of more elaborate observation and experiment, or has led to more marked differences of opinion or more animated controversy, than that of the nature of the influences by which these diseases are transmitted from individual to individual. That many epidemics arise from peculiar conditions of the atmosphere, not in the least as yet understood, can hardly be doubted; and in this case the influence which excites disease simultaneously in many is not dissimilar to that by which contagious diseases are transmitted from individual to individual. Confining ourselves, however, for the moment to this latter mode of transmission, it may be observed that two theories distinctly opposed to each other have long been held on the subject, each of them counting in its advocacy authorities of the very highest character. These may be distinguished as the chemical theory of infection and the germ theory. The chemical theory is founded on a presumed analogy between the propagation of disease in living organisms, and the process of fermentation in certain forms of organic matter without life. This theory assumes a ferment to be an organized substance in a certain state of decay, which possesses the property of exciting the same decay in other organic substances with which it is in contact. Applying this theory to disease, it supposes that infection is communicated by the instrumentality of particles thrown from the person, or from substances proceeding from the person, diseased and borne by the air to other persons in full health, in whom they excite, probably by contact with the membranous linings of the lungs, the same diseased condition which exists in the patient. The opposing theory presumes that the diseased person is suffering from an invasion of his system by microscopic algoid or fungoid vegetative forms having the property of rapid self-multiplication, and that the spores which proceed from these fungi or the cells of the algae are wafted in like manner by the air from person to person, penetrating the systems of the healthy, and establishing new colonies to generate disease in them.[1] . . .

---

[1] The germ theory, as it is here stated and as it is commonly understood, presumes that the minute organisms which cause disease are parasites. Dr. Lionel S. Beale, of London, has put forth a germ theory materially different from this. Holding first that the life of all organisms resides only in that semifluid matter which occupies the interior of living cells, or

THEORIES OF THE ORIGIN OF LIFE

No question at the present day is more sharply debated than that which relates to the origin of life. There is no subject which has been pursued experimentally with more zeal, more earnest solicitude to reach the truth, or more singularly discordant results than this. The notion of spontaneous generation is not, by any means, of modern origin. It has been entertained by naturalists in every age since the dawn of scientific history. But the earlier naturalists, Aristotle and Lucretius, for instance, conceived that organisms of a high order of complexity, such as insects, or fishes, or reptiles might be directly produced out of the moist earth softened by showers, or out of the slime and mud of rivers; whereas those of our time have long since abandoned any such extravagant notions and confine themselves to the assertion that life in its spontaneous origin is manifested only under the simplest forms.

The latest example of an hypothesis resembling the ancient is found in the argument presented in a work entitled "Vestiges of Creation," which appeared about thirty years ago, in which the experiments of Mr. Andrew Crosse upon electric currents of low intensity directed for a long time through a solution of inorganic salt, were supposed to have produced an insect of the Acarus family; such an insect having actually made its appearance during the course of the experiment. But this result has long since been recognized to have been merely accidental, and probably owing to the presence of ova of the insect introduced in some unexplained way into the apparatus. The modern advocates of the theory of spontaneous generation hold, however, or at least most of them hold, only to the certainty of the spontaneous appearance of organisms of a very low type, called bacteria, vibriones, and monads, organisms familiar to the microscopist, and which are sure to make their appearance in every putrefying organic infusion.

---

is seen without an integument in the white globules of the blood, while the cell walls and the structures built up of them are "formed matter" without life; and giving the name *bioplast* to each minute separate mass of this living matter, he shows by the evidence of the microscope, that the bioplasts of the blood multiply by a kind of gemmation, of which the result is to produce other bioplasts resembling the first. In a morbid condition of the blood, however, the process of gemmation is accelerated, and the resulting bioplasts of each generation are more and more minute in size, their numbers becoming incalculably great. These minute bioplasts, escaping from the diseased organism and becoming invested with a protecting coat of "formed matter," may be wafted to great distances and may preserve their vitality for long periods; so that when, by any chance, they are introduced into the circulation of other organisms, where they find material to be assimilated, they multiply once more in this new habitat with the same abnormal rapidity as before; and thus engender disease similar to that in which they originated. This theory is developed by Dr. Beale with great ability in his work entitled, *Disease Germs, their Nature and Origin*, published in 1872. According to this theory, disease germs are not parasitical, but "originate in man's organism, and have descended from the normal bioplasm of his body." The theory avoids many of the difficulties which attend the chemical theory on the one hand, and the theory according to which disease is the effect of a parasitic invasion on the other; but as yet the evidence in its favor cannot be regarded as conclusive.

Less than three centuries ago the belief here spoken of, that living things may originate without eggs, or germs or living parents from which to proceed, may be said to have been universal in Europe. Of the truth of this belief there was supposed to be visible evidence in the invariable occurrence of maggots in putrefying flesh. Curiously enough, scriptural authority was cited in proof of this view, and the Old Testament story of the bees found by Samson in the carcass of the dead lion was presumed to confirm it. The doctrine was therefore held as a matter of faith, and those who first assailed it were naturally accused of impiety and irreverence. Prominent, and perhaps first among these was Francis Redi, an Italian philosopher, scholar, and poet born in 1626. He presented a conclusive disproof of the spontaneous generation of maggots in putrefying flesh, by simply inclosing, in open-mouthed jars covered with gauze, pieces of flesh still sound and leaving them in the sun to putrefy. Putrefaction occurred as before, but no maggots made their appearance. The maggots, nevertheless, did appear on the gauze, and a little observation made their origin manifest. The flies, of which they are the progeny in the larvae state, being attracted by the odor of the flesh, but unable to reach it, laid their eggs upon the covering of the jar, and out of these the larvae were presently developed. Having demonstrated the falsity of the popular belief on this subject in a case so conspicuous, Redi naturally generalized his conclusion and took the ground that no living thing comes into existence without deriving its life from something previously living. He did not say, as it has been said later, "*Omne vivum ex ovo*," but "*Omne vivum ex vivo*." He still believed that out of a living plant may arise a living animal, as the insect within the gall of the oak, or the worm within the fruit which presents no external puncture. His doctrine was, therefore, that which Huxley has named *biogenesis*, in contradistinction to spontaneous generation, called by him *abiogenesis*, and by Bastian *archegenesis*. But archegenesis had been put aside only to return again under a new form. Among the earliest revelations of the microscope was the remarkable fact that whenever a dead organic substance is infused in water, myriads of minute creatures presently make their appearance in the infusion, all possessing most extraordinary, and many of them very varied, powers of reproduction. They multiply by means of *ova*, by means of buds or gemmation, and by means of self-division or fissuration. All this was strongly favorable to the doctrine of biogenesis. Where so many means of reproduction existed, every one of them so effectual and sufficient, to provide that the same forms of life should be produced without any organic antecedents seemed "wasteful and ridiculous excess." This view, however, met here and there with a dissentient. About a century and a quarter ago, John Turberville Needham, an English naturalist, resorted to an experiment which, with various modifications, has been since, many hundreds and possibly many thousands of times, repeated, with the view thoroughly to test the question whether, in its application to infusorial life, the doctrine of biogenesis is universally true. He prepared an infusion, thoroughly boiled it in a flask, corked it tight, sealed the cork with mastic, and covered the whole with hot ashes, designing to destroy by heat any germs which might be in the infusion, as the substance infused, or in the air above the liquid in the flask. After some days or weeks, he found that notwithstanding all these precautions living organisms did make their appearance in the flask, precisely such as in freely exposed infusions habitually appeared earlier. This experiment was immediately repeated by Spallanzani, an Italian eccelsiastic and naturalist; but Spallanzani, instead of corking his flask and cementing his corks, sealed the vessels by fusing the glass, and having thus completely cut off communication with the outward air, kept them at the boiling temperature for three-quarters of an hour. No life appeared in the infusions of Spallanzani, and the doctrine of biogenesis was again apparently triumphant.

The question was, however, not yet universally admitted to be settled. Dissentients made themselves heard from time to time, among them Gleichen, Otho Müller, and Treviranus; the latter of whom pointed out the significant fact, that while the species of infusorial animals found in infusions of the same kind were constantly the same, those which appeared in different infusions were not so. Early in the present century the celebrated naturalist, Lamarck, ranged himself on the side of spontaneous generation. Oken took the same view and, subsequently, Bory St. Vincent, J. Müller, Dujardin, Burdach, and Pineau; while on the opposite side appeared, among others, Schwann, Schultze, and Ehrenberg. The experiments of Schultze and Schwann, undertaken for the purpose of testing the accuracy of those of Spallanzani, were remarkable. Subsequently to the date of Spallanzani's experiments, the importance of air or of oxygen, one of its constituents, to the maintenance of animal life had been discovered, and doubts had arisen whether, in those experiments, the air had not been rendered unfit for the support of life by the operations to which it had been subject. In repeating the experiments, Schultze admitted to the flasks, after boiling the infusions, only such air as had been passed through concentrated sulphuric acid; and Schwann only such as had been conducted through red-hot tubes. No animalcules made their appearance; and these results, reached as long ago as 1836 and 1837, were regarded by the great body of naturalists as finally settling the question.

RENEWAL OF THE CONTROVERSY

The controversy, however, after resting for twenty years, was revived and prosecuted with even more animation than before, by Mr. Pouchet, in the first instance, on the side of spontaneous generation, and Mr. Pasteur, on that of biogenesis; but more recently by many naturalists of distinction, among whom may be named Dr. Jeffries Wyman, of our own country, whose experimental researches tend rather to the support of the archegenetic theory, and Professor Huxley, of London, whose opinion, given on a survey of the whole history of the controversy and expressed before the British Association in 1870, is very decidedly the other way. While the controversy was between Mr. Pasteur and Mr. Pouchet, there can be no doubt that, in the judgment of the world, the former had by far the best of the argument. His experiments, which were substantially repetitions of those of Needham and Spallanzani, but which were variously modified, so as to render his demonstrations, in every possible way, cumulative, seemed to have disposed of the doctrine of spontaneous generation, effectually and forever. In multitudes of instances, infusions hermetically sealed while boiling, remained for indefinite periods of time free from all traces of organic life, while portions of the same infusions exposed side by side with these, but open to the air, were speedily swarming with animalcules. He found that even an unsealed flask, of which the neck had been stopped during the boiling only with a plug of cotton closely pressed together, continued to be equally free from these organisms so long as the stopper remained in its place. This last experiment presented a rather curious resemblance to that of Redi, with his gauze-covered jar; for the cotton forming the plug was found, on a microscopic examination, to contain the germs which its presence had prevented from entering the flask. Mr. Pasteur finally discovered—and this result was long supposed to have furnished an unanswerable reply to all the arguments of the advocates of archegenesis— that flasks containing infusions treated by boiling as before, required neither sealing nor stopping with cotton to prevent invasion of the contained liquids by these low forms of life; provided that only the necks of such flasks had been originally bent over, so as to direct their mouths downward. This result he had predicted as probable, holding, as he did, that the germs by which such infusions are repeopled when the living embryos they may contain have been destroyed by heat, must necessarily subside into them from the air above.

The experiments of Wyman, Bastian, Cantoni, and others, most recent than those of Pasteur, have led to results singularly, and at present, we must say, unaccountably at variance with his. Professor Wyman found that *bacteria* will make their appearance in infusions which have not only been boiled before being sealed up, but which, after being sealed, have been kept at a boiling heat for many hours. He found, moreover, that these same organisms, after their appearance, perish when exposed to a heat not over 134° Fahrenheit. Bastian, in a very extended series of experiments, has pushed the heat in the tubes containing his infusions as high as 300° Fahrenheit, maintaining this high temperature, in some instances, not less than four hours; and has yet found that living forms do not fail subsequently to appear in them. Such forms appear, also, according to him, in solutions containing nothing of organic origin, whatever, but composed entirely of certain salts of soda and ammonia; and he even affirms that in such solutions he has occasionally seen very remarkable fungi to present themselves with their full fructification, drawings of which he has given in his work, recently published, entitled *The Beginnings of Life*.

It seems to me that no one can rise from the perusal of the extraordinary book just mentioned without feeling that, if it does not embrace and contain the conclusion of the whole matter, it is, at least for the present, unanswerable. It leaves us, nevertheless, still perplexed, perhaps more deeply perplexed than before; for it is impossible to understand how the results reached by so many naturalists, all in the first rank of scientific investigators, all conscientiously laboring to elicit the truth of this great question should be, after all, so singularly discordant. And another weighty consideration adds to this perplexity. It is the existence of a practical refutation of the conclusions of the class of experimenters to which Dr. Bastian belongs, which is presented under our eyes every day on the grandest scale, in the operations of one of the most important departments of modern industry. I cannot state this consideration better than in the words of Huxley: "There must," remarks this distinguished physiologist, "be some error about these experiments, because they are performed on an enormous scale every day with quite contrary results. Meats, fruits, vegetables, the very materials of the most fermentable and putrescible infusions are preserved, to the extent I suppose I may say, of thousands of tons every year, by a method which is a mere application of Spallanzani's experiment. The matters to be preserved are well boiled in a tin case provided with a small hole, and this hole is soldered up when all the air in the case has been replaced by steam. By this method they may be kept for years without putrefying, fermenting, or getting mouldy." He argues—and the argument has a weight that must be felt—that there is no mode of explaining this universal and invariable result but the exclusion of germs from these cans. And, in view of the marvelous discrepancy between the results on the small and the grand scale placed side by side, one can hardly repress the suspicion that if there be any such thing as spontaneous generation, it is a thing which occurs only under rare and extraordinary conditions, which conditions Dr. Bastian has unintentionally succeeded in establishing, while as a matter of practical importance or daily interest it is as if it were not. . . .

In order that we may be able to judge of the probability that an infectious disease of which the cause is unknown is a result of the invasion of the blood or the viscera of the patient by a parasitic vegetation, it is important to consider first what has been already ascertained of the effects of such parasitic growths infesting the animal organism. A simple form of fungus, called the *Sarcina ventriculi*, is often found in matters thrown up by persons laboring under disorder of the stomach. It has also been met with in other parts of the body when diseased. But it is likewise found, and not unfrequently, in the stomachs of persons in perfect health; and, as Dr. Carpenter says, it may accumulate there in considerable quantities without causing inconvenience. This parasite, therefore, cannot be regarded as an inciting cause of disease.

The stomachs of many worms and insects are found, moreover, to be frequently infested with fungi, which grow there in great luxuriance. Many of these have been examined and described by Dr. Leidy, of Philadelphia. It does not appear that they occasion inconvenience to the animals within whose bodies they thus establish themselves. On the other hand, some of the dipterous and hymenopterous insects, and some caterpillars, are liable to invasion by fungoid growths which speedily spread through their entire bodies and destroy their lives. In the West Indies, according to Dr. Carpenter, it is not at all uncommon to see individuals of a species of *Polistes* (corresponding to our wasp) flying about with plants of their own length projecting from some part of their surface, the germs of which have been introduced through the breathing-pores at their sides. This fungus growth, however, soon kills the insect, and a similar effect follows a similar cause in the case of certain caterpillars in New Zealand, Australia, and China, of which the bodies become so thoroughly interpenetrated and, as it may be said, replaced by the fungoid vegetation, that when dried they have almost the density of wood, so that, in the language of Dr. Carpenter, "these caterpillars come to present the appearance of twigs, with long slender stalks formed by the projections of the fungus itself." Our common house-fly is a not unfrequent victim of a similar parasitic visitation. A fungus called the *Empusa muscae*, originating from the germination of a single spore brought in contact almost anywhere with the body of the insect, pervades after a time its whole interior, and, while leaving the surface uninjured, emphatically eats out its substance. When the animal's life is nearly exhausted he comes to rest, and fungoid shoots put forth from his body on all sides, clothing him apparently with a kind of fur, consisting of filaments each bearing a fructification of innumerable spores. The harvest of spores becomes very conspicuous when the unfortunate animal makes his last stand upon the window pane, forming a thin film over the glass to a considerable distance around him; and if by any chance a healthy individual of the same species comes within the limit of this infected area, the disease which has destroyed his fellow will be sure to attack him also. There are some forms of parasitic disease affecting insects which have had consequences of serious importance to certain great industrial interests to which these humble forms of animal life are tributary. A fungus called the *Botrytis bassiana* is the occasion of the disease in silk-worms known by the name of *Muscardine*. The spores of this fungus, entering the breathing pores of the worms, soon germinate, and death is the invariable consequence. It is only, or at least rarely however, the case that the cause of the fatality is manifest until after death has occurred; but then the fungus shoots forth luxuriantly, especially at the junction of the rings of the body. A still more destructive epidemic among silk-worms is that which has received the name of *Pébrine*, which is caused by the multiplication of a parasitical organism called *Panhistophyton*, fungoid in its nature. This disease is the more difficult to deal with, in that it is transmissible by inheritance, the *Psorospermiae* entering into the eggs of the diseased worm. It was thoroughly investigated by Mr. Pasteur, who pointed out the means by which it might be extirpated; means which have since been successfully applied. But there are diseases produced by invasions of parasitic fungi in animals of much higher grade than worms or insects. The epidemic among cattle, called in England "the blood," is shown by the researches of Davaine to be occasioned by the presence in the blood of the diseased animals of innumerable living organisms resembling *vibrios*. This disease is communicable to man, producing what is called "malignant pustule," and this is attended with the development of the same organisms in the pustules thus produced. Professor Lister, an eminent surgeon of Edinburgh, long ago observed that when a chronic abscess is discharged by means of a *canula* and *trochar*, the subsequent accumulations of fluid are frequently attended with putrefaction, though none had existed before. The putrid mass is also found to be swarming with *vibrios*, though none had been present in the first discharges. No explanation of this singular phenomenon, according to him, can be given, except that the germs of these organisms were introduced in the original operation with the *canula* and *trochar*. Another remarkable fact noticed by Professor Lister seems strongly to corroborate the theory of inflammation and putrefaction above given. A wound in the chest, producing effusion of blood in the pleural cavity, is attended with great danger, in consequence of the liability of the extravasated blood to putrefy. Yet when the lung is wounded by a broken rib, without any external opening, the blood, though escaping into the cavity in quantity, undergoes no decomposition and excites in the surgeon no concern, even though air at the same time enters in such volume as to inflate the cellular tissue of the entire body. "These facts," says Professor Lister, "involved to me a complete mystery until I heard of the germ theory of putrefaction, when it at once occurred to me that it was only natural that the air should be filtered of germs by the air passages" of the lungs. Now, what Professor Lister conjectured *a priori*, Professor Tyndall, interested by this remark, subsequently proved experimentally. Through the path of the beam of light made visible by his lantern in the dark room described above, he caused the air from his own lungs to pass, by breathing through a tube. The current at first but slightly affected the brightness of the beam; but as the air from the larger passages passed away and that from the deeper network of the lungs succeeded, the light progressively faded, and at length gave place to absolute blackness. The experiment fully confirmed the anticipation of Professor Lister, that the air which passed through the lungs would no longer contain the germs of living things, or any other suspended foreign matter. But what an idea does this give us of our liability, through our lungs, to absorb into our systems anything noxious which the air may contain, no matter how minute in quantity, or how finely divided? If the quantity in given volume is minute, it is to be remembered that the volume we inhale in a limited time is enormous, amounting to two or three thousand cubic feet a day; and the accumulation which must result, from even the partial exhaustion of this great mass of its impurities, must become very considerable.

Having spoken now of the cases in which disease, local or general, in animals, is manifestly occasioned by the presence of parasitic vegetation, it is proper to mention, briefly, similar examples in plants. The smut in wheat, the rust in cotton, the *Oidium* in grapes, and the *Botrytis* in potatoes, are examples of fungi, constantly concomitant with disease, and presumably, almost certainly in the last two instances, its cause. Neither in plants nor animals, however, is it to be supposed that the noxious effects observed are occasioned merely by the presence of these parasites mechanically interfering with and obstructing the vital functions, or by acting directly as poisons in the ordinary sense: but rather by their own vital activity decomposing the substance of the organisms they infest and making them their food. The consequences of their extensive prevalence to the material interests of communities and peoples, and to their means of subsistence, have been occasionally of the gravest character. The *Oidium* may be said to have exterminated the vine from the Island of Madeira; the *Panhistophyton* cut down the product of silk in France from 130,000,000 of francs per annum, to 30,000,000; and the *Botrytis* threatened to depopulate Ireland, by destroying the vegetable which constituted, for the common people, the staple article of their food.

THE GERM THEORY AT LEAST PARTIALLY TRUE

Putting together these, the known, facts regarding this subject, before proceeding to more doubtful cases, we may say that the germ theory has an amount of *prima facie* evidence in its favor which entitles it to careful consideration. In certain instances, and in a certain sense, the evidence is complete that the germ theory is true. But when we come to apply it to infectious diseases in general, we find the analogies which they present with the limited class of examples above enumerated, to be unexpectedly feeble, while the points of dissimilarity are numerous and marked. It is not even enough to discover that in such diseases there are actually present in the blood, or in the tissues, or in the secretions, or in the dejections, of the suffering individuals, living forms of microscopic cryptogams, since the evidence is rarely conclusive either that these minute bodies are injurious to the patient, or that they were present antecedently to the attack. And if, as to the first of these points, the evidence in some cases *is* satisfactory, as to the second it can hardly be pronounced to be so in any.

As to the frequent presence of vegetable organisms in the blood of men or animals suffering under infectious diseases, it is impossible to entertain a doubt. The testimony of all the observers who have occupied themselves with this subject is concurrent to this effect. Coze and Feltz, Klebs, Burdon-Sanderson, Klein, and many others, have found bacteria invariably in the blood of patients suffering under typhoid fever, smallpox, scarlet fever, puerperal fever, pyemia, and septicemia. Dr. J. H. Salisbury, of Cleveland, Ohio, affirms, as the result of his own observations, that in healthy as well as in diseased blood there are always present two species of cryptogams, the one algoid and the other fungoid. In the pustules of smallpox Dr. Salisbury has observed a cryptogam described by him as having both a fungoid and an algoid development, and the spores of this he has also found in the blood. In cowpox, or in the disease produced in the cow by inoculation from a smallpox subject, only the algoid form appears. This the discoverer has named *Ios vacciola*, while the entire plant in its double form he calls *Ios variolosa vacciola*. In typhoid fever the same writer has detected a peculiar algoid vegetation developing itself upon the external surface of the entire body, and upon the mucous membrane of the interior cavities. This he regards as the efficient cause of the disease and the means by which it is propagated. Dr. Ernst Hallier, of Jena, who has published largely on this subject and has made himself prominent as an advocate of the germ theory, has described a large variety of vegetable forms found by him in diseased men and animals, many of which he has subjected to systematic cultivation, in order to study their modes of development. A new and peculiar fungus, found in the rice-water discharges of cholera patients and within the intestinal canal of such persons, has been cultivated by him with special attention. This plant is described as being as marvelous for the rapidity of its development as for its strange forms of growth, and its terribly fatal destruction of the epithelial tissue of the intestine. It is called by Professors Thomé and Klobe the *cylindrotaenium*, but is regarded by Dr. Simon and Dr. Harris as being an exotic member of the family to which belong the *urocystic* and *oidium* blights of cereals and fruits. Among the interesting facts observed in the cultivation, it may be mentioned that the presence of an abundance of nitrogenous matter and the absence of acids in the fluid or substance employed were proved to be essential conditions of the propagation and growth. Also, that when the fungus cells, in the course of their development upon a piece of intestinal membrane, reached a certain stage they rapidly increased, and the epithelium as rapidly wasted away. After reading this, it is rather disappointing to find in the last and recently published edition of Dr. Parkes' *Manual of Practical Hygiene*, the following succinct statement: "As regards cholera, the careful observations of Drs. Lewis and Cunningham, in Calcutta, seem to have disproved the possibility of either fungi or bacteria being the *cause* of cholera."

The disease which appeared in 1868 among the beef cattle brought to this city from the West, and which is known as the Texas cattle disease was investigated at the time by Drs. Harris and Stiles, of the New York Health Department, who found the spores of a peculiar species of fungus both in the blood and in the bile of the diseased animals. Specimens of these cryptogams were sent by these gentlemen to Professor Hallier, by whom they were successfully cultivated, and who succeeded in deriving from them three distinct forms of the fungus. The epizootic, which attacked all the horses of the country twelve months ago, was also marked by the presence of fungi in the blood and the urine of the animals affected, which were described by Dr. Endemann and by Dr. Charles Amende, of Hoboken.

These examples will probably be thought sufficiently numerous to justify the generalization that in infectious diseases the presence of microscopic algoid or fungoid cryptogams is a fact of invariable occurrence. What is the significance of this fact? In all these cases, we find that the fluid in which the cryptogams occur is itself diseased. Is not the disease of the blood the very condition that is necessary to the development of the plant? When mould makes its appearance on the surface of paste, is it the presence of the mould which causes the paste to putrefy, or is it the putrefaction of the paste which provides a congenial nidus for the mould?

About forty years ago, the yeast plant was discovered by Cagniard de la Tour, and almost simultaneously by Schwann. Till that discovery, the chemical theory of disease had a strong support in the imagined analogy of fermentation. To the suggestion, after the discovery, that fermentation is probably a consequence of the rapid growth of the plant, there was at first a very general and natural dissent; but when, in 1843, Helmholtz made a direct experimental test of the question by placing a fermenting liquid side by side with one of the same kind not fermenting, both being contained in the same vessel but separated by a membrane which permitted the mingling of the liquids, but prevented the passage of the plant, that analogy lost its force, for the fermenting liquid continued to ferment, while the quiescent liquid remained quiescent. The case of fermentation assumed now a significance quite the contrary of that which it had before seemed to possess, and it began to be claimed to be quite as conclusive in favor of the germ theory as it had been before in favor of the chemical. This theory, however, though among its advocates have been and continue to be counted many of the most distinguished physicians and physiologists of the past and the present generation, has never met with universal acceptance. Serious difficulties present themselves which it fails to explain, among which are the objections, strongly put by Dr. Bastian, that the theory demands a belief in the existence of about twenty different kinds of organisms never known in their mature state, and whose existence is not demonstrated, but simply postulated; and that these germs, if they exist, are not the germs of any known organisms; because such germs have been experimentally shown to be incapable of producing the particular diseases these are assumed to cause. Moreover, feeding on putrid flesh, as is habitual among the Kalmucks, is followed by no injurious consequences, though such flesh swarms with bacteria; and as the author just referred to affirms, the organisms of ordinary putrefactions may be introduced even into the blood of men and animals without producing any of these specific diseases. The same writer asserts that in sheep-pox the blood and the secretions are not infective, though this disease is allied to, and even more virulently contagious than, human smallpox. . . .

BEARING OF THE QUESTION UPON PUBLIC HYGIENE

As to the bearing of this question upon public hygiene and the principles which should govern sanitary legislation, it is to be observed that if we accept the chemical theory of contagion as exclusively the true one, we can hardly avoid admitting the possibility that contagious disease may originate in a healthy individual without communication with a person already diseased. The causes, whatever they may be, will be found in surrounding conditions. If I have understood what has been said during the present session of this association, the cholera in the West during the season that is past did not originate from without. Somewhere conditions must have existed which favored its origination *de novo* in our own country. In this view of the subject, the business of sanitary science is to discover the nature of the deleterious conditions tending to induce disease, and to prevent their occurrence.

If, on the other hand, infectious disease is propagated by living germs alone, what we have to aim at is to devise measures for promptly extirpating those germs the moment the disease appears. But as the necessary measures of precaution or of extirpation will be substantially the same, whatever may be the theoretic views entertained as to the nature and the origin of the evil to be met, our legislation in any case is likely to be practically the same, however in its motive it may be logically different. Pure air, pure water, wholesome food, thorough drainage, rigidly enforced cleanliness, the severe exclusion from towns and cities of industries which contaminate the air with noxious gases or offensive effluvia, especially such as arise from decaying organic matter, the prevention of overcrowding in dwellings, the prompt and complete disinfection of every spot where pestilence may lift its head, and of every article and substance, including the dejecta of the sick, which may serve as a vehicle of disease, and, finally, a well-organized sanitary police, and untiring vigilance on the part of its members —these are the objects which the guardians of the public health must labor to secure, to whatever school of ethology they may happen to belong. It is, indeed, a fortunate circumstance, a fact observable in no other department of practical human effort that I happen to remember, that here the champions of conflicting theories, however freely they may splinter lances in the arena of controversy, are always found, in the field of actual warfare and in the face of the common enemy, marching harmoniously side by side.

The study of the laws of hygiene is assuming in our time, in the estimation of the public and of the profession themselves, an importance which places it above even the proper business of the profession—that of the science of therapeutics. Drugs, whether remedial or prophylactic, are falling more and more into disrepute; and it is felt that prophylactic action is infinitely better than prophylactic draughts.

Such has been the success of modern measures for closing up all the insidious approaches by which disease has hitherto effected its entrance into the family, the community, or the individual organism, as to encourage a hope, even so seemingly wild and visionary, as that a time is coming in which disease itself shall be utterly extirpated, and men shall begin to live out the days which Heaven intended for them. When that time arrives, if it ever shall, your honorable and learned profession may find, like Othello, its occupation gone; but it will be itself which will have destroyed it, and which will have established, in doing so, a nobler title to the gratitude of mankind than all its untiring labors for the relief of suffering humanity, through centuries of self-sacrificing devotion hitherto, have already won.

DORMAN B. EATON

THE ESSENTIAL CONDITIONS OF GOOD SANITARY ADMINISTRATION

Editor's Note

Dorman B. Eaton (1823–99) was a Vermonter who spent most of his adult life in New York, where he practiced law until 1870. Prior to his retirement he was already actively engaged in the health reform movement. Along with Stephen Smith, he helped draft the Metropolitan Health Bill, and he worked hard for its passage. He preceded Smith in testifying before the legislature in Albany on the necessity for a health department that was independent of party pressures and political spoils.

From 1870 until his death at the end of 1899 Eaton played significant parts in two other reform movements, that of city government and civil service. In recognition of his work to abolish the spoils system in government appointments President Grant named Eaton chairman of the Civil Service Commission in 1873. He then played a major role in drafting the Pendleton Act of 1883, establishing the modern civil service system.

Eaton was one of the original members of the American Public Health Association when it was founded in 1872. Thus it was natural that he should speak on his specialty, public health law, at one of the early meetings. Eaton demonstrated that he was also a student of comparative sanitary legislation in his pamphlet, *Sanitary Legislation in England and New York* (New York: Amerman, 1872.)

Bibliographical Note

A full biography of Eaton is needed. His role in civil service reform has been described by Ari Hoogenboom in *Outlawing the Spoils, A History of the Civil Service Reform Movement, 1865–83*, Urbana: University of Illinois, 1961.

Sanitary administration is relatively good when on the level of the general intelligence, but is absolutely good only when it accomplishes whatever is within the power of government, reasonably exercised, to promote the health and

Reports and Papers, A.P.H.A. 2 (1874–75): 498–514. A discourse at the annual meeting in Baltimore, November 9, 1875.

preserve the lives of a people. Such administration implies and must be sanctioned by judicious and comprehensive sanitary laws.

What, then, in this country are the essential conditions of such administration? I answer, the following three, and I propose to offer a contribution in aid of securing them:

1. That a majority of the people, or those whose advice this majority will follow, have an adequate conception of the true meaning and scope of sanitary laws and administration.

2. That such majority, or its accepted advisers, have faith in sanitary precautions and adequate knowledge how to devise and apply them.

3. That effective methods in harmony with our constitutions, social conditions, and ideas of justice and policy, be provided by statute for securing the coöperation of persons of the most instructed intelligence and the highest *sense* of public duty, in aid of such administration.

These conditions, true theoretically, will be found equally true when considered in reference to the present condition of sanitary intelligence, faith, and administration in this country.

No competent judge, I venture to think, can look into the crude, shallow, arbitrary, and heterogeneous mass of laws and ordinances which are nominally in force in a majority of the municipalities of this country, or compare the statutes recently enacted in various States for creating State Boards of Health, without being painfully impressed with the conviction that the conditions named exist only among a small portion of the people of the United States. Indeed, were it not for the growing spirit of inquiry among the people on the subject of public health, for the more comprehensive legislation and the larger supply of pecuniary means to that end during the last few years, and especially were it not for the enlightened zeal and self-sacrifice of the medical profession, all of which this Association has promoted, and the last of which it nobly illustrates, in aid of sanitary reform, the actual condition in many quarters would be as discouraging as it is disgraceful. In not a small proportion of the states, the condition of the law and administration on the great subject of the public health, and to a large extent on the subject of general morality and prosperity, as dependent upon the public health, is far behind that of the more enlightened states and nations, and is discreditable to our institutions. We must, in view of it, adopt one of these conclusions: either that the majority of the people do not know how great a portion of the premature death and sickness and discomfort among them could be prevented, and how much in other places has been prevented; or else, that they are alike indifferent to health, comfort, and life.

And even when sanitary legislation and administration, more or less satisfactory, have been secured, there is such an absence of any common method—such contrariety of aim, scope, and authority—as indicates pervading immaturity of thought and calls for an examination into the first principles of sanitary administration.

Even the municipal health laws of New York City, which are the earliest and best in the country, while in some particulars superior to any elsewhere, are yet defective as compared with those relating to several European cities. So the laws creating a State Board of Health in Massachusetts, though they are the earliest, and perhaps the best of the kind, in the Union, are yet very feeble and defective as compared with those in force in Great Britain. And perhaps the people of Georgia may have good reason to think—if it shall be well administered—that their law, enacted during the present year, and of which large portions are taken from the health laws relating to the city of New York, is even more comprehensive and enlightened than that of Massachusetts. It is certainly greatly superior to the act creating the State Board of Health in Minnesota, and is beyond all comparison with that moribund pretense of sanitary legislation in Virginia, which at once illustrates the zeal of the medical profession and the lamentable parsimony of its legislators in regard to a subject which vitally concerns the intelligence and prosperity of that venerable state.

But criticism will be more intelligent and appropriate after we have considered some facts and principles. What view, then, shall we take of the scope and aim of sanitary administration?

1. In trying to secure longer life and more comfort and health in our relations with nature and each other, we no more ignore Providence, or attempt to improve upon it or nature, than when we send for a doctor, cook raw meat, or prepare warm clothing and a fire against cold weather, or when we deepen the channel of a river, or grade a roadway track to secure easier and safer transportation. The fact that we are placed in peril of storms and pestilences and miasmata is no good cause for not using our reason to the best advantage for securing good ships, good doctors, good medicines, good food, and good sanitary laws. But the arguments that sickness and death, as they occur, are providentially inevitable, and that pestilence and famine are preordained messengers of God's wisdom and wrath, before which we must dismiss our reason—that our precautions against them are vain floutings of our wisdom in the face of divine Providence—are so nearly monopolized by illiterate grandmamas and superannuated bigots as to be elements of precaution hardly worthy of notice in our sanitary condition on earth. Though Dr. Lyon Playfair, now a professor at Edinburgh, says that in his day Scotch professors dared not preach such heretical doctrines, and it is not very long since an English company was refused the liberty of deepening the channel of the Guadalquivir, because, as it was argued, if God had intended the river to be navigated, He would have made it navigable.

2. We no more assume that human beings can always be preserved in health than that their earthly existence can be made immortal. We no more propose that the hand of the state or the precept of the law shall, at all times and everywhere, assume to instruct or to direct as to our health than as to our habits or our industries; but that, equally as to each, the coercion of the law shall be felt just when and where and to that extent that a sacrifice of individual interest

and preferences will, in harmony with our republican system, promote the general welfare. We ask no new constitutional power and no surrender of individual rights, but only a true application of old principles in a clearer light, in a wider sphere, and for the achievement of a higher good than heretofore. . . .

Stated more specifically, sanitary laws may therefore extend to the following subjects:

1. To the gathering and dissemination of that kind of practical and instructive knowledge relative to the preventable causes of disease and death, and to the cure of sickness, and the building up of the physical system, which, while stimulating individual effort in the same direction, affect the public at large, and cannot be, and are not likely to be, secured by any private effort; and to these ought to be added original and thorough investigations into the science of public health (such as England is causing to be made), to which the world is so much indebted, and which may be made a blessing as valuable and universal as any work which a state can foster.

2. To securing a systematic and complete registry of births, marriages, and deaths; of the particulars of contagions and epidemics, and the other more prevalent and dangerous diseases, and of accidents causing death and inability to labor; whereby life-saving medical knowledge is enlarged and enlightened; the effect of the wisest efforts to protect life and health are brought to a practical test of usefulness; the fatal and bloody secrets of abortionists and corrupt coroners are opened to the light; child murder and secret assassination, and deadly quackery are exposed; land titles, the marital relations, and paternity are made more secure; in short, whereby a nation, and each community in it, is brought face to face with the ugly but admonishing evidence of its ignorance and immorality, and there is provided for posterity the most instructive evidence of past civilization.

3. To securing the highest standard of education and moral tone in the medical profession; but for administrators under laws having such aims, the most suitable members of that profession should be sought, and the pride and sense of duty, which are its honor, should be made the main reliance, as they are to be the great inspiration.

4. To better safeguards through publicity, tests, and penalties, against nostrums and charlatanry—more fatal and costly than the afflictions they pretend to cure; and to the publication of a reliable pharmacopoeia, as is now provided for in England.

5. To providing more severe and certain responsibility on the part of all those who, for love of gain, by negligence, falsehood, or design, make light of, or bring peril to human life, or the health or safety of a people.

6. To all practical measures for securing pure water, pure milk, pure air, and wholesome food; and to this end providing for tests, *inspections*, and penalties which can be promptly and easily enforced and collected.

7. To securing good drainage about villages, and good sewerage in all public streets; and in connection with all public buildings; for the want of which thousands now needlessly sicken, and many die.

8. To adequate ventilation in schools, colleges, hospitals, asylums, court rooms, theatres, public halls, tenement houses, and in any other places used for like public purpose; so that no longer, as now, they shall be the source of universal discomfort and frequent disease.

9. To vaccination in that effective manner which shall disarm both prejudice and peril, and to providing safe vaccine matter, and perhaps other safe and simple medicines for the very poor; and public baths and urinals for general use.

10. To those disinfections and purifications which so generally arrest contagions, and so much limit epidemics.

11. To the regulation and, if needful, to the removal or suppression of occupations and practices dangerous or detrimental to the public health, and to the removal of garbage, offal, and other filthy matter; with suitable provisions for making the expense a lien on property, and a personal charge against those guilty of neglect; and in this regard the *provisions* in force in the City of New York are the best in the country, if not in the world.

12. To the inspection, by the sanitary authorities, of all hospitals, asylums, prisons, schools, and other public buildings and premises, which are within the range of the sanitary laws; and such inspection of private buildings, in presence of epidemics, as may be necessary to protect the public health.

13. To providing for instruction in the art of nursing, to at least that extent which shall secure duly instructed nurses for all asylums, hospitals, and other like public institutions.

14. To preventing over-work, and abuse and neglect of children, as far as practicable, without undue invasion of private rights and the *sanctities* of home.

15. To the supervision of dead human bodies, and to cemeteries, burial grounds, disinterments, inquests, dissections, and morgues.

16. To such provisions as to the width and distances apart of city streets, and the size of city lots, as shall facilitate the erection of separate, small houses for those of small means and tend to keep them out of large tenement houses; and also to rigid requirements as to the height, light, sewerage, and ventilation of buildings offered for rent to the poor; it being in part a consequence of the ground-plan of the city of New York that (so unlike Philadelphia) nearly half her people are in tenement houses.

17. To provisions which shall secure rapid and cheap transit for the poor, so that they may live beyond the densely population parts of cities and work within them.

18. To all this must be added, in places where needed, the usual quarantine authority for preventing the introduction of disease through foreign vessels and external commerce; and also that broad discretionary power necessary in boards

of health, of acting promptly and fearlessly, for subordinating private comfort to public safety, and for making all needful expenditures to avert and alleviate pestilence. . . .

It only remains to make a few suggestions as to the best method of organization for sanitary work:

1. In sections where general intelligence and sanitary appreciation are low, I doubt not that the first organizations and effort will be made almost wholly by the members of the medical profession, and their action will need be confined mainly to inspecting, expostulating, inquiring, and reporting. But this stage soon leads to the next, when restraining power must be exercised and property and persons must be made to bear the cost of removing the sources of disease and death, of which their condition or their neglects have been the cause.

2. The moment we attempt to exercise political power for sanitary purposes, that is, to use the government for compelling citizens to observe the general conditions of public health and to pay penalty of the infringement and the cost of redress, we must not seek our official force wholly from any one profession. No profession is strong enough to wield the power needed to stand up against the vast combination of the ignorant, the greedy, the vicious, and the lawless; nor has any one profession the learning or the wisdom for so difficult a work. Sanitary administration, which has to deal with property, constitutional rights, partisan interests, institutions, buildings, and all the complications of business and commerce, as well as with the abstruse questions of chemical science, hygiene, and medicine, requires the most varied experience and capacity in its official force.

3. As no branch of administration has to do with so varied relations and interests, so in none is continuity of action and length of experience of more importance, and for these reasons, the terms of members of a board of health should be long and they should not all expire at once. It is almost needless to say that where so much discretion must be allowed, where there are the greatest opportunities for corruption, where the want of wisdom and courage in the performance of duty may bring needless death and sickness into hundreds of families and may send many other hundreds to the poor-house, there is as great necessity for pure character as for high capacity in the officers. On these points, as well as in reference to the necessary provisions for securing an efficient and economical sanitary administration, especially in a municipality, the example and the health laws, ordinances, and regulations of the city of New York will be found highly instructive.

And it is important to note that the highest courts of New York have decided that a health board may, under our constitutions, adopt and enforce ordinances, regulate trades and occupations, hold trials, and make and enforce orders which shall be a lien on real property, within the true scope of sanitary legislation, without being arrested by injunctions or delayed by demands for jury trials; but subject, doubtless, to having its action duly reviewed in the courts.

4. It seems to me that this coercive administration must be exercised in part by the nation, in part by the states, and in part by the municipalities, or within such divisions as may be made for sanitary purposes of the rural portion of the people.

Beginning with such divisions as the primary or local unit for administration, there should be a sanitary authority, with adequate power and a clear definition of duties, in each. It is plain that the causes which affect health, and the agencies which counteract disease, have neither their origin nor their sphere of influence confined to mere political divisions; and these facts must be more especially regarded in providing sanitary precautions for the rural districts. Until the public mind is more instructed, however, it will hardly be found practicable to provide those independent agencies of good sanitary administration, which I believe the near future is sure to demand.

At first we must make the best possible use of political divisions and existing officers, and at no time must we forget our legal principles or our constitutional structure.

5. It seems indispensable that there should be a State Board of Health in each state, which shall be a permanent, as it may be made a beneficent, part of the administration.

That board, in addition to the duty of making investigations and reports, and of supplying vigor and high intelligence to the whole system, should have general supervision of vital (and perhaps criminal) statistics, should investigate all cases of extravagant expenditure, of excessive death rate, and of alleged inefficiency or abuses in any local sanitary district; and to this state board all local boards should be required to report.

6. But all this done, and still there would be a sphere of sanitary duty for the federal government. Commerce between the states, and with foreign nations, the territories, the District of Columbia, and many reserved places, are subject to its jurisdiction. The army, the navy, the growing thousands in the civil service, in ships, in ports, in hospitals, in barracks, in the great offices in the cities, are under its control. As population shall grow dense, the impracticability of guarding against disease without this pervading force and varied territory of the federal government being under wise sanitary provisions, in sympathy with state laws, will more and more appear. The army, the navy, and the marine hospital service are now supplied with medical men in the service of the nation. The time may not be remote when the exigencies of foreign commerce will require more uniformity of quarantine regulations than the states now supply. It must be apparent that when the several states shall have active boards of health, there will be a vast amount of instructive sanitary information annually published, with no adequate means for its comparative arrangement or for bringing it before the country at large. Cattle diseases, contagious epidemics, fevers, sweeping on from city to city, from county to county, from state to state, here following rivers and there lakes and mountain ranges, will surely produce the

conviction that a general cause of danger must be met by common arrangements for protection.

Already, in view of the fact that the most fearful contagions and epidemics, originating among degraded nations and on remote continents, threaten the whole commercial world, there is a growing conviction that the question of public health is not merely national but cosmopolitan; and international treaties will, I believe, soon embrace the question of general health as one of the most important subjects.

The federal government has already sanitary laws relating to many subjects, such as the ventilation and overcrowding of ships, hospitals, and asylums; the food, medicines, and housing of soldiers and sailors; and to the facilities to be afforded by federal authorities for the execution of the quarantine and other health laws of the several states. It is not necessary, nor would it be wise, to increase the jurisdiction of the nation at the expense of that of the states, and it would suffice if each within its sphere should wisely exercise that power which it possesses. And how can it be denied that the national jurisdiction over commerce, the authority which extends to every vessel, to every engine, to every passenger, to every package of merchandise on navigable waters; which surveys rivers, harbors, and the depths of the ocean; which searches out the schoolhouses, numbers the scholars, and, with the census, has already published sanitary charts of the whole Union, which on the sea-shore and on the inland hill-tops, gathers the signs of the wind and of the rains, of heat and cold, and sends its bulletins through all the borders to instruct the fishermen and the farmers—in presence of such facts, I say, how can it be denied that it is the right and the duty of the general government to bring the diverse elements of its sanitary jurisdiction, as far as practicable, under one efficient board which shall act in harmony with the health boards of the several states, and gather, arrange, print, and send all over the Union those records of the origin, cause, and progress of disease and death—those instructive and admonishing statistics of vitality and progress which measure the peril and the possibilities of commerce, which illustrate the power and the morality of a nation, which are the measure of our claims to the greatness to which we aspire and of our own fidelity to the religion which we profess. As a republic, proclaiming the common brotherhood of men; in presence of the evidence that the leading monarchies are now surpassing us in the protection given to life and health even among the poor and the humble; in view of the fact that commerce has woven all nations into such a network of dependence that a pestilence in Central Asia alarms the whole commercial world; can we longer as a nation fold our arms and say that we have no duty and will have no part in the sublime Christian work—now elsewhere so high advanced—of building up better physical manhood, of removing to the utmost sorrow and sickness from homes, of increasing, as we may, length of days and days of comfort here on earth?

JOHN SHAW BILLINGS

THE REGISTRATION OF VITAL STATISTICS

Editor's Note

John Shaw Billings (1838–1913) was one of the most versatile and influential physicians of his day. One of his talents lay in planning and administration, another in bibliographical work. After a tour of duty as surgeon in the Civil War, Billings remained in the army to organize the library of the Surgeon-General's office (now the National Library of Medicine). He then became a widely known sanitarian and hospital planner. As vice-president of the short-lived National Board of Health he was responsible for much of its day-to-day administration.

Billings has often been called the father of vital statistics in this country. This perhaps gives him too much credit, but he did play an important role in bringing the subject to the fore. He deserves much credit for urging that vital statistics be included in the United States Census of 1880, and thereafter.

From 1896 until his death in 1913, Billings directed the newly unified New York Public Library. Although noted for many accomplishments, probably the greatest monument to his memory is the massive *Index Catalog of the Library of the Surgeon General* and the *Index Medicus*. These great bibliographical aids are still the first place to turn when one embarks on any project in the history of medicine in America or, for that matter, on the history of almost any medical subject.

Bibliographical Note

Billings wrote many important papers. For a complete list of his works see the biography by Fielding H. Garrison, *John Shaw Billings*, New York: Putnam's, 1915.

For a somewhat more complex and longer discussion of vital statistics by Billings, see his Cartwright Lectures, "On vital and medical statistics," *Medical Record* 36 (1889): 589–601, 617–26, 645–56.

A statistician's view of Billings can be seen in Raymond Pearl's "Some notes on the contributions of Dr. John Shaw Billings to the development of vital statistics," *Bull. Hist. Med.* 6 (1938): 387–93.

For a history of vital statistics in the United States prior to the nineteenth century see James H. Cassedy, *Demography in Early America, Beginnings of the Statistical Mind, 1600–1800*, Cambridge: Harvard University Press, 1969.

Am. J. Med. Sci. 85 (1883): 33–59. This paper contains the substance of a report made to the National Board of Health in October 1882.

The subject of registration of vital statistics is one of the most important, and at the same time most difficult, in sanitary as well as social science. Its difficulties are in part due to its apparent simplicity. Before studying it and attempting to obtain practical results, almost everyone is disposed to think that he understands it and is quite ready, not only to undertake the duties of registrar or census superintendent, but to prepare a law or ordinance regulating the matter.

After one has investigated the matter a little and has become somewhat acquainted with the methods in use, it is not unlikely that he will suppose that he has made some remarkable discoveries of causes of error, imperfect returns, insufficient tabulations, and erroneous conclusions, and will thereupon proceed to prepare a paper criticizing the work of his predecessors and proposing reform. It is probable, however, as he continues his studies, that he will find that his discoveries are not new, that there are various practical objections to his proposed improvements, and that it is much easier to confine his essay to denunciation of that which is, than to point out clearly and definitely that which ought to be and which is at the same time practicable.

Vital statistics, in the widest sense of the term, includes the records of all circumstances affecting the production or duration of human life, corresponding almost precisely with the term "démographie," as used by Guillard and other modern French writers. It includes records of the population living at a given period, such as are obtained by the census; and also a record of the changes taking place in this population by births, marriages, and deaths, such as is obtained by registration. In almost all countries, the census of the population and the system of registration, although depending upon each other for much of their interest and value, are nevertheless kept separate as a matter of administration and are obtained by entirely different methods. It is only where there is no system of registration, as in the United States taken as a nation, that an attempt is made to obtain, through the machinery of the census, the data which should be derived from current records. But while the results thus obtained are certainly better than none at all, they are extremely imperfect and lead to serious errors on the part of those who attempt to use them without bearing constantly in mind their incompleteness and mistakes.

The registration of vital statistics properly includes the obtaining of records of births, marriages, deaths, and disease. The comparison of these records with each other and with those of the living population, form vital statistics proper, and the conclusions drawn from such comparisons form the science of demography.

We have no information that the ancients had any system of registration, although the Jews, Athenians, and Romans took censuses, and it is stated that in China, Japan, and Peru statistical information of this character was collected. In Egypt and in Rome records of births in certain families appear to have been kept, but the first steps toward a general registration were taken through the clergy about the beginning of the sixteenth century. The earliest registers to which I find reference made were those kept at Augsburg and Breslau, which, according to Süssmilch, antedated the order of Lord Thomas Cromwell, in 1538, directing the keeping of parish registers in England.

Little attention, however, seems to have been paid to these English parish registers until 1558, when it was ordered that they should be regularly kept in the churches and for better preservation should be written on parchment.

In France the first legislation on this subject appears to have been the ordinance of Villers-Cotterets, in 1539. In 1579 the ordinance of Blois directed that there should be brought to the courts at the end of each year the registers of baptisms, marriages, and burials of the several parishes, and by the beginning of the seventeenth century such registers seem to have been in general use throughout Western Europe. Bills of mortality for the purpose of preventing the diffusion of the plague were occasionally issued in London during the latter part of the sixteenth century, and a regular series of weekly bills commenced in December, 1603, at the end of the great plague, and were then continued regularly until the present system of the registrar general was established. These bills were under the superintendence of the Company of Parish Clerks of London, first incorporated in 1233, as the "Fraternity of St. Nicholas." In 1625 this corporation obtained a decree from the Star Chamber allowing a press to be kept for the printing of bills of mortality of the city and liberties of London, for which purpose the Archbishop of Canterbury appoints a printer.[1]

In 1629 these bills were arranged to show the distinction of sex and cause of death, and in 1728 the distinction of age was introduced; but the distinction of sex was only shown for the total number of deaths and not for each disease nor for each group of ages.

In 1662 John Graunt, who was subsequently made a Fellow of the Royal Society, published a little work entitled, "Natural and Political Observations Mentioned in the Following Index, and Made upon Bills of Mortality," of which several editions were subsequently issued. In his epistle dedicatory addressed to John, Lord Roberts, the Lord Privy Seal, he says:

> I conceive that it doth not ill become a peer of Parliament, or member of his Majesty's Council, to consider how few starve of the many that beg; that the irreligious proposal of some to multiply people by polygamy is withal irrational and fruitless; that the troublesome seclusions in the plague time are not a remedy to be purchased at vast inconveniences; that the greatest plagues of the city are equally and quickly repaired from the country; that the wasting of males by wars and colonies do not prejudice the due proportion between them and females, etc.

This work of Graunt is the first treatise on vital statistics, and a very good beginning it was.

---

[1] Burrows on Parish Registers, etc., London Medical Repository, 1818, vol. x. p. 277.

The first bills of mortality in which the ages were inserted appear to have
been those of Breslau, which were used by Halley for the construction of his
table of mortality.

In France increased importance was given to the registers kept by the clergy
by the decree of April 16, 1667, section 20, which directs that copies of such
registers should be accepted as legal proof of the facts set forth.

After the revocation of the edict of Nantes, in 1685, it became difficult and
sometimes impossible for Protestants to furnish legal evidence of legitimacy,
etc., and it was not until 1787 that the Protestant registers were made legal.
After the revolution of 1789 registration passed entirely from the hands of the
clergy.

The parochial registers of England were exceedingly imperfect. Even the best
of them showed as a rule only the baptisms and burials, not the births and
deaths. They were not kept by all religious denominations, nor in hospitals or
infirmaries having private burial grounds, and infants dying before baptism were
not registered at all. In the old bills these were sometimes entered under the
name of *Chrisoms*.

The accounts of these registers given by Mr. Bigland,[2] Mr. Lucas,[3] and
others[4] point out in great detail the imperfection of this system. The entries
were irregularly made and illegibly written. There was no special care or responsibility for the books, so that some were lost or stolen, etc. etc. Imperfect as it
was, however, this was the system brought to America by the early settlers of
New England.

In September, 1639, the colony of Massachusetts Bay ordered that births and
deaths should be reported to the town clerk by parents and householders within
one month of the occurrence of the same. Newly married men were also to give
the clerks certificates of their marriage. Similar orders were made by the Ply-
mouth Colony in 1646.

Rhode Island had similar laws prior to 1698, for they are referred to in the
Act of May 3d of that year, and probably all the colonies had somewhat similar
regulations, but they fell into disuse without being formally repealed.

The present system of registration of births, marriages, and deaths in England
dates from the passage of the Act of August 17, 1836. This Act provided for the
creation of the office of registrar general, at a salary of one thousand pounds per
annum, and for the appointment of registrars and deputy registrars throughout
the kingdom; the district of each registrar to be a portion of a union or parish set
apart for that purpose by the guardians of said union or parish, subject to the
approval of the registrar general. The registrars were authorized and required to

---

[2] Observations on Marriages, Baptisms, etc., as preserved in Parochial Registers, 1764.

[3] An Impartial Inquiry into the Present State of Parochial Registers, etc., 1791.

[4] For further history as to early registration consult J. P. Süssmilch, *Die Göttliche Ord-
nung in den Veränderungen des menschlichen Geschlechts*. Editions of 1775 (4th) or 1798.
And the article "Mortality," by Milne, in the Encyclopaedia Britannica.

inform themselves of every birth and death happening within their districts, and to ascertain and register as soon after the event as conveniently could be done, without fee or reward, the particulars required to be registered according to the schedules appended.

This law was followed by the Act, passed in 1837, to explain and amend the previous Acts. This Act placed the establishment of the boundaries of the registration districts entirely within the power of the registrar general, provided for the appointment of deputy superintendent registrars, and, also, that all registrars should be free and exempt from serving on any jury or inquest. The registrar's office was to be provided and furnished at the expense of the Board of Guardians, and for that purpose they were authorized to borrow money and charge it on the future poor-rates; and in case such Board of Guardians neglected or refused to provide such office, then the Commissioners of the Treasury should do so at an expense not exceeding three hundred pounds in each case, and should collect the money from the guardians.

The present system of registrations of births and deaths in England is regulated by the Act passed in August 1874. A copy of so much of the Acts of 1836, 1837, and 1874 as are of special interest in connection with this subject is appended.

A sketch of the early history of registration in the United States is given by Dr. Sutton as an appendix to the second annual report of the registration of births, marriages, and deaths in Kentucky for the year 1853.

From this, and from an examination of the various registration reports which have been published, it is evident that in the great majority of the states the actual registration is exceedingly imperfect, and one would be greatly deceived if he were to judge of these systems by the laws which have been enacted. Copies of nearly all of these state laws are given in an appendix, accompanied with brief memoranda as to the results in the several states; but they are given not so much for the purpose of showing what has actually be done, as to indicate what those who have advocated registration have thought ought to be and could be done.

A brief review of the difficulties and objections which are met with in attempting to provide a complete system of state registration may be useful.

There are four principal objects for a systematic registration of births, marriages, and deaths on the part of a community.

The first is for legal purposes, being intended to identify individuals in their relations to their families and to the community, and rests upon substantially the same grounds as that of the recording of titles of property.

The remark of Dr. Snow, made twenty years ago, that it would probably be impossible for a large portion of the middle-aged men and women in the United States to prove that their parents were ever married and that they have any legitimate right to the name they bear, no doubt still holds good to a great extent.

The second purpose is for the prevention and detection of crime.

The third object, so far at least as births and deaths are concerned, is to furnish data for sanitary purposes, that is, to give warning of the undue increase of disease or death presumed to be due to preventable causes, and also to indicate the localities in which sanitary effort is most desirable and most likely to be of use.

The fourth object is to collect data for scientific purposes as bearing on the laws of human development. It will be seen that the character of the information required differs somewhat for these several objects. For legal purposes the main object is the identification of the individual, the verification of the fact of birth or death, and the ascertaining that the death is due to what are commonly called natural cases. For scientific and sanitary purposes the identification of the individual is of minor importance, as it is required only for the purpose of preventing duplication of the records.

While the importance of all these objects will usually be readily admitted, it will be found in attempting to frame a state law for the registration of vital statistics, that there will be objections urged and that there will be many practical difficulties in its enforcement, no matter what its provisions may be. The principal objection urged by legislators to the passage of such a law will be the cost of the system, and a constant effort will be made to induce those presenting the bill to have the figures for compensation placed at the lowest possible point. As I have stated in a previous report, the attempt to secure complete and satisfactory registration through the voluntary contribution of information by heads of families or by physicians, or by requiring insufficiently paid registrars to obtain the information desired, has always been a failure. As legislators reflect in a general way the state of public opinion in the localities whence they come, it is evident that unless this public opinion has been educated to a certain extent with regard to the importance and value of registration, there is small probability of the passage of any satisfactory law, and still less probability that it will be properly executed if passed.

The first and greatest difficulty in educating the people upon this subject is to get them to understand the objects of the registration. Those who have never given any attention to the subject are apt to suppose that it is merely a hobby of the doctors who want the information for their own private purposes, and that this information can only be obtained by an unjustifiable amount of meddling with private affairs and by a system of espionage which will cause much trouble and difficulty.

These objections are, however, of small importance in comparison with the absolute indifference as to the whole matter which prevails throughout the community, nor do the objections often turn upon the practical difficulties in enforcing such laws, seeing that the objectors are in most cases profoundly ignorant of these difficulties.

Dr. Sutton remarks that legislators will insist upon amending the most carefully drawn bill so as to secure greater cheapness, and what they suppose to be greater simplicity in the machinery, until it sometimes happens that those who have been most active in preparing and urging a law lose their interests in it, and may even become opponents, because they see that it has been so mutilated as to be inefficient or impossible of execution. In this country it has been proved by repeated experiments that it is impossible, by legislation which involves neither payment nor penalty, to induce parents or householders to report the births and deaths which have occurred under their respective jurisdictions to the registrars, whoever they may be. Even in cases where this has been required of them under penalty, no one will attempt to enforce a law which inflicts penalties not sanctioned by public opinion.

A registration law which is, upon the whole, theoretically satisfactory, not unfrequently becomes practically useless, owing to the character of the person who is selected to supervise its execution. It has happened that the person selected to collect and compile the data of registration for a state has been a politician for whom it was desirable to provide an office and who had no other qualifications for the place.

The object of such persons is to do as little as possible and to avoid arousing inquiry or opposition by calling attention to defects. If, for the sake of economy, the duty is placed upon some existing officer of the state, as, for example, the librarian, or the secretary of the senate, or the secretary of state, and no provision of funds is made whereby this officer can employ a really competent man to do the work, the results are certain to be of comparatively little value; for without a properly qualified supervising officer it will not be possible to avoid omissions and errors on the part of the local registrars.

The most difficult of all the problems of registration in this country is how to obtain a complete record of the births in a given locality, nor can we say that it has anywhere been completely and satisfactorily solved. In a report on registration made by Dr. E. M. Snow to the fourth National Quarantine Convention held in Boston in 1860, the best methods of obtaining records of births, especially in cities, were discussed. His conclusion was that requiring parents to furnish the desired information is in this country useless; that requiring physicians to report births occurring in their practice is equally useless; and that the only method by which returns of births can be obtained in cities with any approach to fulness and correctness is by requiring the recording officer to obtain the information personally or by his agents; in other words by sending at periodic intervals some one to call at every house and obtain the data for the births which have occurred there since the last visit. It seems very doubtful, however, as to whether this method would obtain all the births in our large cities, and especially among the floating population. Probably a combination of this method with those pursued in France and Great Britain to obtain the same end would have the best effect. . . .

It is much easier to secure a complete registration of deaths than of births, since it is comparatively easy to enforce a law that a permit shall be necessary for every interment or removal of a dead body, and the community soon learns to consider any attempt at burial without a permit as a suspicious circumstance indicating a desire to conceal either the death or the cause of death and justifying a special investigation by the authorities. When it has been decided to require a burial permit in all cases, there is no difficulty in requiring the data necessary for registration as an indispensable preliminary to the issue of such permit.

A complete system of registration of deaths should include some method of verification of the death and of its cause by a person having the special knowledge necessary for that purpose.

This skilled verification is necessary, first, to insure the fact of a death having taken place. In its absence, in a large city, there is little or no difficulty in having recorded the death of a person who may be either nonexistent or alive and well.

Second, it is necessary to insure the fact of real as opposed to apparent death in any case, and thus to prevent premature burial.

Third, it is necessary to establish the fact that a death has taken place from what may be termed natural causes as opposed to criminal causes. This verification of death and of the cause of death may be made either by physicians employed for that particular purpose, and receiving payment from the state, or by the physician under whose charge the deceased person has been previous to death, only those cases which have not been under the treatment of a physician being referred to a public medical officer or the coroner for verification.

The first system is that employed in France, Belgium, and Austria, the second is the one made use of in England and this country. This matter will be discussed farther in speaking of the methods of ascertaining the cause of death. All registration laws include physicians as an essential part of their machinery. Some do this directly, by requiring that physicians shall keep a list of all deaths occurring in their practice and shall forward this list at stated times to the registrar. This method has always proved a failure, as has the similar requirement of clergymen that they shall furnish lists of marriages. Where burial permits are required, a physician may be made responsible for a certificate as to those matters only about which his special professional knowledge is necessary, such as the cause of death, duration of sickness, etc., or he may be required to certify also to age, birthplace, parentage, etc. To this last class of requirements there are objections which are worthy of consideration, since although it is true that the great majority of physicians furnish the information required without any attempt to question the propriety of the law, still there are always some who will object and a few who will positively decline. The matter can perhaps be best illustrated by taking some of the objections which have been actually urged, and for this purpose we may take first the statement of Sir Dominic Corrigan as to his reasons for refusing in certain cases to fill out death certificates required under the Irish Act. In a paper in the *Dublin Quarterly Journal of Medical Sciences*, vol. li. 1871, p. 341, after stating that he has refused to fill out the certificate required under the Irish Act, he proceeds to give his reasons:

The words of the Act are that the medical practitioner who shall have been in attendance during the last illness and until the death, etc., is to fill up and sign the certificate. No man can be considered as in attendance until the death, unless he was *present at the death*. The interval of an hour equally with that of a month intervening between his last visit and the death puts him out of the category of being in "attendance until death." The certificate requires a medical practitioner to certify to three things; the day of the death, cause of the death, and the length of time the disease had continued. In eight years since the passage of the Act only one case has occurred in which he could certify of his own personal knowledge that death did occur on a particular day. He asks how can a medical practitioner in the majority of instances certify as to duration of disease, information with regard to which must in a great majority of cases be got together on hearsay evidence. A man cannot be compelled to certify to what he is not certain of; therefore, no such acts can be enforced under a penalty. In Ireland the penalty is that of misdemeanor, but no official has ever ventured to bring a recusant into court.

With this may be compared the objections urged by Dr. Buckingham, in the *Boston Medical Journal*, 1868, vol. i, p. 225. He objects to the law, saying the fact that he saw a man during his last sickness, though years before he died, makes him liable to penalty if he refuses to fill a certificate, although no one may have been in attendance when the man died.

Certificates are often filled out by persons with no medical education, but who call themselves physicians. Physicians certify to the cause of death, age, etc., when they should refuse any certificate in cases where they have no data by which to judge either of the age or sickness, except statements of some friend.

The law does not provide that the last attendant shall give it, but any physician having attended a person during his last illness. The undertakers desire certificates because they get a fee, and registrars desire certificates because for each entry they get a fee. The physician is required to give a certificate without fee and liable to fine if he does not give it.

On this letter there was a comment by Dr. Derby, same vol., p. 265.

He replies that with regard to age, duration of disease, etc., they are merely embraced in the certificates signed by the physician for the sake of simplicity of form, that they are practically filled up by the relations or friends, and that no physician need hesitate to certify to them any more than as to the date when he himself was born. We must take the evidence of others as conclusive in circumstances of daily occurrence.

Dr. H. M. Lyman, in the *Chicago Medical Journal*, 1878, p. 252, gives voice to the feeling of passive resistance on the part of a certain number which is felt, but not usually expressed, viz., that registration laws may do very well for countries where people have been trained for generations to acquiescence, but that they are at war with the principles of democratic government and individual freedom.

In this country there is only the curiosity of a few scientific men that can be relied upon for their moral support of a registry law, and it is probable that in Chicago not more than twelve in every thousand would be found to care for the registration of their nativity even in a family Bible. The reason why physicians do not execute the law is because they not only have no personal interest in its execution, but because of an invincible, though not always clearly recognized, feeling or revolt against the injustice of a law which inflicts a special tax on the physician in the shape of postage, time, and trouble, and affords no compensation for the extra labor and expense. People do not like to make a present to government in any shape or form. It is as unjust for the state to add fifty cents to the doctor's tax simply because he is a doctor as it would be to add fifty dollars. The state should pay for all such service and it need not incur any great expense. It might, as in the case of jury duty or military service by conscription, fix its own rate, but the obligation should be recognized. The payment would, of course, require increased general taxation, but the increase would then be levied on all alike. The health officers are trying to get service from the doctors without paying for it.

In the *Chicago Medical Journal* for 1879, vol. 38, p. 148, Dr. Lyman continues this subject by calling attention to the New Hampshire Statute allowing twenty-five cents to each physician for recording. He says: "I am assured that it is perfectly effectual, and that in no part of the world are vital statistics being perfected as in that little old Granite State! In Minnesota, the state values these statistics sufficiently to pay not less than forty cents for registration of each birth and death."

While the views presented by Dr. Lyman are not those of the majority of the medical profession, who in this, as in many other ways, are willing and ready to give gratuitous service for the public good, they are, nevertheless, important in a legal point of view and should be borne in mind in attempting to devise any legislation on the subject. Attempts to compel under penalty physicians to report age and birthplace of their patients are worse than useless. I do not think that the offer of any fee which would be considered reasonable by legislators would have much influence in inducing physicians to report births and deaths, and Dr. Lyman is in error in supposing that New Hampshire or Minnesota have obtained any useful results in this way. The true policy is to call upon medical men to supplement the information that should be demanded from the parent or householder.

As regards births it is bad policy to require under penalty reports of such from medical men, and no sufficient reason exists for so doing. With regard to deaths there is much truth in Dr. Snow's remark that the habit of signing death certificates is incidentally of benefit to physicians as it makes them more careful in diagnosis. . . .

PART **IX**

ANNOUNCEMENT
OF THE
JOHNS HOPKINS
MEDICAL SCHOOL

ANNOUNCEMENT OF THE JOHNS HOPKINS MEDICAL SCHOOL

The Johns Hopkins Medical School was established by the Johns Hopkins University in connection with the Johns Hopkins Hospital in 1893. This Announcement was printed by the Johns Hopkins Press, Baltimore, Maryland.

313

FACULTY

The names are arranged in the several groups in the order in which the members of the staff assumed their duties.

President

DANIEL C. GILMAN, L.L.D.

A.B., Yale College, 1852, and A.M., 1855; LL.D., Harvard University, 1876, St. John's College, 1876, Columbia College, 1887, Yale University, 1889, and University of North Carolina, 1889; Professor in Yale College 1863–72; President of the University of California, 1872–75.

Professors

WILLIAM H. WELCH, M.D.
Professor of Pathology and Dean

A.B., Yale College, 1870; M.D., College of Physicians and Surgeons (N.Y.), 1875; late Professor of Pathological Anatomy and General Pathology in the Bellevue Hospital Medical College, N.Y.; *Pathologist to the Johns Hopkins Hospital.*

IRA REMSEN, M.D., Ph.D.
Professor of Chemistry

A.B., College of the City of New York, 1865; M.D., College of Physicians and Surgeons, N.Y., 1867; Ph.D., University of Göttingen, 1870; Professor of Chemistry in Williams College, 1872–76, and previously Assistant in Chemistry in the University of Tübingen; *Editor of the American Chemical Journal.*

WILLIAM OSLER, M.D., F.R.C.P.
Professor of the Principles and Practice of Medicine

M.D., McGill University, 1872; Fellow of the Royal College of Physicians, London; Professor of the Institutes of Medicine, McGill University, Montreal, 1874–1884; Professor of Clinical Medicine, University of Pennsylvania, 1884–89; *Physician in Chief to the Johns Hopkins Hospital.*

HENRY M. HURD, M.D.
Professor of Psychiatry

A.B., University of Michigan, 1863, and A.M., 1870; M.D., University of Michigan, 1866; Superintendent of the Eastern Michigan Asylum, 1878–89; *Superintendent of the Johns Hopkins Hospital.*

WILLIAM S. HALSTED, M.D.
Professor of Surgery

A.B., Yale College, 1874; M.D., College of Physicians and Surgeons (New York), 1877; late Attending Surgeon to the Presbyterian and Bellevue Hospitals, New York; *Surgeon in Chief to the Johns Hopkins Hospital.*

HOWARD A. KELLY, M.D.
Professor of Gynecology and Obstetrics

A.B., University of Pennsylvania, 1877, and M.D., 1882; Associate Professor of Obstetrics, University of Pennsylvania, 1888–89; *Gynecologist and Obstetrician to the Johns Hopkins Hospital.*

FRANKLIN P. MALL, M.D.
Professor of Anatomy

M.D., University of Michigan, 1883; Fellow of the Johns Hopkins University, 1886–88, and Assistant in Pathology, 1888–89; Adjunct Professor of Anatomy, Clark University, 1889–92; Professor of Anatomy, University of Chicago, 1892–93.

JOHN J. ABEL, M.D.
Professor of Pharmacology

Ph.B., University of Michigan, 1883; Graduate Student, Johns Hopkins University, 1883–84; M.D., University of Strassburg, 1888; Professor of Materia Medica and Therapeutics, University of Michigan, 1891–93.

WILLIAM H. HOWELL, Ph.D., M.D.
Professor of Physiology

A.B., Johns Hopkins University, 1881, Fellow, 1882–84, Ph.D., 1884, Assistant in Biology, 1884–85, Associate, 1885–88, and Associate Professor, 1888–89; Lecturer, University of Michigan, 1889–90, M.D., 1890. and Professor of Physiology and Histology, 1890–92; Associate Professor of Physiology, Harvard University, 1892–93.

Associates

GEORGE H. F. NUTTALL, M.D., Ph.D.*
Associate in Bacteriology and Hygiene

M.D., University of California, 1884; Graduate Student in the Johns Hopkins University, 1885–86, 1890–91, and Assistant, 1891–92; Ph.D., University of Göttingen, 1890.

SIMON FLEXNER, M.D.
Associate in Pathology

M.D., University of Louisville, 1889; Graduate Student in the Johns Hopkins University, 1890–91, and Fellow, 1891–92.

JOHN M. T. FINNEY, M.D.
Associate in Surgery

A.B., Princeton College, 1884; M.D., Harvard University, 1888; Associate in Surgery, Johns Hopkins Hospital.

HUNTER ROBB, M.D.
Associate in Gynecology

M.D., University of Pennsylvania, 1884; Associate in Gynecology, Johns Hopkins Hospital.

J. WHITRIDGE WILLIAMS, M.D.*
Associate in Obstetrics

A.B., Johns Hopkins University, 1886; M.D., University of Maryland, 1888; Assistant in Gynecology, Johns Hopkins Hospital.

B. MEADE BOLTON, M.D.
Acting Associate in Bacteriology and Hygiene

M.D., University of Virginia, 1879; Graduate Student in the Johns Hopkins University, 1886–87, and Assistant in Pathology, 1887–88; Professor of Physiology and Hygiene, South Carolina University, 1888–89; Director of the Department of Bacteriology, Hoagland Laboratory, Brooklyn, 1889–92.

---

*Absent on leave.

ENDOWMENT

The Johns Hopkins Medical School will be opened for the instruction of properly qualified students October 2, 1893. Instruction will continue through the academic year closing about the middle of June. There will be a Christmas recess and a spring recess as announced in the Register of the University. Men and women will be admitted on the same terms. The Medical School will be a department of and under the direction of the Johns Hopkins University, and will derive great advantages from its close affiliation with the Johns Hopkins Hospital. In addition to the resources of these two foundations, the school has an endowment of its own.

The founder of the Johns Hopkins University, in devoting his large fortune to the establishment of the university and the hospital, had in view the organization of a school of medicine. In his letter addressed to the trustees of the hospital, dated March 10th, 1873, these significant words occur:

"It will be your especial duty to secure, for the service of the hospital, surgeons and physicians of the highest character and greatest skill. . . . In all your arrangements in relation to this hospital, you will bear constantly in mind that it is my wish and purpose that the institution shall ultimately form a part of the Medical School of that university for which I have made ample provision by my will."

Delays that could not be foreseen prevented the immediate fulfillment of this purpose of the donor.

Gifts amounting to $111,731.68, most of which were offered to this university in October, 1890, by a committee of women, and an additional gift of $306,977, offered to the university in December, 1892, by Miss Mary Elizabeth Garrett, as contributions toward the endowment of the medical school, on condition that women shall be received upon the same terms as men—now enable the trustees to proceed with the organization of the school.

TERMS OF ADMISSION

The school now established is planned for the professional education of those students who have been especially fitted to receive its instructions by a course of preliminary training in the liberal arts, and especially in those branches of science, like physics, chemistry and biology, which underlie the medical sciences.

As candidates for the degree of Doctor of Medicine the school will receive:

1. Those who have satisfactorily completed the chemical-biological course which leads to the A.B. degree in this university.

2. Graduates of approved colleges or scientific schools who can furnish evidence: (a) That they have a good reading knowledge of French and German;

(b) That they have such knowledge of physics, chemistry, and biology as is imparted by the regular minor courses given in these subjects in this university.

The phrase "a minor course" as employed in this university means a course that requires a year for its completion. In physics, five classroom exercises and three hours a week in the laboratory; in chemistry and biology five classroom exercises and five hours a week in the laboratory in each subject are required.

3. Those who give evidence by examination that they possess the general education implied by a degree in arts or in science from an approved college or scientific school and the knowledge of French, German, physics, chemistry, and biology above indicated.

Applicants for admission will receive blanks to be filled out relating to their previous courses of study.

Hearers, not candidates for a degree, will be received at the discretion of the Faculty.

For the present, no student will be admitted to advanced standing.

Candidates who have not received diplomas of the required character will be examined for admission at the beginning of the session.

THE JOHNS HOPKINS MEDICAL SCHOOL

An Address by Professor William H. Welch, M.D.

DELIVERED AT THE GRADUATING EXERCISES OF THE JOHNS
HOPKINS UNIVERSITY, JUNE 13, 1893

On the twenty-second of last February, at the seventeenth anniversary of the Johns Hopkins University, President Gilman, in behalf of the trustees, announced that the Johns Hopkins Medical School will be opened in October next. In his address on that occasion, he showed that the purpose of the founder of the university and hospital in providing for such a school as a part of the university and in association with the hospital had been kept in view since the beginning of the university, and had influenced the establishment and development of several departments of science in this university. It had been contemplated that the medical department would be fully organized at the time of the opening of the hospital, but when that time came financial difficulties rendered impossible the fulfilment of this long cherished purpose.

This apparently indefinite postponement of the opening of the medical school was the more keenly appreciated because enough had already been done to make clear that here was a great opportunity for medical education. The university had already provided professorships of chemistry, physiology, and pathology; the hospital had secured a staff of able physicians and surgeons, who received from the university the title of professors; many details in construction of the hospital, which added much to its cost, were intended for the use of the medical school; in various ways the resources of these two great institutions, university and hospital, were available for the benefit of the medical school. Additional buildings, laboratories and professorships, however, were needed to complete the organization of a medical department worthy of the university. I need not rehearse how, by the generous gift of Miss Garrett, these difficulties were overcome. This was all told by President Gilman on last Commemoration Day.

It seems appropriate on this occasion to say a few words about what has already been done toward the organization of the medical school and about the aims of the school.

Much needed to be done to prepare for the opening of the school in October, and no time could be or was lost in beginning these preparations. One of the first things to engage the attention of the medical faculty was the determination of the amount and character of preliminary education to be required of students admitted to the medical school as candidates for the doctor's degree. This is, in my opinion, the most perplexing problem concerning medical education, especially in this country. A few words will make the difficulties clear. At present in this country no medical school requires for admission knowledge approaching that necessary for entrance into the freshman class of a respectable college; many schools demand only the most elementary education, and some require no evidence of any preliminary education whatever. Foreign medical schools differ in this respect, but all in Europe have far more rigid requirements for admission than has any school in this country. In Germany, which in recent years has done more than any other country for the advancement of medical science, the student passes from the gymnasium to the university, where, at an average age of nineteen years, he begins the study of medicine with physics, chemistry, and other subjects, which are included in this country in the so-called preliminary medical courses. It is to be noted that training at a classical gymnasium is required and cannot be substituted by that at a real gymnasium, in which a scientific takes the place of a classical course.

For many years in Germany and elsewhere there has been much discussion as to the preliminary education which should be required of students of medicine and there is still great difference of opinion on this subject. In his earlier years DuBois Reymond said Greek by all means should be required; later he cried "More Conic Sections and less Greek." Virchow in his recent rectorate address demands an improvement in methods, especially in such as train the senses, particularly of sight and touch. "At present," he says, "we must complain that the majority of our students have no accurate knowledge of colors, that they make false statements regarding the form of objects which they see, and that they have no sense for the consistence and characters of the surface of bodies," and yet "knowledge of this kind is of the greatest importance for the medical man as often the diagnosis of the most important conditions depends upon it."

Even if there were agreement of opinion as to the best education preparatory for the study of medicine, there would still remain for us very serious and important difficulties peculiar to the system of education in this country. These difficulties result from the anomalous development of those American colleges which are half college and half university, but are neither one thing nor the other, and from which students are graduated at an average age of twenty-two to twenty-three years. The flower of our youth seek a collegiate education and it is eminently desirable that they should have it. We believe that those who have had a liberal education are best fitted for the study of medicine, but it is important that the study of medicine should began at an age not exceeding twenty or at the utmost twenty-one years. The period of professional study should not be less than four years, and after this many will wish to spend a year or a year and a half in hospital service and an equal length of time in special study in this country or in Europe.

How are we to adapt to the embarrassing and anomalous development of American colleges a system of medical education for which a liberal education is demanded as a prerequisite? We are not prepared to recognize a high school training as sufficient, and between this and training in a college or scientific school there is no intermediate grade. We must therefore endeavor to conform to the peculiar conditions in our colleges and scientific schools. We do not claim to furnish an entirely satisfactory solution of the problem, but we have endeavored to do the best we could under all of the circumstances by asking that students who are admitted to the medical school as candidates for the doctor's degree shall possess the liberal education implied by a degree in arts or in science, and shall also have a specified amount of knowledge in certain sciences fundamental to the study of medicine as well as a reading knowledge of French and German. In other words we ask the colleges which keep students two years after the age when the study of medicine should begin, to teach them during these two years such subjects as physics, chemistry and general biology, which in most European schools are included in the medical curriculum, but which can be better taught in the faculty of arts or of science than in a medical school. This means that a student taking a four years' academic course in one of these colleges shall have made up his mind at the end of sophomore year to study medicine. It means that, if compared with European systems of medical education, the course of medical study required for our degree of Doctor of Medicine covers five to six years. We fully realize that the number of students who will meet these rigid requirements is not likely to be large.

I have dwelt thus upon the requirements in education preliminary to the study of medicine, not for the purpose of discussing these requirements for which neither time permits nor is the occasion suitable, but in order to make clear that there are especial difficulties in determining what these requirements should be and that these difficulties are greater in this country than elsewhere. Only experience can determine whether or not the plan which we have adopted is the best one for our purpose. It is to be expected and desired that, with improvements in educational methods and systems in this country, there will be corresponding improvements in the character of the training to be required in preparation for the study of medicine. At any rate we can feel sure that we shall not be subject to the reproach most frequently brought against American medical schools, viz: a low standard of admission, for our standard is not only vastly higher than has ever before been attempted in this country, but is not surpassed in any medical school in the world.

Before opening the medical department it was necessary to fill three professorships, viz: those of anatomy, of pharmacology, and of physiology. The trustees confirmed the appointment of the three men recommended for these chairs by the medical faculty. Dr. Mall has accepted the professorship of anatomy, Dr. Abel that of pharmacology and Dr. Howell that of physiology. We believe that we have been most fortunate in securing these young men, who are enthusiastic and well trained in their special departments, and who have shown distinguished ability both as teachers and investigators. Each relinquished, in order to come here, important professorships with brilliant prospects in other institutions: Dr. Mall in the University of Chicago, Dr. Abel in the University of Michigan, and Dr. Howell at Harvard. It is a source of no slight gratification that these three new professors were all formerly connected with this University—Dr. Mall as fellow and assistant in pathology, Dr. Abel as a graduate student, and Dr. Howell first as student and ultimately as associate professor of physiology.

By Dr. Martin's resignation of the professorship of biology, we have been deprived of his aid in the organization of the medical school. He had formed a part of the small nucleus of a medical faculty which had existed in the university for many years. He had looked forward for years to helping to start the new school from which so much was expected. It was largely by his scientific work in this university that the Johns Hopkins Medical School had a distinguished reputation before it really existed. He has done a great work not for this university alone, but for the whole country, in the advancement of higher physiology; and the medical school should not and will not forget Dr. Martin's services in lighting here the flame of one of the chief medical sciences. That this flame will be kept bright by his successor in the chair of physiology, we all believe.

At present the Pathological Building on the grounds of the Johns Hopkins Hospital is receiving two additional stories, which will accommodate the departments of anatomy, physiological, and chemistry until other buildings of the medical school are constructed.

The length of time required to complete the course of study in the medical school will be four years. The first year will be devoted chiefly to the study of anatomy, physiology, and physiological chemistry. At the end of this year the student will have reached about that point in the course which corresponds to the *examen physicum* in the German universities. With us, however, there will follow three years of strictly professional, mostly practical, study, instead of two years of such study in the German system. Pathology, pharmacology and the general principles of medicine and surgery will be taken up in the second year, and during the last two years the work will be very largely clinical, that is bed-side and dispensary instruction. At present only the details of the first year's course have been worked out and announced, as students at the beginning will be admitted only to the first year of study.

In the methods of instruction especial emphasis will be laid upon practical work in the laboratories and dissecting room and at the bedside. There will be close personal contact between teacher and student. Graduates of the school may look forward to securing places as internes in the Hospital.

The aim of the school will be primarily to train practitioners of medicine and surgery, that is to qualify persons to take care of diseased and injured conditions of the human body. We hold that the medical art should rest upon a thorough training in the medical sciences and that, other things being equal, he is the best practitioner who has this thorough training. The medical sciences have made great progress in the last quarter of a century, greater than has the practice of medicine with which alone the general public has much concern. The prevention and treatment of disease have, however, also made important advances, and it cannot be doubted that they will derive still greater benefits in the future from the discoveries which have been made and are to come in physiology and pathology.

But medical education is not completed at the medical school; it is only begun. Hence it is not only or chiefly the quantity of knowledge which the student takes with him from the school which will help him in his future work; it is also the quality of mind, the methods of work, the disciplined habit of correct reasoning, the way of looking at medical problems.

In order to cultivate in the student this habit of thought, this method of work, I believe that there is no one thing so essential as that the teacher should be also an investigator and should be capable of imparting something of the spirit of investigation to the student. The medical school should be a place where medicine is not only taught but also studied. It should do its part to advance medical science and art by encouraging original work, and by selecting as its teachers those who have the training and capacity for such work. In no other department of natural science are to be found problems awaiting solution more attractive, more significant than those in medicine; and certainly these problems do not lose in dignity because they relate to the physical well-being of mankind.

The Johns Hopkins Medical School will start unhampered by traditions and free to work out its own salvation. It will derive inestimable advantage from being an integral and coördinate part of this great university, which will see to it that university ideals and methods are not lost sight of in the new school. It will have the support of a great hospital, the trustees of which have already shown the most enlightened spirit in the encouragement of medical research. May the Johns Hopkins Medical School not only receive lustre from the university and the hospital, but may it also add to the renown and usefulness of both these institutions, of which it is to form a part.

GENERAL PLAN OF INSTRUCTION

The course of instruction will continue through four years. Anatomy, including normal histology and embryology, physiology, and physiological chemistry will be the principal studies of the first year. The study of anatomy will be continued in the second year, and, in addition, pharmacology, general pathology and pathological anatomy, bacteriology, and the general principles of medicine and surgery will be taken up. During the last two years, clinical instruction will be given in medicine, surgery, obstetrics and gynecology, and the various special branches of practical medicine and surgery, such as ophthalmology, dermatology, laryngology, neurology, pediatrics. Instruction in hygiene, psychiatry, legal medicine and medical history will be provided during the course.

Abundant clinical material is afforded by the Johns Hopkins Hospital and Dispensary. The clinical amphitheatre and the clinical laboratories are in the hospital buildings. A four story building on the grounds of the hospital, intended for a pathological laboratory, affords accommodation also for the departments of anatomy and physiological chemistry. Physiology will be taught in the biological laboratory of the university.

In the main building of the hospital is a good medical library with full sets of medical periodicals. This, as well as the libraries and reading room of the university, will be available without charge for the use of medical students.

Practical work in the dissecting room, in the laboratory, and at the bedside, demonstrations, clinics, and recitations will form the most prominent features of the methods of instruction. Conferences or seminary methods will also be employed.

First-Year Courses

Inasmuch as for the coming year students, who are candidates for the degree of Doctor of Medicine, will be admitted only to the medical course of the first year, the statement for the curriculum of this first year is the only one which is announced in detail at present. Similar statements regarding the courses for the second and following years will be made hereafter.

A. ANATOMY

The instruction in anatomy will be under the charge of Dr. Franklin P. Mall, professor of anatomy, with the aid of the demonstrator and assistant demonstrators of anatomy.

The course in anatomy will consist of vertebrate embryology, histology and histogenesis, and human anatomy. It is the intention to cover most of the field in one academic year.

The course in embryology and histology will be continuous during the year, although either course may be taken by itself.

During the first half-year histology will be taught by lectures, demonstrations, and laboratory work. In the spring, vertebrate embryology will be taught. The aim of the latter course will be to throw as much light as possible upon the structure and development of tissues and organs, and human anatomy in general.

Parallel with the above course that on human anatomy will be given.

Beginning in the autumn with lectures, recitations, and demonstrations in osteology, the study of human anatomy will be continued with practical work in the dissecting room as soon as cool weather sets in. The aim will be to teach as much as possible of human anatomy by work in the dissecting room and by demonstrations, leaving only certain general and special topics for the lecture room. Surgical anatomy, as well as a share of topographical anatomy, will be given during the second year in connection with the department of surgery.

B. PHYSIOLOGY

Instruction in physiology will be given by Dr. William H. Howell, professor of physiology, by means of lectures, experimental work in the laboratory, demonstrations, recitations, and conferences. The lectures will be given three times a week throughout the year and will be fully illustrated by experiments and demonstrations given in the lecture room. Weekly recitations will be held upon the subject matter covered by the lectures, and in the latter half of the year weekly conferences will also form part of the class work.

The laboratory courses will be arranged so as to occupy two afternoons a week for about twelve weeks. This work will include the study of the properties of muscle and nerve, the physiology of blood and digestion, circulation, respiration, and special senses. It is intended to give the student an idea of the methods used in experimental physiology, and to furnish also that basis of actual acquaintance with facts which is so necessary for intelligent reading.

In the conferences special topics will be assigned to a certain number of students to form the subjects of conference papers to be read before the class. The preparation of these papers will involve the reading of the more important recent literature, and whenever possible the student will be given opportunities to do special laboratory work in connection with his paper.

In addition to the foregoing exercises, which comprise the required work, students will be given opportunities to participate in the more advanced courses carried on in the laboratory, and intended primarily as graduate work. These courses are as follows: A biological journal club meets weekly to discuss the recent literature in the various fields of biological research, including animal physiology. A physiological seminar meets weekly during the first half of the year to read and discuss some one or more of the older contributions to physiology, which are of interest because of their bearing upon the historical development of the science. In the latter half of the year the same hour will be given up to a series of advanced lectures upon special topics in physiology, in which the subjects presented will be treated exhaustively from the standpoint of the most recent contributions. An advanced course of laboratory work will be arranged— intended to teach the methods of physiological demonstration and research. This course will be under the control of the professor of physiology, and will not be limited as to time or amount of work, with the exception that assistance from the professor must be arranged for by definite engagements. This course is designed for those who expect to become teachers or investigators in physiology, pathology, or pharmacology, and the number permitted to take it will necessarily be limited. For purposes of research the laboratory is well equipped. Those who are prepared to do special investigations will be given every opportunity for work, including shop facilities for the construction of new apparatus.

C. PHYSIOLOGICAL CHEMISTRY

The instruction in physiological chemistry will be for the present under the charge of Dr. John J. Abel, professor of pharmacology, with the aid of an assistant.

Instruction in this branch will be given by illustrated lectures, conferences of a less formal character and recitations, and laboratory work.

In the lectures the substances that have been isolated from the fluids and tissues of the body will be considered chiefly with regard to their connection with physiological processes. The physical and chemical properties of these substances and their chemical relationships will also receive due attention whenever they promise to throw light on animal metabolism, for it is thought that a treatment of the subject which emphasizes the chemical properties of the constituents of the body will best prepare the student to meet important questions that will arise later in his study of pathology and practical medicine.

The laboratory instruction will cover the following ground:

1. The isolation of the more important constituents of the various tissues and fluids of the body, of its secretions and excretions in health and in disease, and the study of such of the physical and chemical properties of these constituents as are of most importance from the physiological point of view.

2. The synthetic formation of some of these constituents, such as urea, uric acid, hippuric acid, cholin, and leucin.

3. Selected qualitative and quantitative methods employed in the study of the various tissues, the urine, blood, bile, biliary and renal calculi, milk, pus, and feces.

The separation of poisons from the tissues and fluids of the body and their identification will be taken up in the second year in connection with toxicology. A special course in clinical chemistry adapted to the needs of the hospital student will also be offered later in the course.

CHARGES FOR TUITION

The charge for tuition will be two hundred dollars per annum, payable at the treasurer's office, in semi-annual instalments, October 1 and February 1. There will be no extra charges for instruction in any department or for laboratory courses except for materials consumed. A deposit of ten dollars as caution money will be required from each student at the time of his enrollment. The caution money is repaid to the student when he leaves, if there are no charges against him. Special charges are made for breakage and for damage to apparatus.

Inquiries may be addressed to the Registrar of the Johns Hopkins University.

June 1893

Special Courses for Physicians

A statement of the courses open to physicians in the year 1893–94 is issued as a separate pamphlet, and can be obtained upon application to the registrar of the Johns Hopkins University.

APPENDIX

THE TERMS OF MISS GARRETT'S GIFT

AS COMMUNICATED BY HER TO THE BOARD OF TRUSTEES,
FEBRUARY 20, 1893

Miss Mary Elizabeth Garrett, in order to make up the sum of $500,000, which the Board of Trustees required should be secured as an endowment before the medical school of the university was opened, has contributed to that fund the sum of $306,977 upon the following terms, which have been agreed to by the university:

1. That women shall enjoy all the advantages of the medical school of the Johns Hopkins University on the same terms as men, and shall be admitted on the same terms as men to all prizes, dignities or honors that are awarded by competition, examination, or regarded as rewards of merit.

2. That not more than $50,000 of the original endowment of $500,000 shall be expended on a building or buildings; and that in memory of the contributions of the committees of the Women's Medical School Fund, this building, if there be but one, or the chief building, if there be more than one, shall be known as the Women's Fund Memorial Building.

3. That the medical school of the university shall be exclusively a graduate school as hereinafter explained, that is to say: That the medical school of the Johns Hopkins University shall form an integral part of the Johns Hopkins University, and like other departments of the university, shall be under the management and control of the trustees of the said university; that it shall provide a four years' course, leading to the degree of Doctor of Medicine; that there shall be admitted to the school those students only who by examination or by other tests equally satisfactory to the faculty of the medical school (no distinction being made in these tests or examinations between men and women), have proved that they have completed the studies included in the preliminary medical course (Group Three, Chemical-Biological Course) as laid down in the University Register (but this condition is not meant to restrict the trustees from receiving as hearers, but not as candidates for the degree of Doctor of Medicine,

327

those who have received the degree of Doctor of Medicine, or its equivalent in some school of good repute); and that the degree of Doctor of Medicine of the Johns Hopkins University shall be given to no doctors of medicine who have not proved by examination or by other tests equally satisfactory to the faculty of the medical school that they have completed the studies included in the preliminary course, besides completing the course of instruction of the medical school of the Johns Hopkins University.

The aforegoing provisions shall not be construed as restricting the liberty of the university to make such changes in the requirements of the admission to the medical school of the Johns Hopkins University or to accept such equivalents for the studies required for admission to this school as shall not lower the standard of admission specified in this clause: provided that the requirements in modern languages other than English shall not be diminished, and provided also that the requirements in nonmedical scientific studies shall include at least as much knowledge of natural science as is imparted in the three minor courses in science now laid down in its university register, the subjects and arrangements of these scientific studies being subject to such modifications as may from time to time seem wise to its board and to the faculty of the medical school, but being at all times the same for all candidates for admission. (For such requirements always see University Register.)

4. That the terms of this gift and the Resolutions of October 28th, 1890, by which the trustees accepted the gift of the Women's Medical School Fund, will be printed each year in whatever annual calendars may be issued announcing the courses of the medical school.—See appended Resolutions.

5. That there shall be created a committee of six women to whom the women studying in the medical school may apply for advice concerning lodging and other practical matters, and that all questions concerning the personal character of women applying for admission to the school, and all nonacademic questions of discipline affecting the women studying in the medical school shall be referred to this committee, and by them be in writing reported for action to the authorities of the university; that the members of this committee shall be members for life; that the committee, when once formed, shall be self-nominating, its nominations of new members to fill such vacancies as may occur being subject always to the approval of the Board of Trustees of the university.

6. That in the event of any violation of any or all of the aforesaid stipulations, the said sum of $306,977 shall revert to her, or such person or persons, institution or institutions, as she by testament or otherwise may hereafter appoint.

It will be observed that by the tenor of the aforegoing terms no university course will be in any way modified by any conditions attached to her gift. Those conditions relate exclusively to preparation for the medical school, and have received, in the shape in which they are now presented, the unanimous approval of the medical faculty of the university.

The terms of admission to the medical school of the university as formulated and interpreted by the medical faculty of the university, February 4, 1893, and here subjoined, are therefore in entire accordance with the terms of her gift.

(Signed) Mary E. Garrett

REQUIREMENTS FOR ADMISSION TO THE MEDICAL SCHOOL OF THE JOHNS HOPKINS UNIVERSITY, UNANIMOUSLY APPROVED BY THE MEDICAL FACULTY, FEBRUARY 4, 1893

A course of four years' instruction will be provided leading to the degree of Doctor of Medicine.

To this course there will be admitted as candidates for the degree:

1. Those who have satisfactorily completed the chemical-biological course which leads to the A.B. degree in this university.

2. Graduates of approved colleges or scientific schools who can furnish evidence: (a) that they have a good reading knowledge of French and German; (b) that they have such knowledge of physics, chemistry, and biology as is imparted by the regular minor courses, given in these subjects in this university.

3. Those who give evidence by examination that they possess the general education implied by a degree in arts or in science from an approved college or scientific school, and the knowledge of French, German, Physics, Chemistry, and Biology, already indicated.

By approved colleges and scientific schools are meant those whose standard for graduation shall be considered by this university as essentially equivalent to its standard for graduation in the undergraduate department.

It is to be understood that at least one year's study in the chemical and biological sciences in their immediate relations to medicine shall be required from students after their entrance to the medical school.

MINUTE ADOPTED BY THE BOARD OF TRUSTEES, OCTOBER 28, 1890, IN ACCEPTING THE WOMEN'S MEDICAL SCHOOL FUND

The President and Board of Trustees of the Johns Hopkins University have received from Mrs. Nancy Morris Davis, chairman of one of the committees formed for the purpose of raising a fund to procure the most advanced medical education for women, the gratifying intelligence that $100,000 has been raised for the use of their intended medical school, and is at their disposal, if they will, by resolution, agree to the terms upon which the money was contributed by its donors.

These terms are that this board, if it accepts the funds thus raised, shall agree, by resolution, that, when its medical school shall be opened, women whose training has been equivalent to the preliminary medical course prescribed for men, shall be admitted to such school upon the same terms as may be prescribed for men.

The offer to this university of the particular fund is the free voluntary act of women residing in this state and in other states, made without the suggestion or solicitation of this board, and we accept it under and subject to the terms which are made a part of the gift, with the understanding and declaration, however, that such preliminary training in all its parts shall be obtained in some other institution of learning devoted, in whole or in part, to the education of women, or by private tuition.

The fund so contributed shall be invested and known as "The Women's Medical School Fund," and that fund, and all interest to accrue thereon, and all additions made thereto for the same purpose, shall remain invested for the purposes of increase only until, with its aid as a foundation, a general fund has been accumulated amounting to not less than $500,000, and sufficient for the establishment and maintenance of a medical school worthy of the reputation of this university and fully sufficient as a means of complete medical instruction. Then, and not until then, will a medical school be opened by this university; and then, and not until then, will the gift now offered be used by this university; and then, and not until then, will the terms attached thereto be operative.

The utility of a training school for women nurses has been demonstrated by the experience of practice of the Johns Hopkins Hospital, and by the necessities of home life among our people.

This board is satisfied that in hospital practice among women, in penal institutions in which women are prisoners, in charitable institutions in which women are cared for, and in private life, when women are to be attended, there is a need and place for learned and capable women physicians; and that it is the business and duty of this board, when it is supplied with the necessary means for opening its proposed medical school, to make provision for the training and full qualification of such women for the abundant work which awaits them in these wide fields of usefulness.

Nothing contained in this minute shall be construed as abridging, in any manner, the right of the Board of Trustees of the Johns Hopkins University to make such rules and regulations as they may deem necessary for the government of its school of medicine, when it is organized; and in making such rules and regulations, the terms of this minute shall always be respected and observed.

WOMEN'S COMMITTEE OF THE MEDICAL SCHOOL, APPOINTED
BY MISS GARRETT, DECEMBER 22, 1892

Their duties are stated in paragraph 5 of the letter printed above.

MRS. HENRY M. HURD	MISS M. CAREY THOMAS
MRS. IRA REMSEN	MISS MARY M. GWINN
MRS. WILLIAM OSLER	MISS MARY E. GARRETT

INDEX

INDEX

Abel, John J., 315, 231, 325
Abell, Irvin, 166
Abel-Smith, Brian, 236
Ackerknecht, Erwin H., 115, 165, 233, 279
Ambulance, 242, 244
Amende, Charles, 290
American Journal of the Medical Sciences, 45, 107
American Medical Association, 38, 62–63, 127; Committee on Literature, 45–54; Committee on Medical Education, 4–5
American Medico-Psychological Association, 222–29
Anatomy, 25–27, 40, 323–24
Anderson, James, 265
Andral, Gabriel, 104
Andrews, Edmund, 176–81
Anemia, 138
Anesthesia, 163, 169–75, 188, 203–4, 234
Aneurysm, 101, 163
Animal magnetism, 73
Antimony, 93, 125
Antisepsis, 163, 188, 190, 193, 198–200, 203–4, 249
Apprenticeship, 3, 5, 17
Aristotle, 282
Asepsis, 237
Ashurst, John, Jr., 234
Association of Medical Superintendents of American Institutions for the Insane, 217, 222–29
Autopsy, 115

Bacteria, 199, 278. *See also* Germ theory
Bard, Samuel, 6, 233
Barnard, Frederick A. P., 278–92
Bartlett, Elisha, 115–26, 163
Bastian, Henry C., 283, 286
Bauer, Louis, 59–60

Beach, Wooster, 51
Beale, Lionel S., 281–82
Beddoes, John, 171
Bell, John, 54
Bell, Luther V., 218
Bellevue Hospital, 39–40, 148, 186, 201–9, 234–35, 242, 244
Bellevue Hospital Training School for Nurses, 242, 247
Berman, Alex, 88–89
Bigelow, Henry J., 164, 169–75, 189
Bigelow, Jacob, 98–106, 128, 130, 134
Billings, John Shaw, 6, 45–46, 165, 301–9
Billroth, Theodore, 194
Blane, Gilbert, 106
Blanton, Wyndham B., 88–89
Bleeding, 89, 92, 95, 111, 123–25, 127, 132, 137–39, 141, 182
Blisters, 95, 112, 132, 137, 139
Blood-letting. *See* Bleeding
Bloomingdale Asylum, 219
Boardman, Andrew, 24–36, 37
Bockoven, J. S., 214
Bolton, B. Meade, 315
Bond, Thomas, 37
Bonner, Thomas N., 60, 88, 128
Boston Medical and Surgical Journal, 45
Broussais, Francois, 137
Brown, John, 133, 137
Brown, Lucille, 6
Bryan, Leon S., 89
Bryce, James, 182
Buck, Gurdon, 39, 265
Buley, R. Carlyle, 89
Bulkley, Henry D., 39, 265
Bulloch, William, 279
Burdon-Sanderson, John, 289
Burrage, Walter, 170
Butterfield, Lyman H., 90

333

Cabanis, Pierre, 115–17
Cagniard de la Tour, Charles, 291
Caldwell, Charles, 89
Calomel, 58, 112, 182. *See also* Mercury
Camac, C. N. B., 235
Caplan, Ruth B., 214
Carr-Saunders, A. P., 60
Cassedy, James H., 301
Cathartics, 137, 139
Census, 164, 302
Certainty, in medicine, 77, 96, 115–26
Chadwick, Edwin, 253, 255
Chapin, John B., 222–23
Chapman, Nathaniel, 46–47, 107–14
Chaptal, Jean A., 93
Charity Hospital, Blackwell's Island, 247
Charles, Steven T., 237
Cheesman, John C., 39
Chemistry, 26
Cherry bounce, 168
Childs, S. Russell, 40
Cholera, 104, 145, 253–54
Chomel, A. F., 138
Churchill, Edward D., 236
Cinchona, 131
Citizens' Association (New York), 253–54, 263–77
Civil service, 293
Civil War, 176–77, 187, 201, 217
Clark, Alonzo, 37, 40, 265
Cleanliness, in surgery, 209
Clinical instruction, 37, 39, 186
Clysters, 95
Cock, Thomas F., 40
Coe, Rodney M., 60
Coffer, William, 168
College of Physicians and Surgeons, 37–42
Combe, George, 59
Compton, T. A., 146
Conservative surgery. *See* Surgery, conservative
Cooper, Astley, 185
Corner, George W., 3, 90
Corrigan, Dominic, 308
Corvisart, Jean V., 101
Corwin, E. H. L., 234
Counterirritation, 139–41
Coze, Leon, 289
Crawford, Jane Todd, 166–68
Crosse, Andrew, 282
Curability, cult of, 215
Currie, James, 102

DaCosta, Jacob, M., 148
Dain, Norman, 214
Dalton, John C., 38
Dana, Charles L., 143
Davaine, Casimir, 287
Davies, John D., 24
Davis, Nathan Smith, 5, 60, 127–33, 176
Davy, John, 144, 146
Death certificate, 310
DeFoe, Daniel, 195
Delafield, Edward, 38
Delafield, Francis, 152–59
Dennis, Frederic S., 165
Derby, George, 309
Deutsch, Albert, 214–15
Diarrhea, 107–14, 254
Diet, 113
Disease, 50, 119–20, 129–33
Dissection, 34, 40, 67, 186
Dix, Dorothea, 213, 216
Doremus, R. Ogden, 265
Drake, Daniel, 8–23, 24, 54
Draper, John W., 265
Draper, W. H., 146, 148
DuBois-Reymond, Emil, 319
Duffy, John, 60, 88–89, 264
Dunglison, Robley, 107, 163
Dyspepsia, 109, 113, 116, 152–59, 259

Earle, A. Scott, 165–66, 169
Earle, Pliny, 215–21
Earnest, Ernest, 222
Eaton, Dorman B., 213, 293–300
Eaton, Leonard K., 235
Ebert, Myrl, 47
Ellis, George E., 98
Emetics, 92, 95, 111, 139
Erichson, John Eric, 60, 190, 198, 234, 242, 249
Erysipelas, 147. *See also* Hospitalism
Ether, 168–75
Ethics, medical, 51, 75–76, 79
Evans, A. S., 134
Exercise, 114

Faxon, Nathaniel W., 236
Fees, student, 40, 70, 89, 92
Feltz, Victor T., 289
Fevers, 115
Finney, John M. T., 315
Flexner, Abraham, 4
Flexner, James T., 8, 166, 169

Flexner, Simon, 315
Flinn, Michael W., 255
Flint, Austin, 54, 134–42, 143, 148, 152
Forbes, John, 116, 118, 128, 130, 137
Fordyce, William, 241
Foster, S. Conant, 40
Fothergill, John, 102
Francis, John W., 59
Frankford Asylum, 219
Franklin, Benjamin, 235
Freidson, Eliot, 60

Gallagher, Thomas M., 38
Garrett, Mary E., 316, 327–30
Garrison, Fielding H., 301
Geneva College, 25–28
Germ theory, 190, 197, 200–1, 278–92
Gilman, Chandler R., 40
Gilman, Daniel C., 314, 318
Glaab, Charles N., 253
Godkin, Edwin L., 75–83
Goodman, Nathan G., 90
Goodman, Walter, 62
Goulden, Henry, 265
Graduation, requirements, 40–41
Graham, Sylvester, 256
Grant, Ulysses, 293
Graunt, John, 303
Great Britain, medical education, 7
Green, Caleb, 5
Greene, Isaac, 40
Griscom, John H., 39, 253–54
Grob, Gerald, 214
Gross, Martin L., 62
Gross, Samuel D., 8, 89, 134, 164–65, 183, 189, 190–97
Gynecology, 208

Hahnemann, Samuel, 116, 133, 137
Hale, Enoch, 54
Hallier, Ernst, 290
Halsted, William S., 314
Hammond, William Alexander, 127
Handlin, Oscar, 182
Harris, Elisha, 263, 265, 290
Hartford Retreat, 216–17
Hartley, Robert H., 254
Harvard Medical School, 98
Hayes, Rutherford B., 264
Hays, Isaac, 107
Hayward, George, 170, 174
Helmholz, Hermann, 291

Henschel, Charles, 265
Hippocrates, 83, 108, 127
Hodges, Richard M., 189
Hoffman, Richard K., 39
Holmes, Oliver Wendell, 45–54, 88, 127–31
Holmes, Timothy, 234
Homeopathy, 58, 73, 75–76, 78–81, 87–88, 116, 121
Hoogenboom, Ari, 293
Hooker, Worthington, 5, 58, 60, 87, 127–28
Hopkins, Johns, 316
Horine, Emmet F., 8, 166
Hospital construction, 235
Hospitalism, 188, 191–92, 197, 234–35
Hospitals, 105, 233–50
Hospital training, 26, 67
Hotel Dieu, 238
Howard, John, 241
Howell, William H., 315, 321, 324
Hudson, Robert, 4
Hufeland, Christian W., 71
Hume, Edgar E., 237
Hunter, John, 205
Hurd, Henry M., 214, 236, 314
Huxley, Thomas, 283–84, 286
Hygiene, 134, 253–310
Hypochondriasis, 158

Immigration, 275
Insanity, 213–29, 259
Intemperance, 19
Iron, 131
Isaacs, Charles, 39

Jackson, Charles T., 169, 175
Jackson, James, 137
Javert, Carl T., 37
Jefferson, Thomas, 163
Jewell, Wilson, 274
Johns Hopkins Hospital, 323
Johns Hopkins University, School of Medicine, 6, 313–30
Johnson, Samuel, 92
Johnston, Christopher, 189
Jones, John, 237–41
Journal of the American Medical Association, 127

Kaufman, Martin, 88
Keen, William W., 227

Kelly, Howard A., 170, 314
Kett, Joseph F., 60, 88
Keys, Thomas E., 169
King, Anthony, 236
King, Lester, 115
Kircher, Athanasius, 280
Klebs, Edwin, 289
Klein, Emanuel, 289
Koch, Robert, 279
Kraft, Ivor, 143

Laennec, Rene, 101, 123, 134, 233, 235
Lambert, Royston, 255
Lancet, The, 185
Language, foreign: in medical education, 15-16, 24, 31
Laudanum, 95, 168
Lee, Charles A., 46
Lefanu, W. R., 45
Leidy, Joseph, 286
Levine, Norman D., 8
Ligature, 163, 204-6
Lind University, 127, 176
Lister, Joseph, 193, 198-201, 249, 288
London, death rate, 273
Louis, Pierre, 105, 123-25, 134, 233
Lucretius, 282
Lyman, H. M., 309-10
Lynn, Kenneth S., 60

Mall, Franklin P., 315, 320-21, 324
Marshall, Mary Louise, 47
Martin, H. Newell, 321
Martin, J. R., 234
Massachusetts General Hospital, 98, 188
Massachusetts Medical Society, 98
Matas, Rudolph, 88
McClean Asylum, 216, 218
McCready, Benjamin W., 40, 253, 255
McDowell, Ephraim, 166-68
McDowell, James, 167
Mease, James, 237-41
Measles, 100, 102
Mechanic, David, 60
Medical education, 65, 127, 186; in Europe, 66, 68
Medical ethics. *See* Ethics, medical
Medical journals, 45-50
Medical jurisprudence, 26
Medical profession, status of, 57-65
Medical students, examination of, 33, 35; preparation of, 9; qualifications of, 10, 13-14, 30-31, 35, 329; selection of, 9

Mercury, 100, 109, 112, 137, 140, 167. *See also* Calomel
Metcalf, John T., 40
Microscope, 39, 45, 143
Miller, Edward, 48
Miller, Genevieve, 3
Miller, Zane L., 9
Mitchell, Arthur, 219-20
Mitchell, John Kearsley, 222
Mitchell, Samuel L., 48
Mitchell, S. Weir, 222-29
Moliere, Jean, 83
Morehouse, George R., 227
Morgan, John, 6
Morse, John T., 47
Mortality, bills of, 91
Mott, Frank Luther, 47
Mott, Valentine, 265
Moxa, 139
Multhauf, Robert P., 115

Nation, the, 75-83
National Association for the Protection of the Insane and the Prevention of Insanity, 213-14
National Board of Health, 264, 301
Nature, 93, 98-106, 127-34
Needham, John T., 283, 285
Neuburger, Max, 128
New England Journal of Medicine, 45
Newman, Charles, 7
New York Academy of Medicine, 263
New York City: death rate, 273; health laws, 295, 298; hospitals, 242-50; medical colleges, 67; medical education in, 6; medicine in, 88; sanitary conditions, 263-77; streets, 267-68; tenements, 269-70
New York Eye Infirmary, 39-40
New York Hospital, 39, 146, 202
New York Medical Repository, 48-49
Nightingale, Florence, 235, 237
Nitrous oxide, 170-71
Northhampton Lunatic Hospital, 215, 219
Northwestern University, 176. *See also* Lind University
Norwood, William F., 3, 6
Numerical method, 105, 123, 137
Nuttall, George H. F., 315

Opium, 141
Orfila, M. J. B., 172
Osler, William, 88, 115, 152, 314

Packard, Francis R., 165
Paine, Horatio, 250
Palliation, 100, 105
Pancoast, Joseph, 189
Paré, Ambroise, 105
Parent-In Chatelet, A. J. B., 253
Parish registers, 303
Paris school, 90, 104, 115, 233
Parker, Willard, 37, 40, 189, 234, 265
Parkes, Edmund A., 290
Pasteur, Louis, 190, 284–87
Pearl, Raymond, 301
Pennsylvania, University of, 107
Pennsylvania General Hospital, 185
Peruvian bark. *See* Cinchona
Philadelphia, death rate, 273–74
Philadelphia Journal of the Medical and Physical Sciences. See *American Journal of the Medical Sciences*
Phrenology, 24, 59
Physiological chemistry, 325–26
Physiology, 39, 324–25
Pickard, Madge E., 89
Plague, 195
Playfair, Lyon, 275, 295
Pleurisy, 137
Pneumonia, 120–25, 137
Post, Alfred C., 39, 265
Post mortem, 35
Pouchet, Felix, 284–85
Poynter, F. N. L., 7
Preceptors, qualifications of, 17–19
Pregnancy, 167
Premedical education, 319
Prescriptions, 93
Priestley, Joseph, 48, 241
Pringle, John, 239–40
Prudden, T. Mitchell, 152
Psora, 100
Public health, 253. *See also* Hygiene
Pus, 205
Puschmann, Theodor, 7
Pusey, William A., 89

Quackery, 58, 68, 71, 76

Ray, Isaac, 215
Reader, W. J., 60
Redi, Francisco, 283, 285
Remsen, Ira, 314
Research, 226
Richman, Irwin, 107
Richmond, Phyllis Allen, 279

Rideing, W. H., 242–50
Ringer, S., 148
Robb, Hunter, 315
Rodgers, J. Kearny, 39
Rogers, D. L., 27–28
Rogers, Frank B., 46
Rokitansky, Carl, 140
Roosevelt, James H., 250
Roosevelt Hospital, 242, 244, 249–50
Rosen, George, 89, 165, 255
Rosenberg, Carroll S., 253
Rosenberg, Charles E., 59–60, 88, 165, 214, 253, 255
Rush, Benjamin, 57–58, 90–97, 107, 223, 240–41

St. Bartholomew Hospital, 238
St. Thomas Hospital, 238
Salisbury, J. H., 289
Sanborn, F. B., 215
Sanctorio, Sanctorio, 240
Scarlet fever, 102
Schneider, David M., 214
Schuppert, Moritz, 198
Schwann, Theodor, 284, 291
Seguin, Edouard, 143–51
Seguin, Edward C., 143, 148
Seguin, Jules, 144
Selden, W., 54
Shafer, Henry B., 6, 165
Shaftel, Norman, 134
Shapiro, Henry D., 9
Shattuck, George C., Jr., 54
Shattuck, Lemuel, 253–55
Shaw, George Bernard, 278
Shrady, John, 38
Shryock, Richard H., 24, 59–60, 87–90, 165, 256
Simon, John, 234, 255, 279
Sims, J. Marion, vii, 89
Small pox, 100, 254, 271
Smillie, Wilson G., 255
Smith, Elihu H., 48
Smith, Henry Nash, 98
Smith, Joseph M., 39, 265
Smith, Southwood, 102
Smith, Stephen, 165, 176, 182, 201–9, 234–35, 242, 263–77
Smith, Sydney, 47
Snow, Edwin, 305, 307, 310
Spallanzani, Lazaro, 284–86
Specialism, 58–59, 165, 184

Spontaneous generation, 282–86
Stevens, Audrey D., 165
Stevenson, Lloyd G., 89, 115, 278
Stewart, Dugald, 260
Stewart, F. Campbell, 62–74
Stiles, Henry R., 2
Stille, Alfred, 63, 107
Stone, John O., 40
Stretcher, 245
Strychnine, 131
Surgeons, 21–22
Surgery, 77, 126, 163–209; conservative, 135, 182–83
Sussmilch, Johann P., 303–4
Swett, John A., 39
Sydenham, Thomas, 111
Syphilis, 100

Taylor, Isaac E., 265
Temkin, Owsei, 115
Thacher, James, 49
Therapeutic nihilism, 127
Therapeutics, 58–59, 87–142
Thermometry, 143–51
Thomas, L., 145
Thomson, Anthony Todd, 172
Thomsonianism, 73, 139
Thurnam, John, 219–20
Tilton, Eleanor M., 47
de Tocqueville, Alexis, 182
Todd, Eli, 216–17
Tomes, Robert, 256–62
Toner, Joseph M., 234
Traube, Ludwig, 145
Tuberculosis, 141, 148
Tucker, D. A., Jr., 9
Tunley, Roul, 62
Tyndall, John, 288
Typhoid fever, 105, 147
Typhus, 147, 240–41, 254, 271

Uhle, J. P., 145

Van Buren, William H., 40, 189, 242
Viets, Henry R., 169
Virchow, Rudolf, 319
Vital forces, 141
Vital signs, 148
Vital statistics, 301–9

Walsh, James J., 38, 88
Walter, Richard D., 222
Ware, John, 24, 137
Warren, John C., 170
Water supplies, 254
Watson, John, 39
Watt, James, 171
Weir, Robert F., 198–200, 242, 249
Welch, William H., 6, 314, 318–22
Wells, Horace, 169
Whipple, Allen O., 165
White, Andrew D., 263
White, James P., 37
Whooping cough, 101
Williams, J. Whitridge, 315
Wilson, P. A., 60
Wiltshire Asylum, 219
Wood, James R., 40, 189, 242, 265
Woodward, Samuel B., 216–17
Worcester State Hospital, 216–17, 219
Word, R. C., 61
Wunderlich, C. A., 144–45, 147, 150
Wylie, W. Gill, 208, 234–35
Wyman, Jeffries, 284–85
Wyman, Rufus, 216

Yager, Sanford C., 61
Yellow fever, 91–92
York Retreat, 220
Young, J. Harvey, 59